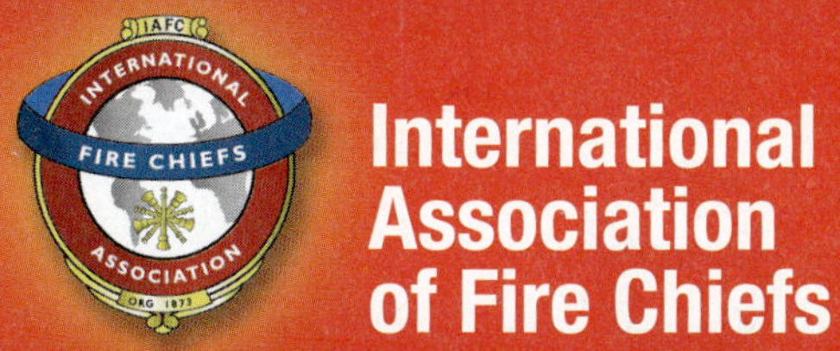

International Association of Fire Chiefs

Emergency Vehicle Operator

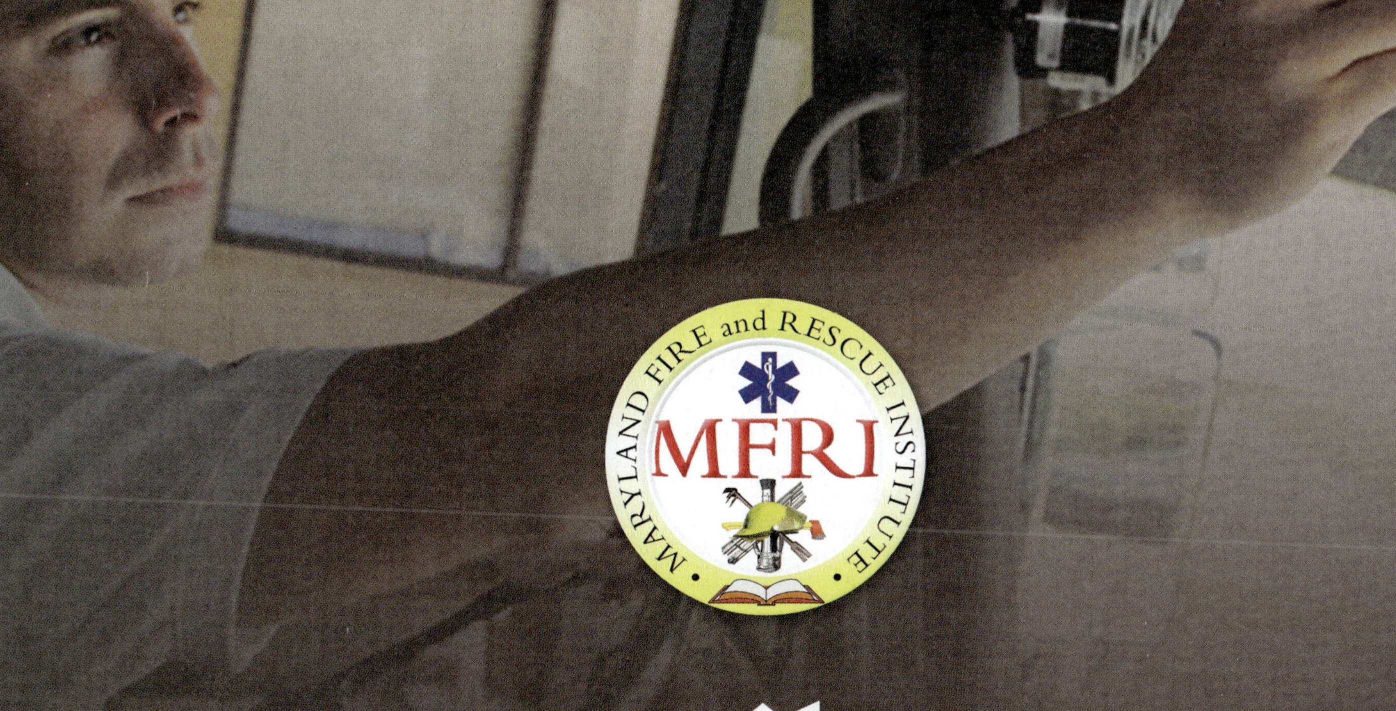

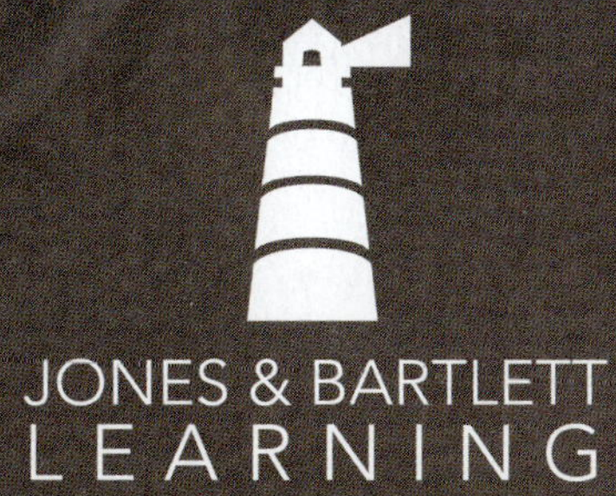

JONES & BARTLETT LEARNING

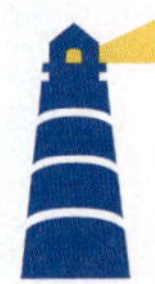

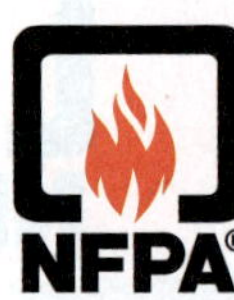

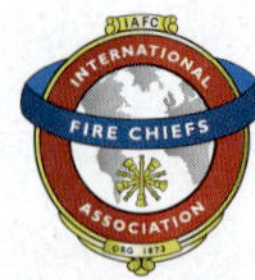

Jones & Bartlett Learning
World Headquarters
5 Wall Street
Burlington, MA 01803
978-443-5000
info@jblearning.com
www.jblearning.com
www.psglearning.com

National Fire Protection Association
1 Batterymarch Park
Quincy, MA 02169-7471
www.NFPA.org

International Association of Fire Chiefs
4025 Fair Ridge Drive
Fairfax, VA 22033
www.IAFC.org

Jones & Bartlett Learning books and products are available through most bookstores and online booksellers. To contact the Jones & Bartlett Learning Public Safety Group directly, call 800-832-0034, fax 978-443-8000, or visit our website, www.psglearning.com.

18192-0

Production Credits
General Manager and Executive Publisher: Kimberly Brophy
VP, Product Development: Christine Emerton
Senior Managing Editor: Donna Gridley
Executive Editor: William Larkin
Director of Production: Jenny L. Corriveau
Project Specialist: Robert Furrier
Director of Marketing Operations: Brian Rooney
VP, Manufacturing and Inventory Control: Therese Connell
Composition: S4Carlisle Publishing Services
Cover Design: Kristin E. Parker
Text Design: Scott Moden
Cover Image (Title Page, Part Opener, Chapter Opener):
© Jones & Bartlett Learning. Photographed by Glen E. Ellman.
Printing and Binding: LSC Communications
Cover Printing: LSC Communications

Library of Congress Cataloging-in-Publication Data
Names: University System of Maryland. Maryland Fire and Rescue Institute, issuing body.
Title: Emergency vehicle operator / Maryland Fire and Rescue Institute.
Description: First edition. | Burlington, Massachusetts : Jones & Bartlett Learning, [2020] | Includes bibliographical references and index.
Identifiers: LCCN 2018053958 | ISBN 9781284181920 (pbk.)
Subjects: | MESH: Emergencies | Motor Vehicles | Automobile Driving | Emergency Responders | Accidents, Traffic--prevention & control | Safety Management--methods | Risk Management--methods | United States
Classification: LCC TL235.8 | NLM WX 215 | DDC 629.225--dc23
LC record available at https://lccn.loc.gov/2018053958

6048

Printed in the United States of America
22 21 20 19 18 10 9 8 7 6 5 4 3 2 1

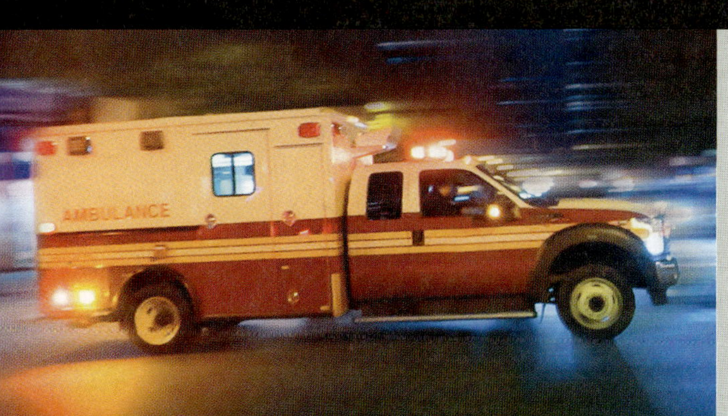

Brief Contents

CHAPTER **1** **Driver Attributes, Training, and Selection** **1**

CHAPTER **2** **Making Safety a Priority** **27**

CHAPTER **3** **Mental, Emotional, and Physical Preparedness** **39**

CHAPTER **4** **Emergency Vehicle Operation and the Law** **49**

CHAPTER **5** **Vehicle Inspection and Maintenance** **57**

CHAPTER **6** **Driving Emergency Vehicle Apparatus** **69**

CHAPTER **7** **Emergency Vehicle Driving** **91**

CHAPTER **8** **Emergency Services Communications** **125**

CHAPTER **9** **Technological Aids** **147**

CHAPTER **10** **Standard Operating Procedures** **153**

APPENDIX **A** **Daily/Weekly Inspection Check Sheet** **163**

GLOSSARY **168**

INDEX **173**

CHAPTER 1

Driver Attributes, Training, and Selection

KNOWLEDGE OBJECTIVES

After studying this chapter, you will be able to:

- Describe the role of the driver/operator when promoting safety, educating crew members, and promoting team building.
- Describe the driver/operator's responsibility in maintaining a safe work environment.
- Describe the functions and limitations of the fire apparatus and its equipment.
- Identify the general requirements of a driver/operator as stated in NFPA 1002. (**NFPA 1002, 5.1.1**)
- Identify the medical and physical requirements of a driver/operator as stated in NFPA 1500.
- Describe the driver training requirements as stated in NFPA 1451.
- Describe the testing and selection process for a driver/operator.

Pump/Water Supply Operator

- List the major causes of death and injury for fire fighters. (**NFPA 1002, 5.1.1**)
- Describe the 16 Fire Fighter Life Safety Initiatives. (**NFPA 1002, 5.1.1**)
- Describe some of the organizations that set the regulations, standards, and procedures intended to ensure a safe working environment for the fire service.
- Describe the connection between physical fitness and fire fighter safety.
- Describe the components of a well-rounded physical fitness program.
- Explain the practices fire fighters should take to promote optimal physical and mental health and well-being.
- Explain the role of a critical incident stress debriefing in preserving the mental well-being of fire fighters.
- List signs and symptoms of behavioral and emotional distress.
- Describe the purpose of an employee assistance program.

SKILLS OBJECTIVES

There are no skills objectives for driver/operator candidates. NFPA 1002 contains no driver/operator Job Performance Requirements for this chapter.

Additional NFPA Standards

- **NFPA 1001**, *Standard for Fire Fighter Professional Qualifications*
- **NFPA 1250**, *Recommended Practice in Fire and Emergency Services Organization Risk Management*
- **NFPA 1451**, *Standard for a Fire and Emergency Service Vehicle Operations Training Program*
- **NFPA 1500**, *Standard on Fire Department Occupational Safety, Health, and Wellness Program*
- **NFPA 1582**, *Standard on Comprehensive Occupational Medical Program for Fire Departments*

Emergency Call

Whether you have worked as a fire fighter for several years or you have been given the opportunity to serve your department as a non-sworn driver/operator, you must be prepared for the responsibility that comes with this position. After completing the required driver training that your department offers to its members, you are now eligible for promotion to the driver rank. Your department has a testing process, and you must score well to be placed on the list of eligible candidates. As you prepare for the promotional exam, you think about the following questions:

1. What is the driver/operator responsible for?
2. Which training is required to operate different fire apparatus in the department?
3. What are the qualities that the department is looking for in a driver/operator?

Introduction

As a **driver/operator**, you have obligations to yourself, to your crew, and to the community that you serve. Both internal and external expectations depend on your ability to perform and complete your initial response assignments, as well as to fulfill any extra duties that arise at the scene. You know the ones—those little problems that occur at almost every call. You hear about them time after time: the generator that is difficult to get running or the power unit that will not start. You are charged with the responsibility to prevent, manage, or rectify those little requests that can make or break the ongoing operations at the scene.

To be successful in your new role, you must first understand and accept the responsibilities that come with the job. You may have moved from the attack crew to the driver/operator position, but that transition does not remove you from any frontline responsibilities. As a driver/operator, you now assume a greater role in ensuring the efficiency and success of your crew. Preventive maintenance, regular inspections of apparatus and equipment, and adherence to jurisdictional operating guidelines will support your own and your crew's success and offer some relief from the pressures created by your new challenges.

New driver/operators may not always realize the responsibilities inherent in this position. Fire fighters are injured or killed every year as a result of accidents that occur while responding and returning from emergency and nonemergency incidents. You must first acknowledge the hazards associated with driving and operating apparatus, and then you must accept the responsibility to prevent these hazards. The position itself is not hazardous; rather, it is the risks associated with driving and operations that are hazardous. You have a responsibility to meet the demands of this role through the "lead by example" process.

When you complete regularly scheduled fire apparatus and equipment inspections, you instill confidence in the other crew members that the fire apparatus and equipment will function when needed. Suppression, rescue, hazardous materials, and emergency medical crews have enough to deal with during the normal course of an emergency. If they have confidence in your ability and the reliability of the fire apparatus and equipment, the fireground situation becomes much easier to manage.

Despite your best inspection and preventive maintenance efforts, situations may still arise in which the equipment fails. If you have a solid foundation of knowledge, experience, and skill, however, a variety of backup plans and alternative methods for accomplishing specific assignments will be readily available to you. Simply stated, more knowledge offers more options, and more options lead to better outcomes.

Pump/Water Supply Operator

Safety Is Everyone's Responsibility

Injury prevention, steps to reduce fire personnel injuries and deaths, and the safety and health measures needed during all activities performed by fire personnel, from training to fireground operations to fire station duties, are everyone's responsibility. Firefighting and other emergency responses are, by their very nature, dangerous. However, many fire personnel are injured off the fireground. Each individual must be aware of the risks inherent in all job responsibilities and activities and learn safe methods of confronting all possible risks. Every fire department must do everything it can to reduce the hazards and dangers of the job and help prevent injuries, illnesses, and deaths. Each fire department must have a strong commitment to health and safety, with the members of that department taking the lead to ensure their own health and safety. When fire personnel understand the various risks associated with their job responsibilities and activities, and the actual threats that they present, safety measures can become routine, consistent, and fully integrated into every activity, procedure, and job description.

Advances in standards, technology, and equipment require fire departments to review and revise their health and safety policies and procedures regularly. Safety officers are responsible for evaluating the hazards of various situations and recommending appropriate safety measures to the incident commander (IC). Each accident, injury, or near miss must be thoroughly investigated to learn why it happened and how it can be avoided in the future. Postincident reviews and research by designated health and safety officers can identify new hazards as well as appropriate safety measures to deal with those hazards. In addition, reports of accidents, fatalities, and near misses from other fire departments can help identify common problems and lead to the development of effective preventive actions.

Because fire personnel must be ready to react immediately to an alarm, preparations for the response begin long before the alarm sounds. These preparations include verifying physical and mental readiness, checking personal equipment, ensuring that the fire apparatus is ready, and confirming that all equipment carried on the apparatus is ready for use. Fire personnel also should be familiar with their response district, know the buildings under their protection, and understand their department's SOPs.

Response actions for the apparatus driver/operator also include considering road and traffic conditions, determining the best route to the incident, identifying nearby hydrant locations or water sources, and selecting the best position for the apparatus at the incident scene.

The Many Roles of the Driver/Operator

The driver/operator is a vital crew member and a safety advocate. When you fill this position, you may be expected to fix components that are broken, offer alternative methods, maintain a state of constant readiness, and support every function that your apparatus can provide. In addition, you have a duty to educate other crew members on their roles and responsibilities to support you, much in the same way that you support their efforts on an emergency scene. For example, if you drive a ladder apparatus, you should ensure that all of the fire fighters in your company understand how to assist in the setup and deployment of the aerial device.

Crew members may not always understand the problems created by their small and seemingly insignificant actions during the response and return phases of an assignment. Consider what happens when fire fighters remove a tool from the fire apparatus and do not inform you. If you do not know the tool has been taken away, you may not account for it when the fire apparatus leaves the scene—and then you have a missing tool. It is your job to bring these problems to light so that success is shared by all.

To build crew confidence and efficiency, you must demonstrate your commitment to the department, the crew, your officer, and the community. You can accomplish this goal by following operating guidelines and applicable laws and regulations, creating and maintaining a safe work environment, and following sound risk-management principles. Team synergy begins with confidence and trust. These attributes initially begin with your words and are later demonstrated through your actions.

DRIVER/OPERATOR TIP

You and your fire officer are a team. By working together and being on the same page, you set an example of teamwork and leadership for the entire department.

Promoting Safety

An effective driver/operator plays several key roles in the company, before, during, and after the response. As with all of the positions within the fire service, safety is always your first priority. Your safety and the safety of your crew and the community serve as an important motivating factor for the manner in which you conduct yourself.

Getting to the incident is important to the operation, but you should also consider the events that occurred prior to your response. Were the required preventive maintenance actions taken? Is the fire apparatus in a proper state of readiness? These are all good questions—but what are the real answers?

Driver/operators greatly influence the safety and efficiency of fire service operations. Indeed, you can take many steps to support a safer work environment. You begin by recognizing the associated hazards and then taking measures to reduce or eliminate these hazards.

Many fire departments utilize standard operating procedures (SOPs)/standard operating guidelines (SOGs) to maintain work-safe environments. In most cases, SOPs were developed to prevent injuries, establish uniformity, and serve as a basic foundation for effective operations at an incident. As a driver/operator, you have an obligation to acknowledge the importance of these SOPs/SOGs. Additionally, acceptance and demonstration of these procedures are critical to the overall safety of the crew and the community.

Seat belts are one safety device that is all too often underutilized by many crew members. According to chapter 4 of National Fire Protection Association (NFPA) 1002, *Standard for Fire Apparatus Driver/Operator Professional Qualifications*, it is the driver/operator's responsibility to ensure that passenger restraints are used. You can demonstrate the importance of wearing a seat belt by being the first one to buckle up and by insisting that your crew members follow suit. A variety of excuses may be cited for not using these safety devices;

however, if you educate crew members on the consequences of ignoring this safety measure, compliance is usually achieved, and safety is maintained FIGURE 1-1. Safety is an attitude, and changing attitudes may not come easy. Your job is to demonstrate the importance of utilizing vehicle safety systems by being the first to comply with them. Driver/operators should also emphasize the importance of passive safety systems such as seat belt monitoring systems.

Another area of concern is the equipment carried on the fire apparatus to support its function. This equipment, including heavy tools, is often stored in elevated areas that may present a significant risk to fire fighters when they are retrieving or restoring this equipment by themselves during preventive maintenance activities, training activities, and emergency response activities FIGURE 1-2. You should demonstrate to crew members the safest technique to accomplish this task with proper use of the fire apparatus' mounted steps, ladders, and rails.

Heavy equipment, regardless of the location in which it is stored, can present a significant safety problem for fire fighters. To minimize their risk of injury, you can educate crew members on the proper removal and lifting techniques for specific pieces of equipment. Mounting devices such as racks, brackets, or trays are not standardized; consequently, each device may have a specific process for tool and equipment removal. It is your role to explain and demonstrate the proper techniques for removing and restoring equipment to its proper location.

SAFETY TIP

Many older apparatus built on both commercial and custom chassis did not include seats and seat belts that would accommodate the extra bulk of fire fighters' personal protective equipment (PPE) and clothing. Restraint systems should be evaluated with fire fighters wearing full PPE while seated in the apparatus. Older apparatus may need to be retrofitted with longer-than-normal seat belts; however, steps should be taken to make certain that any conversions are approved by the chassis and/or seat manufacturer.

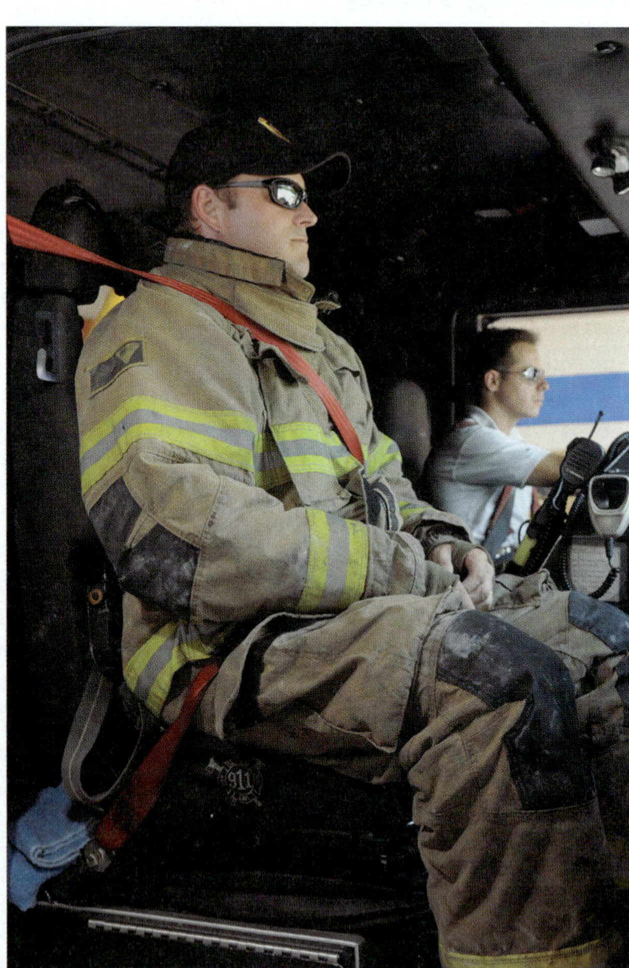

Figure 1-1 Seat belts have saved many fire fighter lives; you can promote safety by being the first crew member to buckle up.

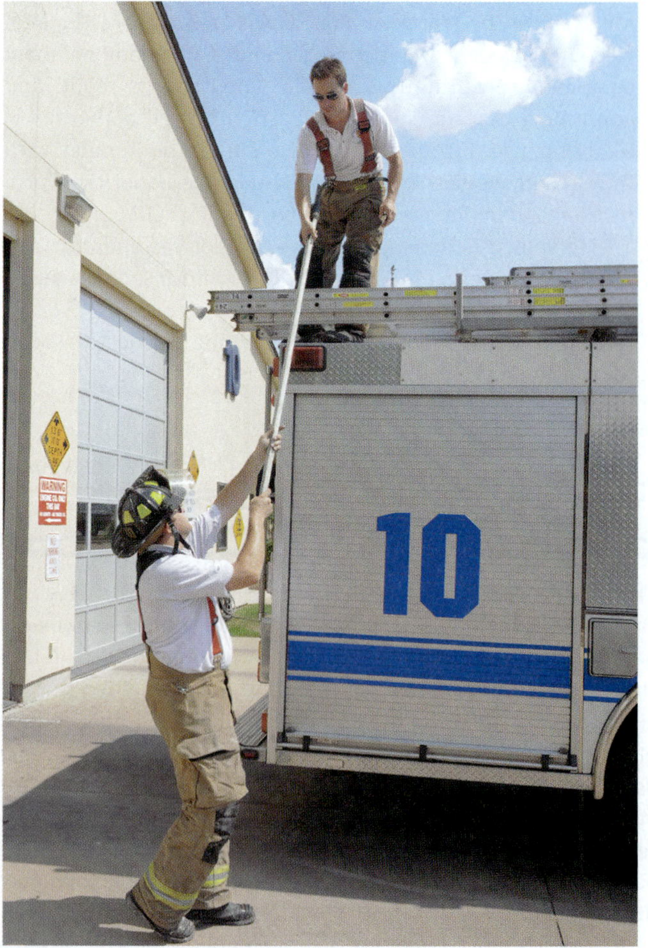

Figure 1-2 Equipment and heavy tools are often stored in areas that present a significant risk to fire fighters.

As a safety advocate, you can play an important role in influencing future fire apparatus and equipment purchases as well as modifications to existing equipment. Explaining and demonstrating the potential hazards to management is a proactive approach toward maintaining a safe work environment. For example, you might demonstrate what can be accomplished by installing the proper rails and steps on the fire apparatus so that fire fighters can safely retrieve equipment. By considering fire apparatus design needs, your department will save in the long term on injury and lost-time compensation costs.

Educating Crew Members

As a driver/operator, you must educate your crew members on the many potential hazards associated with the fire apparatus and its equipment. All too often, fire fighters have been injured while working around fire apparatus–mounted equipment, such as pike poles and ground ladders that stick out on the apparatus.

Here is one simple philosophy that can increase safety: Knowing the "why" makes the "how" come easy. In other words, determining why hazards or dangerous conditions exist makes it easier to reduce or prevent these conditions. As a driver/operator, you can offer many safety tips to your crew members; knowing which information to present is the key to ensuring an effective and safe response. For example, when you are positioning the fire apparatus at an emergency scene, you are observing the traffic conditions while approaching the scene. In contrast, the rest of the crew members do not have the luxury of viewing mirrors and facing forward all of the time. The crew may be unaware of hazards as they exit the fire apparatus—and it is up to you to make sure they are properly informed of any dangers before they leave the cab.

In addition, you must address issues with rider positioning with the crew members. Crew members may inadvertently create a hazard during the response or return phase simply by blocking your view. For example, if a crew member attempts to don self-contained breathing apparatus (SCBA) in the front cab area while en route to a call, his or her actions may obstruct your view of the side-view mirror. By placing an arm out the open window while sitting in the front passenger position, a fire fighter may obstruct your view of a spot mirror during critical apparatus positioning maneuvers. Explaining or demonstrating the hazards created makes other crew members aware of such dangerous conditions so that these situations are not repeated in the future.

Riding assignments are used by many fire departments, where each seat or riding position represents a specific task or function. For example, most fire departments designate the front passenger seat for the fire apparatus fire officer in charge (OIC). Other assigned positions may include the fire fighter on the nozzle, backup line, ventilation, or forcible entry (irons). Assigned riding positions represent a proactive means to ensure that critical functions are assigned to team members prior to arrival. You can extend the responsibilities of these riding positions by explaining to the crew members the response and return hazards associated with driving the fire apparatus. Fire fighters positioned in the other seats can communicate when they see vehicles attempting to pass the fire apparatus or vehicles hanging back in one of the fire apparatus' many **blind spots**. Taking advantage of the existing riding positions is an effective safety measure to make the response safer.

Sometimes communicating on the fireground or en route to the scene can be difficult. You can educate crew members on the various distractions that hinder effective communications, such as sirens, engine noise, equipment noise, and other radio traffic. Collectively, this barrage of noise can make effective communications almost impossible; it may also contribute to long-term hearing loss. Having prior knowledge of these possible conditions allows the crew members to develop a backup plan to reduce possible delays in critical communications during emergency situations. Some apparatus are equipped with a **vehicle intercom system**, which provides a headset and microphone for each rider on the fire apparatus. Such a system enables the fire fighters on the fire apparatus to communicate clearly, without interference from outside noise. The intercom system may also be connected to the fire department's communication system, allowing company personnel to listen to and transmit information over a radio channel. Some intercom systems are hardwired, whereas others are wireless; wireless systems enhance the ability of the driver and spotters to communicate while backing up or positioning the apparatus at emergency scenes.

You must be familiar with SOPs regarding emergency communications such as mayday, emergency traffic, urgent communications, or emergency evacuation signals. In many cases, fire departments rely on air horns from the fire apparatus to signal an emergency evacuation of the structure. If you are not familiar with this process or if you are not fully focused on the events of the incident, the outcome could be catastrophic. Paying strict attention to the **tactical benchmarks** of the incident will keep you ready to initiate life-preserving actions.

Trust and Team Building

The more the crew knows about the driver/operator's roles and responsibilities, the stronger the crew synergy becomes. The best way to impart this knowledge and ensure cohesiveness is to educate the other members of the crew on what you do. Show them how you operate the aerial device, the fire pump, and other features of the fire apparatus. The crew members may not be responsible for the actual operation of the equipment at a fire scene, but better-educated personnel will have a better appreciation of what you and the rest of the team are trying to accomplish.

Staying focused on the tasks at hand makes for a more effective effort. Team building begins with confidence and finishes with trust. Trusting someone means that you believe in that person's abilities. In the fire service, crew members must believe in your ability as a driver/operator. They must believe that you have prepared the fire apparatus, the equipment, and yourself to the best of your abilities. They must believe that your decisions are calculated and that your actions are precise. This all sounds good, but how do you make it a reality? Trust is built through your communications and your actions. Consistency is the foundation needed to gain someone's trust. The more consistent your decisions and your actions, the more trust you will gain.

Building a solid team takes time and patience. It is important to have support when you need it most. A working team makes successful outcomes look easy, even though that is not always the case. Consider this scenario: Do you and your crew perceive packing hose as a meaningless task, or do you perceive it as an action of readiness to meet the demands of the next alarm, thereby making your job easier at the next call? If you have ever pulled a "spaghetti mess" hose load, you can relate to the importance of team building—effective teams do not demonstrate such carelessness.

How does this issue relate to the roles and responsibilities of a driver/operator? All members of the crew must be able to perform their assignments without reservation or hesitation. As the nozzle operator at a fire scene, have you ever stood at the front door of a burning building waiting for the driver to charge the hoseline? When you are in this position and ready to make an attack on the fire, it is frustrating to not have the line immediately charged with water. Crews want a driver whom they can trust to deliver a sustained water supply quickly and efficiently. As the driver/operator, you are obligated to provide your crew members with the best possible on-scene support that you can muster up. Members of sports teams rely on one another to win championships; fire fighters rely on one another to survive.

SAFETY TIP

No nonessential conversation should be allowed while responding to an emergency call. All communication should be limited to mission-critical information, and crew members should be instructed to listen for essential radio messages.

Pump/Water Supply Operator

Causes of Fire Fighter Deaths and Injuries

Deaths and injuries are not stopped by titles or ranks. The term "fire fighter" is used in this section to identify *all* fire personnel who respond to emergencies. The NFPA reports that 69 fire fighters were killed in the line of duty in 2016. These deaths occurred during fireground operations, at nonemergency incident scenes, in nonemergency situations such as in fire stations, during training, and while responding to or returning from emergency situations **FIGURE 1-3**.

The largest number of deaths occurred from stress, overexertion, and medical issues **TABLE 1-1**. Cardiac events accounted for 38 percent of these deaths. The second leading cause of death was vehicle crashes. In 2016, 19 fire fighters died in vehicle accidents, a majority of which occurred while responding to or returning from incidents **FIGURE 1-4**.

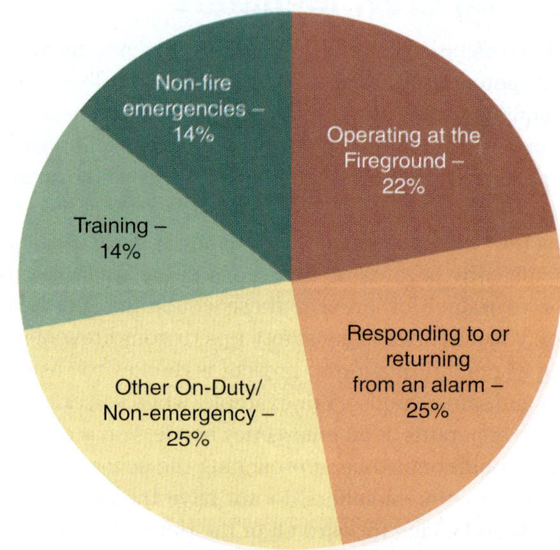

Figure 1-3 Fire fighter deaths in the United States by type of duty. A total of 69 fire fighters died in the line of duty in 2016.
National Fire Protection Association, Firefighter Fatalities in the United States—2016 (June 2017).

Table 1-1 Fire Fighter Deaths by Cause of Injury

Cause	Percent
Overexertion, stress, medical	42%
Vehicle accidents	25%
Falls	10%
Struck by objects	6%
Other	6%
Fatal assault	4%
Structural collapse	4%
Struck by vehicles	3%

Source: National Fire Protection Association, Firefighter Fatalities in the United States—2016 (June 2017).

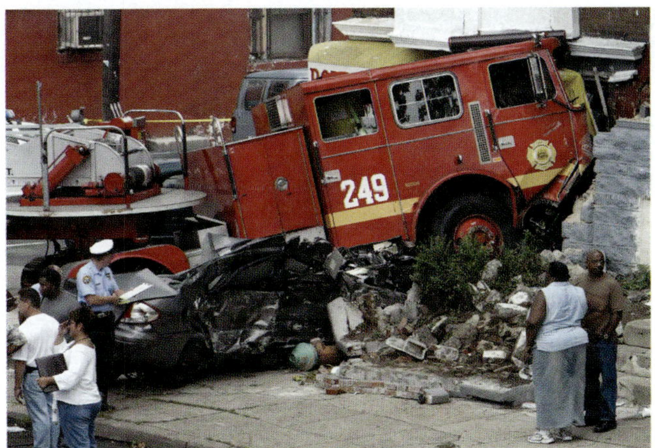

Figure 1-4 Motor vehicle collisions are one of the leading causes of death for fire personnel.

The NFPA estimates that 62,085 fire fighters were injured in the line of duty in 2016, an 8.8 percent decrease from the previous year. Fewer than half of the injuries occurred on the fireground. The leading cause of fireground injuries was overexertion or strain.

Reducing Fire Fighter Deaths and Injuries

In 1992, Congress created the National Fallen Firefighters Foundation to lead a nationwide effort to remember U.S. fire fighters who died in the line of duty. In the years since then, this foundation has expanded its programs to sponsor the annual National Fallen Firefighters Memorial Weekend, offer support programs for family members and other survivors, award scholarships to fire service members' survivors, and work to prevent line-of-duty injuries and deaths.

Most fire fighter injuries and deaths are the result of preventable situations. Recognizing this fact, organizations such as the International Association of Fire Chiefs (IAFC) and the National Fallen Firefighters Foundation have developed programs with the goal of reducing line-of-duty deaths. For example, the Near-Miss Reporting System, developed in 2005, provides a method for reporting situations that could have resulted in injuries or deaths. This system, which is accessible via the Internet, provides a means for all fire personnel to learn from situations that occur both rarely and frequently.

In an effort to do more to prevent line-of-duty deaths and injuries, the first National Firefighter Life Safety Summit convened in 2004, uniting fire service leaders and organizations across the United States. The result was the creation of the Everyone Goes Home Program and a set of key initiatives, the 16 Firefighter Life Safety Initiatives. The goal of the Everyone Goes Home program is to raise awareness of life safety issues, improve safety practices, and allow everyone to return home at the end of his or her shift. The 16 Firefighter Life Safety Initiatives describe steps that need to be taken to change the current culture of the fire service to help make it a safe work environment **TABLE 1-2**.

Reducing fire fighter injuries and deaths requires the dedicated efforts of every fire fighter, of every fire department, and of the entire fire community working together. It also requires a safety program that integrates important components such as regulations, standards, procedures, personnel, training, and equipment.

SAFETY TIP

Injury and illness prevention is a responsibility shared by each member of the firefighting team. Fire fighters must always consider three groups when ensuring safety at the scene:

- Their personal safety
- The safety of other team members
- The safety of everyone present at an emergency scene

Regulations, Standards, and Procedures

Safety is the highest priority in the fire service. Ensuring a safe working environment for the members of the fire service is a challenge that has been and continues to be addressed by several professional organizations and is the goal of various regulations, standards, and procedures related to fire fighters' work.

Standards are issued by nongovernmental entities and are generally based on consensus. The NFPA develops standards that help to ensure the consistency of training courses, apparatus, equipment, and operations. The NFPA's mission in creating these standards is focused on safety: The standards are intended to save lives and reduce loss by arming fire fighters with information, knowledge, and passion. Ultimately, they are designed to help you become a safe, efficient, and competent fire fighter. You will see many NFPA standards referenced throughout this course. Most fire departments have access to the full text of these standards.

To reduce the risks of accidents, injuries, occupational illnesses, and fatalities, a successful health and safety program that complies with NFPA 1500, *Standard on Fire Department Occupational Safety, Health, and Wellness Program*, must be established. NFPA 1500 includes

Table 1-2 16 Fire Fighter Life Safety Initiatives

1. **Cultural Change:** Define and advocate the need for a cultural change within the fire service relating to safety and incorporating leadership, management, supervision, accountability, and personal responsibility.
2. **Accountability:** Enhance the personal and organizational accountability for health and safety throughout the fire service.
3. **Risk Management:** Focus greater attention on the integration of risk management with incident management at all levels, including strategic, tactical, and planning responsibilities.
4. **Empowerment:** All fire fighters must be empowered to stop unsafe practices.
5. **Training and Certification:** Develop and implement national standards for training, qualifications, and certification (including regular recertification) that are equally applicable to all fire fighters based on the duties they are expected to perform.
6. **Medical and Physical Fitness:** Develop and implement national medical and physical fitness standards that are equally applicable to all fire fighters based on the duties they are expected to perform.
7. **Research Agenda:** Create a national research agenda and a data collection system that relates to the 16 Firefighter Life Safety Initiatives.
8. **Technology:** Utilize available technology whenever it can produce higher levels of health and safety.
9. **Fatality and Near-Miss Investigations:** Thoroughly investigate all fire fighter fatalities, injuries, and near misses.
10. **Grant Support:** Grant programs should support the implementation of safe practices and procedures and/or mandate safe practices as an eligibility requirement.
11. **Response Policies:** National standards for emergency response policies and procedures should be developed and championed.
12. **Violent Incident Response:** National protocols for response to violent incidents should be developed and championed.
13. **Psychological Support:** Fire fighters and their families must have access to counseling and psychological support.
14. **Public Education:** Public education must receive more resources and be championed as a critical fire and life safety program.
15. **Code Enforcement and Sprinklers:** Advocacy must be strengthened for the enforcement of codes and the installation of home fire sprinklers.
16. **Apparatus Design and Safety:** Safety must be a primary consideration in the design of apparatus and equipment.

Source: National Fallen Fire Fighters Association. Everyone Goes Home. 16 Fire Fighter Life Safety Initiatives.

guidance on several key aspects of health and safety, including policies, training and education, apparatus operation, PPE, emergency operations, station safety, medical and physical requirements, and health and safety programs. This chapter addresses each of these areas briefly.

NFPA 1500 provides a template for implementing a comprehensive health and safety program. Additional NFPA standards focus on specific subjects directly related to health and safety—for example, NFPA 1582, *Standard on Comprehensive Occupational Medical Program for Fire Departments.*

Regulations are issued and enforced by governmental bodies. The federal **Occupational Safety and Health Administration (OSHA)**, along with a variety of state and provincial health and safety agencies, develops and enforces government regulations on workplace safety and, in some cases, responder safety. NFPA standards often are incorporated by reference in government regulations.

Each state in the United States has the right to adopt and/or supersede workplace health and safety regulations put forth by the federal agency OSHA. States that have adopted the OSHA regulations are called state-plan states. California, for example, is a state-plan state; its regulatory body is called Cal-OSHA. Approximately half of the states in the United States are state-plan states. States that have not adopted the OSHA regulations are considered non-plan states. Non-plan states are called EPA (Environmental Protection Agency) states because they follow Title 40 of the **Code of Federal Regulations (CFR)**, Protection of the Environment, Part 311, Worker Protection. The CFR is a collection of permanent rules published by the federal government; it includes 50 titles that represent broad areas of interest that are governed by federal regulation.

LISTEN UP!

It is important to understand the relationship between OSHA regulations and NFPA standards. OSHA regulations are the law; NFPA standards are generally utilized as guidelines that under some circumstances have the force of law.

Every fire department should have a set of SOPs or SOGs that provide specific information on the actions that should be taken to accomplish a certain task. These procedures are vital because they enable everyone in the department to function properly and know what is expected for each task. Each member is responsible for understanding and following these procedures, thereby enabling fire personnel from different stations or companies to work together safely and smoothly. The fire department chain of command also enforces safety goals and procedures. In particular, the command structure keeps everyone working toward common goals in a safe manner. An Incident Command System (ICS) is a nationally recognized plan to establish command and control of emergency incidents. The ICS is flexible enough to meet the needs of any emergency situation, so it should be implemented at every emergency scene—from a routine auto accident to a major disaster involving responders from numerous agencies.

Many fire departments have a health and safety committee that is responsible for establishing policies and monitoring fire fighter safety. Members of this committee should include representatives from every area, component, and level within the department, from fire fighters to chief officers. The health and safety officer and the fire department physician also should be members of the committee.

Personnel

A health and safety program is only as effective as the individuals who implement it. Safety officers are members of the fire department whose primary responsibility is safety. At the emergency scene, the designated safety officer reports directly to the IC and has the authority to correct or stop any action judged to be unsafe. Safety officers observe operations and conditions, evaluate risks, and work with the IC to identify hazards and ensure the safety of all personnel. They also determine when fire fighters can work without SCBA after a fire is extinguished.

Safety officers can enhance safety in the workplace, at emergency incidents, and at training exercises. Even so, it is important to remember that each and every member of the fire department shares the responsibility for promoting safety, both as an individual and as a member of the team.

Teamwork is an essential element of safe emergency operations. On the fireground and during any hazardous activity, members must work together to get the job done. Freelancing has no place on the fireground; it poses a danger both to the fire fighter who acts independently and to every other person on the emergency scene. **Freelancing** is acting independently of a superior's orders or the fire department's SOPs.

A team member who freelances can easily get into trouble by being in the wrong place at the wrong time or by doing the wrong thing. For example, a fire fighter who enters a burning structure without informing a superior may be trapped by rapidly changing conditions. By the time the fire fighter is missed, it may be too late to perform a rescue. Searching for a missing fire fighter exposes others to unnecessary risk.

Training

Adequate training is essential for fire fighters' safety. Fire personnel must avoid sloppy practices or shortcuts that might potentially contribute to injuries and learn how to identify hazards and unsafe conditions.

The knowledge and skills developed during training are essential to maintain safety at actual emergency scenes. The initial training course is just the beginning—all members must continually seek out additional courses to keep their skills current.

Equipment

A driver/operator's equipment ranges from power and hand tools to PPE and electronic instruments. When filling this role, you must know how to use equipment in the correct manner and then operate it safely at all times. Equipment also must be properly maintained. Poorly maintained equipment can create additional hazards to the user or fail to operate when needed.

Manufacturers usually supply operating instructions and safety procedures for their equipment. These instructions cover proper use of the equipment, its limitations, and warnings about potential hazards. All personnel must read and heed these warnings and instructions. In addition, new equipment must meet applicable standards to ensure that it can perform under the difficult and dangerous conditions often encountered on the fireground.

Personal Health and Well-Being

Safety and well-being are directly related to personal health and physical fitness. Although fire departments regularly monitor and evaluate the health of fire personnel, each department member is responsible for his or her own personal health, conditioning, and nutrition. To be an effective driver/operator, you must exercise regularly, eat a healthy diet, get an adequate amount of sleep, and take preventive measures to avoid illnesses such as heart disease and cancer.

Physical Fitness

All personnel—whether career or volunteer, sworn or civilian—should spend at least an hour each day in physical fitness training FIGURE 1-5. Personnel should be examined by either a personal or departmental physician before beginning any new workout routine. An exercise routine that includes weight training, cardiovascular workouts, and stretching with a concentration on job-related exercises is ideal. For example, many people use a stair-climbing machine to focus on the muscle groups used for climbing.

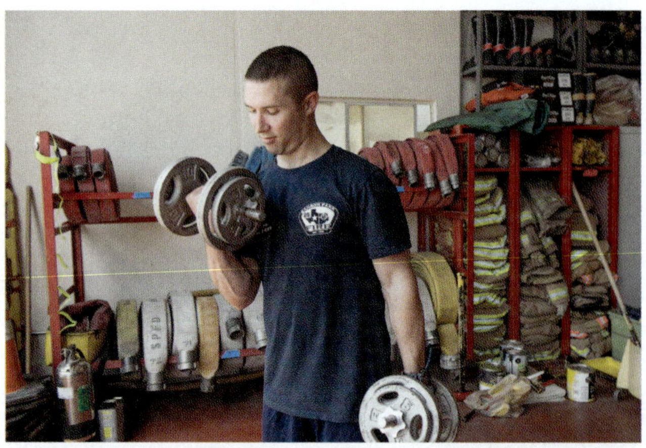

Figure 1-5 Regular exercise will help you to stay healthy and perform your job effectively.

Although this type of exercise builds cardiovascular endurance for the fireground, other muscle groups should not be neglected. Physical fitness must be a career-long activity. Operating fire apparatus is a stressful activity that demands you maintain a good fitness level throughout your career.

Nutrition

Diet is another important aspect of personal health. A healthy diet includes fruits, vegetables, healthy fats, whole grains, and lean protein. Pay attention to portion sizes—unfortunately, most people eat larger portions than their bodies need. Substitute healthy choices (such as fruit) for high-calorie desserts.

Hydration

Hydration is an important part of staying healthy. A good guideline is to consume 8 to 10 ounces (0.2 to 0.3 liter) of water for every 5 to 10 minutes of physical exertion. Do not wait until you feel thirsty to start rehydrating. In fact, fire personnel should drink up to a gallon of water each day to keep properly hydrated. Being adequately hydrated before an emergency occurs will enable you to better maintain adequate hydration and continue to function as an effective and healthy fire fighter.

The amount of water needed to maintain adequate hydration depends on the type of work you are doing and the ambient temperature. Whenever you are working in full PPE, however, you should recognize that your internal environment will rapidly become hot, and you cannot dissipate body heat to the outside environment.

Proper hydration enables muscles to work longer and reduces the risk of illness and injuries at the emergency scene. Some recent studies have indicated that maintaining a good level of hydration while engaged in firefighting activities may also reduce your chance of having a heart attack.

LISTEN UP!

Maintaining proper hydration is essential to performing at your peak physical level.

Sleep

Good health requires that you get an adequate amount of uninterrupted sleep to maintain alertness, prevent stress, and avoid illnesses and injuries. Because it is not always possible to get adequate sleep during long work shifts, it is important that you get adequate amounts of uninterrupted sleep during your off-duty time. Establish a consistent sleep schedule and sleep routine, such as turning off all electronic devices a half hour before bedtime to allow your mind to wind down and prepare for sleep.

Heart Disease

Heart disease is the leading cause of death in the United States as a whole and a leading cause of death among fire personnel in particular. A healthy lifestyle that includes a balanced diet, weight training, and cardiovascular exercise can help reduce many risk factors for heart disease and enable fire fighters to meet the physical demands of the job.

Research projects are now under way that are seeking to use advanced technology as a means to improve health and safety in the fire service. For example, the SMARTER project (Science, Medicine, Research, Technology for Emergency Responders) uses specially designed, wearable monitoring equipment to measure the physiological stress of fire fighters while they perform on-the-job duties. Participants' heart rates, core body temperatures, respiratory rates, and more are recorded, allowing for early detection of abnormalities and real-time monitoring of atmospheric conditions (Smith, 2017).

Cancer

An increase in the use of synthetic products has led to an increase in the toxicity of today's modern fires. Cancer—now the second leading cause of death among fire fighters—can be caused by a wide variety of cancer-causing substances (carcinogens) entering the body (International Association of Fire Fighters, 2017). These include exhaust from diesel engines, poisonous gases in smoke, and a wide variety of chemical particles. The dirt and soot that become attached to a fire fighter's turnout gear and uniform contain large quantities of substances known to cause cancer. Fire personnel's hoods and gloves are thought to contain especially high concentrations of carcinogens. In general, carcinogens can be ingested through the mouth, injected into the body, absorbed through the respiratory system, or absorbed through the skin. Fire personnel, however, are most likely to absorb carcinogens through their skin and through their respiratory systems.

The Firefighter Cancer Support Network (2017) estimates that fire fighters have a 9 percent higher risk of being diagnosed with cancer than the general U.S. population. Along the same lines, a study conducted by the National Institute for Occupational Safety and Health (NIOSH) concluded that the nearly 30,000 fire fighter participants had a greater number of cancer diagnoses and cancer-related deaths than the general U.S. population. These diagnoses consisted of mostly digestive, oral, respiratory and urinary cancers. When comparing fire fighters in this study to each other, researchers found that the chance of lung cancer increased with the amount of time spent at fires, and the chance of leukemia deaths increased with the number of fire incidents to which fire fighters responded (Centers for Disease Control and Prevention, 2016).

The Fire Fighter Cancer Support Network suggests actions you can take to protect yourself, as a fire fighter, from developing cancer:

1. Use SCBA from the initial attack to the end of overhaul.
2. Do gross field decontamination of PPE to remove as much soot and particulates as possible.
3. Use Wet-Naps or baby wipes to remove as much soot as possible from head, neck, jaw, throat, underarms, and hands immediately and while still on the scene.
4. Change your clothes and wash them immediately after a fire.
5. Shower thoroughly after a fire.
6. Clean your PPE, gloves, hood, and helmet immediately after a fire.
7. Do not take contaminated clothes or PPE home or store it in your vehicle.
8. Decontaminate the interior of the fire apparatus after fires.
9. Keep bunker gear out of living and sleeping quarters.
10. Stop using tobacco products.
11. Use sunscreen or sunblock.

Notably, contaminated objects that are placed in the cab of a fire engine or in the trunk of a member's personal vehicle will continue to release cancer-causing substances into the area around them. The longer contaminated objects are present, the longer these objects will continue to release toxic substances. Remove bunker gear and all other contaminated clothing as soon as possible. Bunker gear should be transported away from the riding compartment in a fire apparatus and be thoroughly washed immediately according to the manufacturer's instructions FIGURE 1-6.

Some cancers do not present for twenty years or more after exposure to a carcinogen. Given this reality, it is important to reduce your exposure to cancer-causing substances starting on your first day of service as a fire fighter.

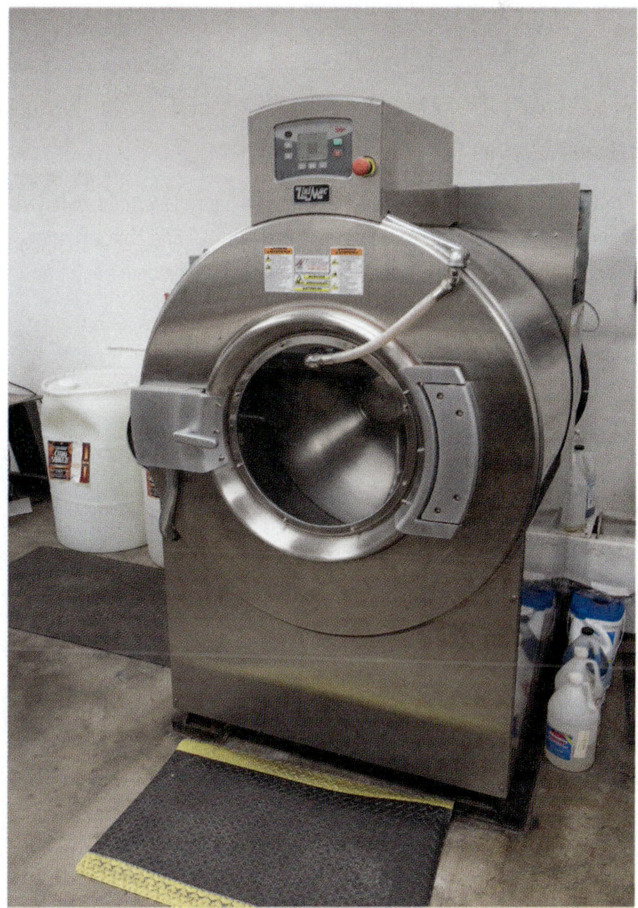

Figure 1-6 Special washing machines are available to launder personal protective clothing.

Tobacco, Alcohol, and Illicit Drugs

Many fire departments have adopted policies that prohibit the use of tobacco products by fire personnel, both on duty and off duty. Smoking is a major risk factor in cardiovascular disease, reduces the efficiency of the body's respiratory system, and increases the risk of lung and other types of cancer. You should avoid tobacco products entirely for both health and insurance reasons.

Alcohol is another substance that fire personnel should avoid. Alcohol is a mood-altering substance that can be abused. Excessive alcohol use can damage the body and affect performance. Driver/operators who have consumed alcohol within the previous 8 hours must not be permitted to engage in training or emergency operations. In addition, alcohol use increases the risk of mouth, throat, larynx, esophagus, liver, colon, and breast cancers (American Cancer Society, 2017).

Illicit drug use has absolutely no place in the fire service. Many fire departments have drug-testing programs to ensure that personnel do not use or abuse drugs. The illegal use of drugs endangers your life, the lives of your team members, and the public you serve.

SAFETY TIP

Everyone is subject to an occasional illness or injury. Operating safely as a member of a team, however, requires both fitness and concentration. Do not compromise the safety of the team or your personal health by trying to work while you are ill or injured.

Counseling and Critical Incident Stress

Fire personnel are often exposed to stressful situations and work in an environment in which they are subject to unscheduled and unexpected emergency events. Many fire personnel see more traumatic situations in a short time than most other citizens see in their entire lifetime. Fighting fires involves not only the stresses directly connected to firefighting and to rendering emergency medical care but also the added burdens of disrupted sleep patterns, rotating work schedules, unscheduled overtime, and interrupted meal schedules. High levels of stress can produce a variety of symptoms. Some people are not able to sleep well; others tend to gain or lose weight. Many people become irritable when stressed. Overeating, increased consumption of alcoholic beverages, and use of nonprescribed drugs may be some individuals' responses to stress. In still others, stress may produce depression or suicidal thoughts.

To diminish the negative effects of these stressors, it is important to get adequate sleep, consume a healthy, balanced diet, and engage in adequate exercise. It is also important for you to balance your work schedule with other activities and monitor your behavioral health. Finally, it is essential to identify and utilize the resources that are available to assist in maintaining behavioral health. Some of these resources are provided by employers, such as the employee assistance programs discussed later in this chapter. Other resources and assistance are provided by professional organizations. For example, the International Association of Firefighters (IAFF) has information available through its website, as well as the inpatient IAFF Center of Excellence for Behavioral Health Treatment and Recovery.

DRIVER/OPERATOR TIP

Find time for yourself and your family as a mental buffer from the stressors of the job.

Critical Incident Stress Management

Critical incidents challenge the capacity of most individuals to deal with stress. It is important to understand what the stressors in this job are and to learn how to work to diminish their effects. Examples of critical incidents include the following:

- Line-of-duty deaths (police, fire/rescue, emergency medical services [EMS])
- Suicide of a colleague
- Serious injury to a colleague
- Situations that involve a high level of personal risk to fire fighters
- Events in which the victim is known to the fire fighters
- Multiple-casualty/disaster/terrorism incidents
- Events involving death or life-threatening injury or illness to a victim, especially a child
- Events that are prolonged or end with a negative or unexpected outcome

This list is not complete, nor is it necessarily a fact that any of these situations will seriously trouble every individual. Normal coping mechanisms help many fire personnel to successfully handle many situations. Some individuals have a high capacity to deal with stressful situations by engaging in exercise, talking to friends and family, or turning to their religious beliefs. These are healthy, nondestructive ways to deal with the pressures of being exposed to a critical incident.

Sometimes, however, individuals react to critical incidents in ways that are not positive—such as alcohol or drug abuse, depression, the inability to function normally, or a negative attitude toward life and work. These symptoms can occur in anyone, even individuals who usually have healthy coping skills. Reactions will vary from one individual to the next, both in type and in severity. Many times fire personnel do not realize they are affected in a deeply negative manner. A somewhat routine incident, however, may trigger negative reactions from a critical incident that occurred in the past. Critical incident stress can also be cumulative, building up over time. This condition, which is called burnout, cannot be traced to any one incident.

The recognized stages of emotional reaction experienced by fire fighters and other rescue personnel after a stressful incident can include the following:

1. Anxiety
2. Denial/disbelief
3. Frustration/anger
4. Inability to function logically
5. Remorse
6. Grief
7. Reconciliation/acceptance

These stages can occur within minutes or hours, or they can take several days or months to unfold. Not all of the steps will occur for every event, and they do not necessarily occur in the order given here.

Fire personnel should recognize the resources available to them and know how they can access them. Maintaining good emotional health is a simple but important part of fire personnel survival. The aim of counseling, peer support teams, employee assistance programs, and **critical incident stress management (CISM)** programs is to prevent these emotional reactions from having a negative impact on fire personnel's work and life, over both the short term and the long term **FIGURE 1-7**. The major difference between CISM and peer support teams is that CISM teams usually respond immediately after a crisis incident, whereas peer support teams provide continuous, ongoing support. For example, a **critical incident stress debriefing (CISD)** is held as soon as possible after a traumatic call; it provides a forum for fire and EMS personnel to discuss the anxieties, stress, and emotions triggered by a difficult call. Follow-up sessions can be arranged for individuals who continue to experience stressful or emotional responses after a challenging incident. With peer support teams, specially trained department members help those struggling with day-to-day issues by communicating with them regularly and recommending resources to assist them.

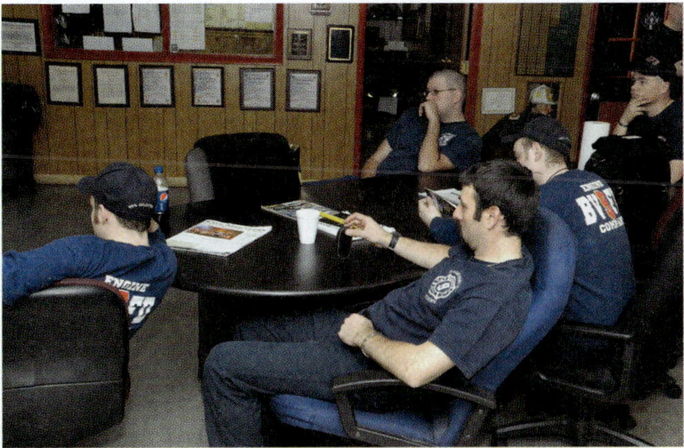

Figure 1-7 Group stress debriefings are sometimes used to alleviate stress reactions generated by high-stress emergency situations.
© Tom Carter/Getty Images.

Everyone handles stress differently, and new fire personnel need time to develop the personal resources necessary to deal with difficult situations. If any incident proves mentally or emotionally disturbing to you, and it is beyond your ability to deal with it alone or with those closest to you, ask your supervisor for assistance. Your supervisor should be familiar with the resources available to fire fighters and may refer you to a qualified professional. Signs that you may need assistance include having trouble sleeping or having difficulty dealing with your thoughts or feelings. Some departments are proactive and include training in topics such as stress first aid.

Firefighting is a job that requires close teamwork. It is the responsibility of all fire personnel to monitor themselves and other members of their team for signs of mental stress. All fire fighters are all interdependent on other members of their team to accomplish the team's goal. This team needs to function well not only at emergency scenes but also when performing routine tasks or relaxing between runs. As a fire fighter, it is important that you respect each member of your team. Bullying or discrimination should never be tolerated. It is also everyone's job to be on the lookout for signs of unhealthy behavior or stress. If you think a fellow member is exhibiting signs of stress or suffering from depression, there are several ways in which you may be able to help. Although those approaches may vary, the overall purpose remains the same.

Sometimes it may be helpful to sit down with a coworker and ask how the individual is doing or to let your coworker know that you are concerned about him or her. Encourage your coworker to seek help, if necessary. If you see signs of stress, talk with your officer or someone who can help that person receive assistance.

Suicide Awareness and Prevention

In recent years, there have been more fire personnel suicides than line-of-duty deaths. In 2016, there were 99 reported fire fighter deaths as a result of suicide (Firefighter Behavioral Health Alliance, 2017). Recent estimates suggest that a fire department is three times more likely to experience a suicide in any given year than a line-of-duty death

(National Fallen Fire Fighters Association, 2017). This ratio reveals that stressful occupations may experience a higher rate of suicides than the general population, and many people are concerned about the relatively high incidence of suicide in fire fighters and other emergency care providers.

The Firefighter Behavioral Health Alliance (FBHA) recommends that organizations discuss the negative effects of "cultural brainwashing" among department members. This term describes how fire fighters are "supposed to act" so they do not look weak or burden others. While fire personnel are trained to be the best they can be, many are not prepared for the ill effects or aftermath of stress or a traumatic situation. It is important to understand that by recognizing signs of stress or depression in a team member, you may be able to help that person get assistance for the problem before it becomes worse.

DRIVER/OPERATOR TIP

According to the Firefighter Behavioral Health Alliance, the top five warning signs of job-related stress include the following:

- Recklessness/impulsiveness
- Anger
- Isolation
- Loss of confidence in abilities or skills
- Sleep deprivation

If you are suffering from these issues, please seek help from your employee assistance program, chaplain, peer support team, or a qualified counselor in your community.

Employee Assistance Programs

Many formal programs have been developed to support fire personnel behavioral health. These programs are maintained by fire departments, unions, local governments, and even charitable organizations. Support is provided through special events, projects, peer support, chaplain programs, and education. A traditional and common form of support for fire fighters is **employee assistance programs (EAPs)**, which provide confidential help with a wide range of problems that might affect performance. Many fire departments have established EAPs so that fire fighters can get counseling, support, or other assistance in dealing with physical, financial, emotional, or substance abuse problems. EAPs include a variety of helpful resources, including access to qualified counselors and chaplains who have a working knowledge of the fire service. Some fire departments have qualified counselors available around the clock. The initial counseling may consist of a group session for all fire personnel and rescuers; alternatively, it can be done on a one-on-one basis or in smaller groups. A fire officer may refer a member to an EAP if a problem starts to affect the individual's job performance. Members who take advantage of an EAP can do so with complete confidentiality and without fear of retribution.

According to the FBHA, many fire fighters do not seek help when they need it, mainly due to confidentiality concerns, job promotion concerns, or counselors' lack of familiarity with the fire service culture. The FBHA recommends inviting counselors to the station and including them on ride time, in training, and during meals. Another suggestion is to have the EAP counselors create a video biography so department members and their families can see who they are and get to know them.

Maintaining a Safe Work Environment

Maintaining a safe work environment is a tough job. As part of that environment, keeping fire apparatus and equipment service-ready can be a challenge for the newly appointed driver/operator. To make the process flow seamlessly, experienced driver/operators should start training future candidates for this position early in their careers.

Educating crew members is a major responsibility for any driver/operator. You must teach them how to recognize operational errors or equipment malfunctions that occur at emergency and nonemergency events. In addition, you should help them understand the **stressors** that challenge the driver/operator on a regular basis and emphasize that everyone plays a role in maintaining a safe work environment. Obtaining team buy-in is your goal; you want to have the entire crew onboard with your work-safe philosophy. Over time, your efforts will create a work-safe ethic that will accommodate future changes in emergency and nonemergency operations.

Safety is embedded in all aspects of firefighting. As a driver/operator, you are charged with performing apparatus and equipment inspections and undertaking basic preventive maintenance operations. When the hydraulic rescue system will not start, things can become very stressful, very quickly. Regularly scheduled inspections, operational service checks, and scheduled preventive maintenance actions will make major contributions to ensuring the reliability of the fire apparatus and equipment carried onboard. Routine inspections must be taken seriously. Fire apparatus and equipment operational checks must not only be performed but also documented by the driver/operator—after all, that is part of your job.

What should you be doing in the course of a day? First, you should actively promote the work-safe philosophy by completing daily inspections of equipment and fire apparatus systems such as tank, tank water, and fuel levels; hydraulic rescue systems; electrical power plants and cables; pneumatic equipment and supply hoses; portable and mobile radios; fire pump operation; gas detection meters; ladder main or boom operation; thermal imagers; SCBA; hand lights; apparatus braking systems; tires and wheels; and audible and visual warning devices. The key to completing a thorough inspection is to develop a routine that allows the driver/operator to conduct the inspection the same way every time. **Job aids**, such as checklists or inspection sheets, are critical to ensuring the accuracy and consistency of inspections. If supported by a thorough inspection process, these inspection sheets or checklists will quickly become routine parts of the job. Their ongoing use will provide the consistency that supports and confirms fire apparatus and equipment reliability. Cutting corners has no place in the fire service. An upfront commitment to completing the full scope of your assigned responsibilities is paramount.

Other informational sources that should be used during routine inspection and preventive maintenance processes include operating and general service manuals. These manuals are required to be provided by the manufacturer with the purchase of its fire apparatus or equipment. Operating manuals are key resources for any preventive maintenance and general service program. The purchasing of fire apparatus and equipment is a competitive market for manufacturers; the continuing stream of apparatus system upgrades, equipment functionality revisions, product design changes, and newly introduced safety features makes it imperative for you to stay on top of the ongoing process of upgrading and redesigning equipment and fire apparatus. Unfortunately, not all fire pumps, rescue and suppression equipment, and apparatus systems are created equal. Different manufacturers require specific procedures, service and maintenance schedules, and lubricants to comply with their warranty obligations and life-cycle expectations. The task of keeping fire apparatus and equipment in good working order becomes much easier when you remember to refer to the manufacturer's recommendations—in other words, always check the manual.

After completing your inspections, your day is not done. Training and education continue at the fire station. In the firehouse, you should educate crew members on the importance of using the safety equipment. Demonstrate how to preset, start, and operate specialized equipment. This task can be accomplished during the daily inspection and maintenance process. Get everyone involved—after all, their involvement supports their own personal safety. Teach company members how to troubleshoot problems in the field and how to correct problems as they occur through the use of a process or routine.

Consider the gasoline-powered equipment carried on the apparatus. "I started it this morning but it wouldn't start at the rescue scene"—does that complaint sound familiar? Give crew members something to work with, something to remember. In basic training, fire personnel are taught the PASS mnemonic as a tool to help them execute the procedure for operating a fire extinguisher: Pull the pin, Aim the nozzle, Squeeze the handle, and Sweep the base of the fire. Even to this day, you should remember that memory aid. If this technique works for fire extinguishers, it should also work for starting power units. Try something like FCSP ("fire fighters can save people") to help crew members remember the right sequence: Fuel, Choke, Switch, and Pull. This acronym may help fire fighters remember to first check the fuel level and fuel shut-off valve, then set the choke, then turn the start/engine cutoff switch to "start" or "run," and finally pull the cord or engage the start/ignition switch. To reinforce this sequence, you might write the acronym on the top of the engine cover.

Tools such as mnemonics and acronyms are used often in the fire service to help fire fighters remember important information. Commercial driving instructors use ABCDE to emphasize key points to be covered in fire apparatus tire inspections: Abrasions, Bulging, Cuts, Dry rot, and Even-wear inspection. Remember the "everything under pressure is worse" philosophy? That statement holds true for fire personnel whether they are attempting to do 10 things at once while people are screaming for help or whether they are performing routine preventive maintenance procedures. Your role is to relieve some of the stress on the job by educating the crew on the basic mechanics of how equipment operates and functions.

DRIVER/OPERATOR TIP

You can make a difference by educating your crew, maintaining your knowledge and skill levels, and following the rules that are in place for your safety.

With experience, you may discover other roles and responsibilities attached to the driver/operator position. For example, while operating at the scene of a motor vehicle accident, you may not only position the fire apparatus so as to protect the scene but also act as a lookout for the crew in heavy traffic conditions. If you anticipate and prepare for these additions and changes in your role, you will maintain your consistency and reliability while completing your assignments. Know your fire apparatus, your equipment, and your community—how you perform will reflect your knowledge of these three areas. In time, you will gain confidence and experience. Your reliability will be acknowledged, and your consistency will be steadfast.

Lead by Example

As a driver/operator, you must lead by example. Follow the rules yourself. SOPs are for everyone—so lead by adhering to them. Follow and promote compliance with all SOPs. For example, by completing and documenting your fire apparatus inspections as part of your normal routine, you demonstrate to the crew your commitment to everyone's success. This will give you credibility with the other crew members and keep you safe at the same time. SOPs cover many fire department service areas, such as responding to and departing from incidents, required personal protective equipment for highway incidents, fire apparatus positioning, and general company assignments. Examples of such procedures include having the first-due engine company lay a supply line and connect to the fire department connection (FDC)

SAFETY TIP

Always follow the rules of your fire department to the best of your ability. Whether you are driving, pumping, or operating a specialized piece of equipment, your actions invariably fall under a law, regulation, local ordinance, or SOP. Do the right thing; exercise **due regard** on and off the street. You should always advocate safety and compliance with SOPs to others.

and having the first-due ladder company go to the address side of the structure.

As a driver/operator, you must know many critical, life-preserving guidelines. Evacuation signals, mayday or urgent communications, and water supply hand signals are a few examples. Remember, each fire department operates in a manner intended to best meet the needs of its community and the situation at hand. You must fully understand the strategies and tactics used by your department's fire officers. For example, some fire departments may have their driver/operators perform horizontal ventilation of a structure fire by breaking a window while the attack team calls for ventilation.

If you put a concerted effort into learning the fire apparatus and equipment systems and acknowledge and comply with SOPs, you will be recognized as a leader and a valued crew member. Your colleagues will respond to your successes and actions by following your example. Over the long haul, equipment may begin to run a little better, or the tactical operations may be executed a little more smoothly.

LISTEN UP!

Personal protective equipment requirements for driver/operators always seem to be a point of discussion, but this debate can be easily resolved by following your department's SOPs. Get involved in the process of developing these SOPs. Demonstrate safety concerns as they relate to the process of evaluating the effectiveness of each SOP.

Fire Apparatus and Equipment: Functions and Limitations

Successful driver/operators understand the primary function of each fire apparatus they are expected to operate, and they recognize the limitations of the apparatus and the specialized equipment that it carries. For example, the primary mission for a pumper is to supply water to attack lines or other units. Water tenders haul large volumes of water, whereas brush units are primarily used to suppress vegetation fires. Regardless of the fire apparatus' function, you must know the expectations of the crew and the fire officers. Missing an assignment or not completing an assignment properly is not an option in the firefighting business. You must communicate immediately if a problem arises that cannot be quickly managed in the field. The only way to accomplish this is to fully understand the functions and limitations of the fire apparatus.

Consider the different water supplies that may be available at incident: onboard supplies, municipal water supplies, and static water supplies. How many hoselines or gallons per minute (liters per minute) can be deployed until the demand for water surpasses your available water supply? Will your process for supplying water change with different types of water supplies? The fireground is not the place to seek out the answers to these questions. Although the answers are in reach, it takes the proper training to identify them. Before these questions arise on the fireground, take the fire apparatus out and flow some water with the equipment that you have on it. Try out different scenarios that you and your crew might face, such as a broken hydrant or a burst hoseline. The complexity of knowledge and skills needed to become proficient in the driver/operator position is high, but great driver/operators should be able to troubleshoot a problem and find a way to resolve it.

Have you ever seen a fire fighter use a tool for something other than the purpose for which it was intended? For example, a pike pole with a fiberglass handle would be a poor choice of equipment for trying to pry open a door or window. This application would be using the wrong tool for the job and would create a safety hazard. Because safety is critical to a successful operation, you must know the functions and limitations of the equipment and the onboard systems. What can each rescue tool cut—and what can it not cut? What are the stabilization limitations and restrictions on the operation of the aerial device? You need to know the answers to these questions or, at the very least, know where to find them quickly. Operating manuals are the best sources when seeking answers to specific operational questions. Educate your crew members on the limitations of the equipment established by the manufacturers. Over the long term, this kind of education and training will save your fire department money by keeping the equipment in proper working condition. It will also reduce the risk that personnel will be exposed to avoidable hazards because they have used the equipment for unintended assignments or an otherwise improper manner.

Not all restrictions are associated with the fire apparatus' equipment and systems, however; the fire apparatus itself presents some challenges. What happens when you cross a bridge with a 6-ton (5.4-metric-ton) weight limit while driving a 15-ton (13.6-metric-ton) truck? Knowing the height and weight restrictions for each fire apparatus is always helpful. This is easily accomplished by displaying the height and weight in the cab so that it is visible to the driver/operator and the fire officer in charge of the unit. **Vehicle dynamics** are also critical to the safe operation of the fire apparatus. Weight added or subtracted will change the handling characteristics of the fire apparatus as well as the vehicle dynamics. Simply stated, a fire apparatus may not handle in the same way with a full tank of water as it does when

Voice of Experience

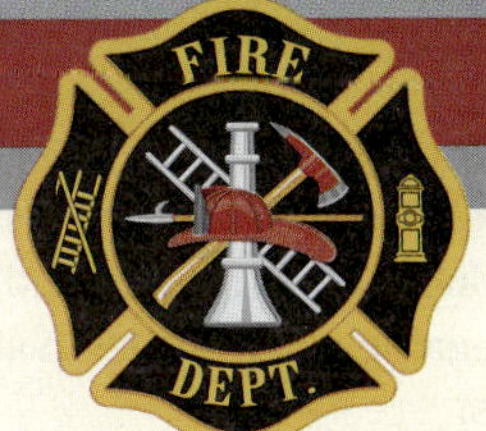

I remember the first pump operations class I attended as a fire fighter. The instructor was a veteran engineer/operator and took enormous pride in his skill. He informed me and my fellow fire fighters that anyone can be a driver/operator, but only a few select individuals truly earn the title of Engineer. I remember feeling overwhelmed by all the gauges, levels, and lights. I never thought that I would truly be able to earn the title of Engineer. After a few years, however, I was promoted to Engineer and was determined to truly earn the title. I made it my mission to learn my way around a pump panel—not just the physical skill set but also the science and hydraulics of being an Engineer.

A number of years later, I was the Engineer on the first-due truck company to a large (36,000 ft^2 [3345 m^2]) commercial-occupancy fire. The building was located in a part of our district that had just had fire hydrants installed by the local taxing district. Prior to the installation of the hydrant system, our prefire plans had us establish a water shuttle as well as draft from a large community pool.

Upon our arrival, there was heavy smoke showing. We initiated an aggressive interior attack. I set up the aerial device in preparation—in the event the incident commander decided he wanted it. Fortunately, the incident commander remembered the new fire hydrants and had the second-in company lay a supply to me. The interior attack was not successful due to a large fire load inside the building, and we had to go defensive. Two more truck companies were requested and set up in opposite locations to us, and we began extinguishing the fire. Although we had the one fire hydrant, it was not enough. Additional supply lines had to be laid from nearby hydrants, along with water being shuttled to the scene.

This fire taught us the value of understanding hydraulics. If we had been better prepared in regard to understanding our potential water supply, we would have known that additional supply lines could have been attached to the hydrant, providing more water in the terms of volume. From that point forward, as a department, we began attaching a shut-off valve to the 2½-inch (64-mm) outlet of the hydrant when connecting large-diameter hose (LDH) to a hydrant in preparation for additional water if the need arose.

We eventually extinguished the fire. The contents were a complete loss due to either fire or smoke damage, but the Fire Marshal's Office felt that the building was salvageable.

Captain Robert Barron
Prairie View Fire Department
Prairie View, Texas

it carries a quarter tank of water. Prior knowledge of these conditions will provide for a much safer return.

Keeping all of these details in your head sounds like a tall order; however, it makes perfect sense. You should know the capabilities and limitations of the fire apparatus that you drive and operate, as well as the equipment that it carries and the systems that support operations. The driver/operator is the crew's "go-to person." When you fill this position, you always need to be on your game—to have the correct answers or the perfect backup plan. Education, training, and repetition will support your ability and enable you to develop alternative options during critical situations.

DRIVER/OPERATOR TIP

You should know your response area well so that there are no weight limitation or vertical clearance surprises. Also, be aware of hills or dips where the fire apparatus could potentially "bottom out" from a low chassis clearance.

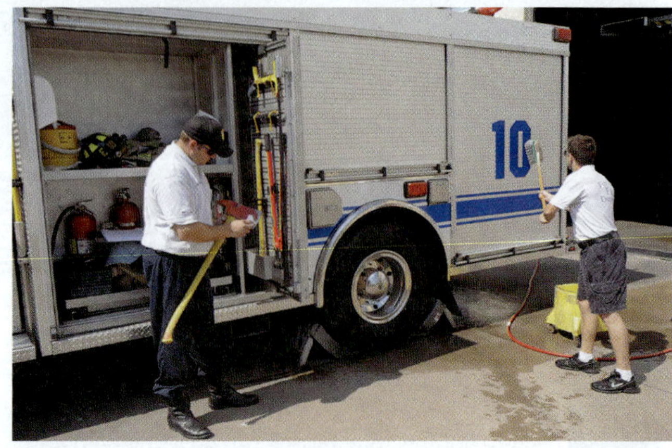

Figure 1-8 Encourage fire fighters to inspect equipment as they clean it. This "double duty" saves time and offers another level of protection from personal injury.

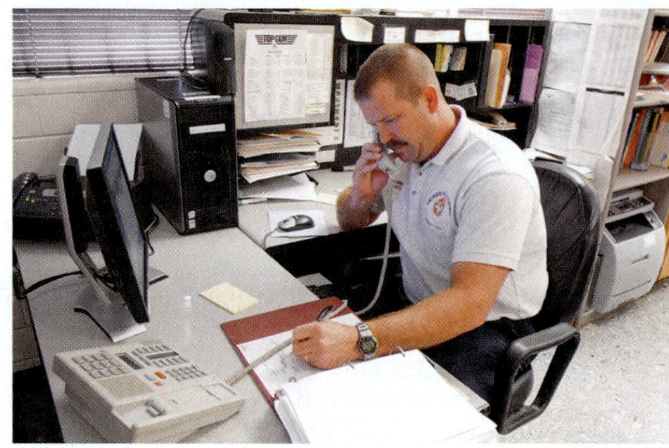

Figure 1-9 Specific information on maintenance schedules and indications of component wear can be obtained from a certified emergency vehicle technician.

Fire Apparatus and Equipment Inspections

All onboard systems and all equipment carried on the fire apparatus should be subject to routine inspections. If equipment is not used on a regular basis, it may be forgotten. As a consequence, it may not always be in service-ready condition.

The best place to start is with a complete inventory of the fire apparatus. This exercise will provide you with a working document; at the same time, it will ensure that you and your crew learn where the equipment is kept and how to perform operational checks for each device. Although this inventory process sounds basic, it really is not. You may be surprised by the knowledge and skill levels of your crew members when it comes to the equipment carried on the rig; it is not always at the level you might expect.

Cleaning equipment is another method of inspection. Teach crew members to inspect the equipment as they clean it FIGURE 1-8. This "double duty" saves time and offers another level of protection from personal injury.

As a driver/operator, you are responsible for performing routine inspections and basic preventive maintenance procedures pertaining to the fire apparatus and the equipment it carries. To assist in this effort, you should identify resources from which you can retrieve accurate information, proper specifications, and timelines for periodic inspections or maintenance schedules. For instance, when should you bring the fire apparatus in to have the transmission fluid changed? When does the pump need to be tested? At what point does tire wear become a major concern? Other areas of fire apparatus safety include coolant systems, steering components, batteries and charging systems, engine lubrication, and fuel systems. Driver/operators should always consult the operator's manuals provided by the apparatus manufacturer as well as service and maintenance manuals. Certified emergency vehicle technicians are also a good source of information and advice FIGURE 1-9.

The driver/operator must also ensure that tools and equipment are in good repair. Making sure handles are secure to the tool head, tools are sharp and free of rust, nozzles operate correctly, battery packs are charged, and air cylinders are full are just a few areas that require attention.

Safety Across the Board

Many different types of fire apparatus are used in the fire service. Some fire apparatus, such as the vehicles used by engine companies, are equipped with the water and hoselines necessary to extinguish a fire. Ladder companies' apparatus are equipped to help crew members gain access to structures and effect support functions at a fire scene. A heavy rescue company will be equipped for technical rescue and special operations.

No matter what the fire apparatus is used for or which type of emergency scene it may respond to, all fire apparatus are operated in two basic ways:

1. **Driving operations.** This includes all operations when the apparatus is traveling. It may include both emergency and nonemergency responses.
2. **On-scene operations.** This includes the operation of the apparatus and any of the apparatus equipment at the incident.

Both operations are critical components of fire services and will dramatically affect the outcome of the incident.

As the driver/operator, you set the tone for the rest of the team members with your response to the incident. If you drive the fire apparatus in a calm, defensive, and safe manner, your behavior will have a positive effect on the other members of your crew. The fire officer will be able to focus on the communications and scene size-up instead of worrying about your driving abilities. The fire fighters in the back of the apparatus will be less likely to get too excited and lose focus on the upcoming tasks. Conversely, if you drive in an erratic, out-of-control manner and allow your emotions to get the best of you, the entire crew may be in jeopardy. If the crew does not get to the call safely, they will not be able to help anyone. When responding to an emergency, remember this mantra: It's not my emergency. Always respond in a safe manner no matter what the situation is.

Once at the scene, you will have to effectively operate the equipment found on the fire apparatus. You must be capable of operating alone. While the other members of the crew may be tasked with various duties at the scene, your job is to support the crew. If you are part of an engine company, you may need to establish a water supply and charge the attack lines for the crew. Members of a ladder company may rely on you to set up the aerial device so that the ladder company can perform vertical ventilation. Whatever the circumstance, your job is not done once you reach the scene. You must be well trained and use your equipment effectively to support the crew.

NFPA 1002 Requirements

According to NFPA 1002, the driver/operator is responsible for getting the fire apparatus to the scene safely, setting up, and operating the pump or aerial device. In the fire service, a driver/operator may also be referred to as an engineer, chauffeur, or technician FIGURE 1-10. This function is a permanently assigned role in some fire departments; in other fire departments, it is rotated among the fire fighters.

The operation of fire apparatus and equipment is a critical life-safety issue for all fire fighters. Too many lives are lost every year as a result of fire apparatus accidents. In fact, driving to and from the scene can be as dangerous as operating on the fireground itself. In addition, if the equipment fails on the fireground, the consequences can be disastrous. An unexpected loss of water could jeopardize the safety of an attack line crew, an overextended aerial device could suddenly fail with fire fighters on the device, or difficulty in troubleshooting a mechanical problem could result in the inability to prime a pump. For all these reasons, the driver/operator has a tremendous responsibility for the success and safety of the entire company.

As the driver/operator, you will be responsible for all aspects of the call, including the following issues:

- Preparing the fire apparatus and equipment for a safe response
- Driving the fire apparatus in an emergency response mode to a call FIGURE 1-11
- Placing the fire apparatus at the scene in such a way as to ensure fire fighter safety and the maximum effectiveness of the equipment
- Safely and properly operating the equipment to support all operations on the fireground
- Securing the equipment and safely returning the fire apparatus and members of the company to the fire station

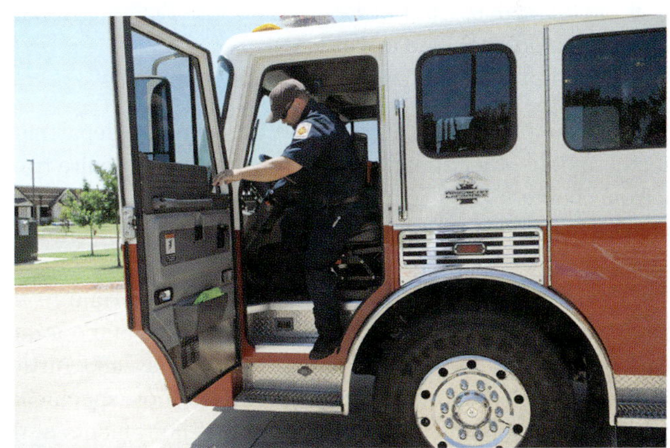

Figure 1-10 A driver/operator in action at the scene of a fire.
© Jones & Bartlett Learning. Photographed by Glen E. Ellman.

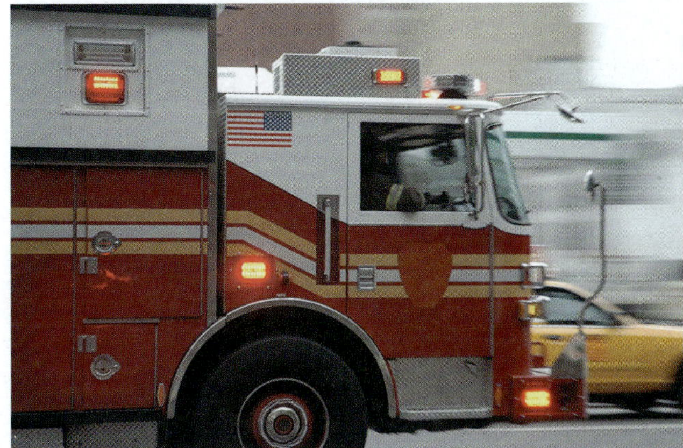

Figure 1-11 Fire apparatus responding to a call with lights activated.
© Maciej Korzekwa/Getty Images/iStockphoto/Thinkstock.

NFPA 1002: General Requirements of a Driver/Operator

All drivers must meet the general requirements of NFPA 1002 before they are allowed to operate a **fire department vehicle**, which includes all apparatus and vehicles operated by the fire department. NFPA 1002 also outlines the minimum job performance requirements (JPRs) for personnel who will drive and operate specific types of fire apparatus. The purpose of this standard is to ensure that each member meets these minimum requirements before he or she is allowed to operate a specific fire apparatus. The following NFPA 1002 chapters identify requirements to operate specific fire apparatus:

- **Chapter 4**: General Requirements (all members who operate fire department vehicles must meet these requirements)
- **Chapter 5**: Apparatus Equipped with a Fire Pump
- **Chapter 6**: Apparatus Equipped with an Aerial Device
- **Chapter 7**: Apparatus Equipped with a Tiller
- **Chapter 8**: Wildland Fire Apparatus (not included in this text)
- **Chapter 9**: Aircraft Rescue and Fire-Fighting Apparatus (not included in this text)
- **Chapter 10**: Mobile Water Supply Apparatus

For example, if a department has only one fire department pumper and no other apparatus, the drivers would require training from chapters 4 and 5 of NFPA 1002. Each department should ensure that its members are properly trained and authorized before they operate the apparatus.

Personnel must meet those provisions that pertain to the types of apparatus they will be expected to drive and operate, and the authority having jurisdiction (AHJ) may add further requirements. Driver/operators of vehicles not specifically identified are expected to meet the general requirements of the standard—chapter 4 of NFPA 1002. These vehicles may include staff or command vehicles and rescue or utility vehicles **FIGURE 1-12**. This text covers the general requirements of NFPA 1002, apparatus equipped with a fire pump, apparatus equipped with an aerial device or a tiller, and mobile water supply apparatus.

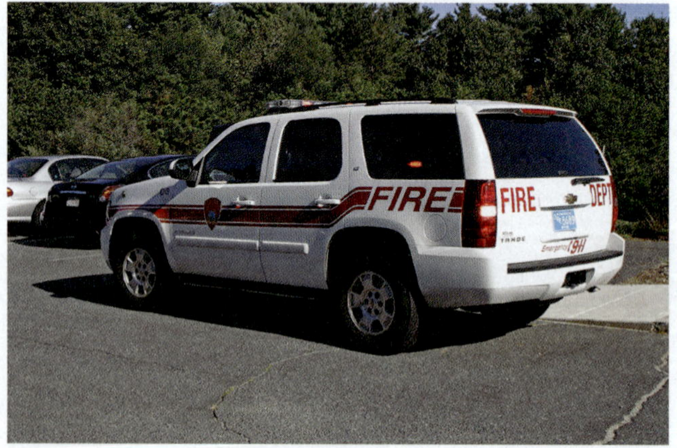

Figure 1-12 A command or chief's vehicle.

To meet the general requirements of NFPA 1002, the fire department vehicle driver/operator must be licensed to drive the vehicle that he or she is expected to operate. Some states may require driver/operators to have a **commercial driver's license (CDL)**; others may exempt their drivers from certain licensing requirements altogether. A CDL ensures the driver has met the requirements to operate certain types of commercial vehicles depending on the weight of the vehicle, the number of passengers, and the presence (or not) of any hazardous materials. The U.S. Department of Transportation (DOT) and Canadian Ministry of Transportation (MOT) have established requirements for licensing drivers, but each state or provincial/territorial government usually dictates the licensing requirements needed to meet its own requirements. Each fire department is responsible for ensuring that its members are properly licensed at the appropriate level for the jurisdiction. All fire fighters should be familiar with their department's requirements. For example, some departments require their driver/operators to hold a CDL, even though those personnel are not mandated to do so by state law.

NFPA 1002 also requires that driver/operators meet the requirements of NFPA 1001, *Standard for Fire Fighter Professional Qualifications*, for Fire Fighter I, if they will be responsible for operating a fire pump or aerial device on the fire apparatus. Any fire fighter who has been qualified as a Fire Fighter I should review the requirements related to fire hose, nozzles, appliances, fire streams, water supplies, and sprinklers, as they may be tested on this information to confirm that they meet the requirements of NFPA 1002. All of the requirements in this standard should be evaluated using a vehicle that is similar in weight, wheelbase, and function as those expected to be operated in the performance of the driver/operator's normal duties **FIGURE 1-13**.

NFPA 1002: Medical and Physical Requirements of a Driver/Operator

According to NFPA 1002, the driver is subject to a medical evaluation, as required by NFPA 1500, to verify that the driver/operator is medically fit to perform the duties required. Just as fire fighters need to be in good physical condition to perform their job, so the driver needs to be physically ready to meet the challenges of this position. NFPA 1500 states that the driver shall be medically evaluated and qualified for duty by a physician, with this medical evaluation taking into account the risks and the functions associated with the individual's duties and responsibilities. All drivers who will engage in fire suppression should meet the medical requirements specified in chapter 8 of NFPA 1582. These medical requirements include, but are not limited to, a medical history review, physical examination, and several laboratory tests.

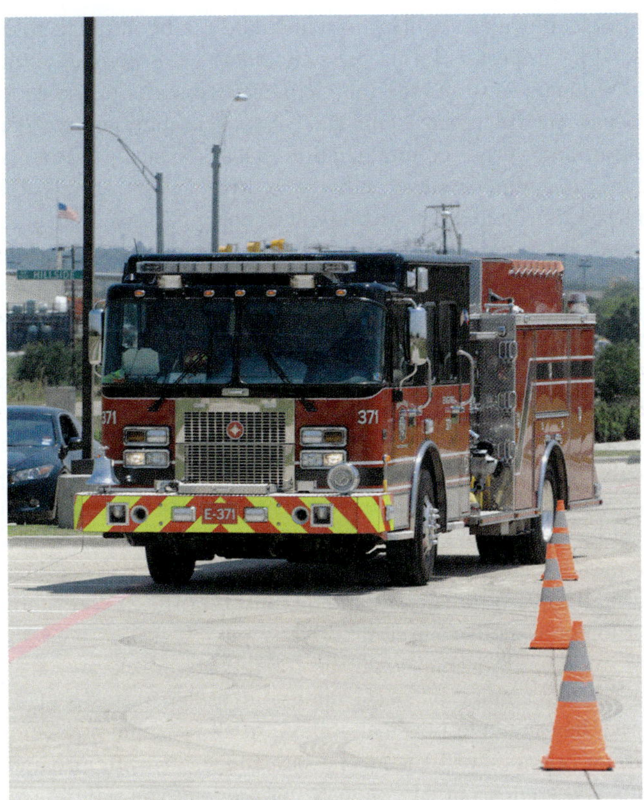

Figure 1-13 Apparatus on a fire department training ground completing a cone course or driver course.

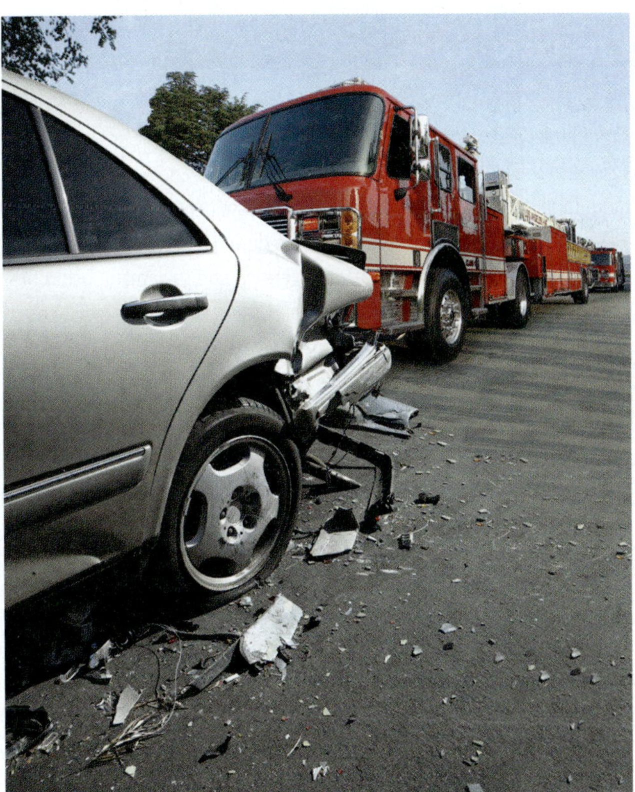

Figure 1-14 A fire apparatus and civilian vehicle crash scene.

Driver/Operator Training

Training drivers to operate their apparatus safely and efficiently is critical to the success of any fire department. NFPA 1451, *Standard for a Fire and Emergency Service Vehicle Operations Training Program*, contains the minimum requirements for such programs, including the organizational procedures for training drivers, maintaining vehicles, and identifying equipment deficiencies. According to NFPA 1451, each fire department should:

- Establish and maintain a driver training program with the goal of preventing vehicle crashes, deaths, and injuries to its members and the public.
- Institute a program of post-crash drug and alcohol testing for any driver involved in a crash involving an injury or fatality **FIGURE 1-14**.
- Adopt a risk management plan, which includes risk reduction, risk evaluation, risk control techniques, and risk management monitoring.
- Evaluate the effectiveness of the vehicle training program once every 3 years.
- Establish written SOPs for safe driving of, riding within, and operating vehicles during emergency and nonemergency responses.
- Ensure all members are trained to operate specific vehicles before being authorized to drive the vehicle.
- Ensure all members are reauthorized annually for all vehicles they are expected to operate.
- Provide driver training for all members as often as necessary, but no less than twice each year, with at least one training session to include actual hands-on exercises with the vehicle the member is expected to drive.
- Ensure all members receive training when new or unfamiliar vehicles are placed into service.

Driver/Operator Selection

What makes a good driver/operator candidate? Knowledge, skill, and attitude are some key attributes. Driver/operators must be knowledgeable in the services provided by their fire departments. They must understand how consistent delivery of excellent services provides for a safe and successful outcome. Driver/operators must also be educated and trained in operating at emergency scenes. They must possess the required skills to complete critical, life-preserving actions, and these skills must be developed through a continuing process of performance and repetition. Reviewing the JPRs identified in NFPA 1002 will give potential candidates a better understanding of their fire department's expectations regarding their performance.

LISTEN UP!

To gain and maintain proficiency in the role of the driver/operator, you should take every opportunity to engage in skill exercises or training sessions requiring the use of the onboard systems and equipment. The more familiar you are with the related processes, the more effective you will be in solving any problems that arise during emergency responses.

Always attempt to train as if you were on an assignment, using the same crew sizes, same fire apparatus, and same equipment resources as you would on a real call. During these training sessions, you may discover better methods that will make you and your crew more efficient. Be sure to pass on the lessons that you learn to other driver/operators and other crew members.

Remember—do not just train for the large-scale or unusual incident. It is usually the basic skills needed at the bread-and-butter responses that cause the most problems.

An effective driver/operator is also a good problem solver. When fire apparatus or equipment malfunctions arise, he or she must be able to quickly evaluate all possible solutions to rectify the problem and seamlessly implement a backup plan. To attain this level of efficiency, driver/operators must understand the basic and complex systems of the fire apparatus and the equipment that it carries. Just as driver/operators need a working knowledge of fireground hydraulics to achieve positive results during fire suppression efforts, so they must be well versed in all of the onboard devices and systems carried on the fire apparatus. The modern fire apparatus is a multitasking unit that performs many functions to support fire department services to the community, and many of these functions require a variety of support and power systems—hydraulic, electrical, and pneumatic. Driver/operators, in turn, must be proficient in correcting the problems that are related to all of these onboard systems. One of the best sources for understanding these systems is the manufacturer's operating manual, many of which are available in an electronic format **FIGURE 1-15**.

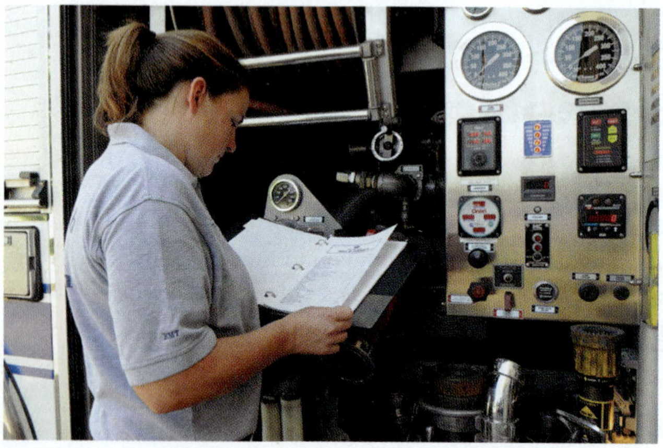

Figure 1-15 One of the best methods for understanding apparatus systems is to reference the manufacturer's operating manual.

Selecting a driver/operator candidate can be difficult, so the selection process is based on a candidate's knowledge, ability, and willingness to pursue the challenge. To start this selection process, fire officers may consider a few basic qualities: excellent written and verbal communication skills, physical and mental fitness, basic mechanical ability, and attitude. Driver/operators must be thorough when completing reporting forms, inspection forms, and documentation of deficiencies or corrective actions. Reporting is a major job function of the driver/operator. Do you remember being told sometime in your career, "If it's not documented, it didn't happen"? This assertion holds true for the driver/operator. Undocumented events, conditions, or actions may lead to disaster. Crews cannot be expected to perform their assignments without the required equipment, in proper working condition. For this reason, driver/operators must explain the importance of reporting to their respective crews. Educating the other crew members will make your job easier and begin to shift the paradigm away from the notion that "reporting is complaining" and toward the understanding that "reporting is preventing a problem or dangerous situation."

Another desirable quality is for the driver/operator to be physically capable of performing the assigned tasks. Good vision, hearing, and physical ability are all personal assets that a driver/operator will need to be safe and successful. Fire apparatus and equipment can be very unforgiving; you will be challenged both mentally and physically by the malfunctions and errors that occur on scene. Your patience will be tested and your reactions watched. Remaining focused on your assignment and being acutely aware of the ongoing operation will better position you to handle the various stressors headed your way.

Next on the list of preferred driver/operator qualities is mechanical ability—driver/operators should have a basic understanding of mechanics. Familiarity with basic preventive maintenance processes such as lubricating components, adding fluids, and inspecting equipment and onboard systems for proper operation forms an essential skill set for driver/operators **FIGURE 1-16**. Driver/operators are charged with handling minor system repairs and preventive maintenance servicing only; qualified

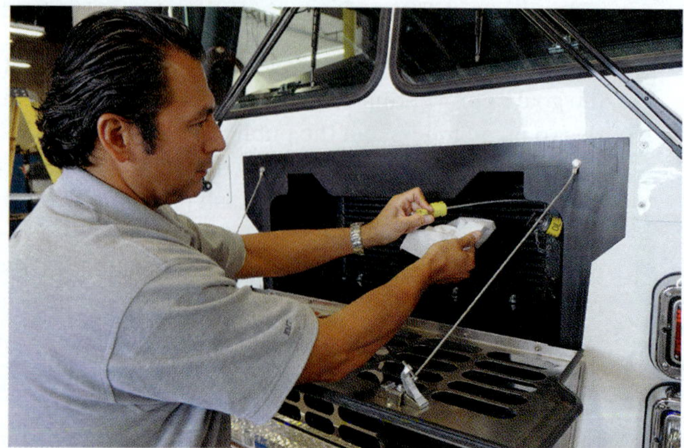

Figure 1-16 A driver inspecting the engine compartment area.

emergency vehicle technicians should perform major repairs or adjustments.

Finally, attitude is a key consideration for the driver/operator. The right attitude demonstrated by the driver/operator is critical for building a successful team, instilling confidence in crew members, and promoting positive response outcomes. Driver/operators must take their roles and responsibilities seriously. Many variables hinge on the ready availability of a well-maintained apparatus and service-ready equipment. Having a positive attitude toward the job will breed additional support and confidence from your crew members. You will inevitably experience operational setbacks; these come with the job. However, a driver/operator who is committed to the mission of the fire department and dedicated to providing excellent service to the community will be able to meet these challenges and make a difference when it counts.

Each department is unique in its selection process for drivers. In some departments, the driver may be a senior fire fighter assigned to the apparatus or a promoted position within the department, while other departments may rotate all fire fighters' driving duties. If the driver position is considered a promotion, a testing process for this position is usually required.

The testing process may involve a written examination and sometimes an **assessment center**, which is a series of simulation exercises **FIGURE 1-17**. Such written examinations usually include information from the department's policies, procedures, and guidelines concerning driving and positioning apparatus, hydraulic calculations, emergency vehicle driving, vehicle maintenance and operation, and material pertaining to the position of apparatus driver. The assessment center may include several practical skill exercises that determine how well a candidate can perform the essential skills required for the position. These tasks may include driving and positioning the apparatus, performing maintenance checks, pumping water from the apparatus, or operating aerial devices. Once the testing process is completed, candidates are usually placed on a promotional eligibility list, which ranks them according to how well they scored. The department then promotes members of the list as positions become available. Such a testing process can be very expensive to administer, so many departments offer such tests only once every few years. If your department has a testing process for the rank of driver, you should make sure that you know how the process works and what is required to be eligible for the testing process.

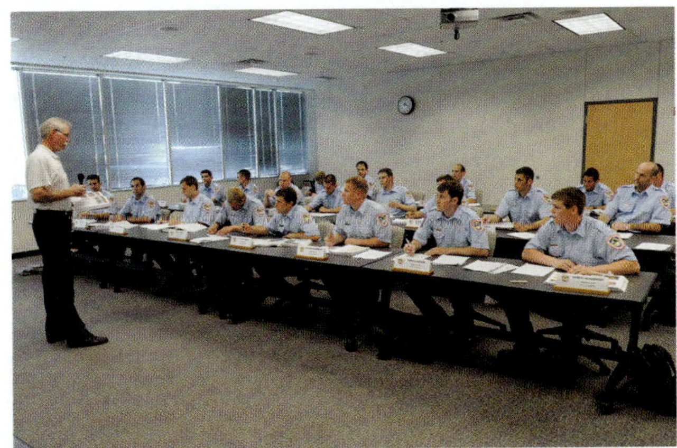

Figure 1-17 A large group of fire fighters completing a written exam.

After-Action Review

IN SUMMARY

- To be successful in your role as a driver/operator, you must fully understand and accept the responsibilities that come with the job.
- As a driver/operator, you have many obligations to your crew and to the community. Both internal and external expectations depend on your ability to perform your initial response assignments.
- Every member of the fire department must have a strong commitment to safety and health. Safety must be fully integrated into every activity, procedure, and job description.
- The majority of all fire fighter deaths are caused by stress, overexertion, and medical issues. Cardiac events account for 38 percent of these deaths.
- Motor vehicle collisions are the second leading cause of fire fighter fatalities. Always wear your seat belt each and every time you are in a motor vehicle.
- A successful safety program includes four major components: regulations, standards, and procedures; personnel; training; and equipment.
- Safety and well-being are directly related to personal health and fitness. You should eat a healthy diet, maintain a healthy weight, exercise regularly, stay hydrated, and sleep for 7 to 8 hours whenever possible.

- Employee assistance programs are available to provide fire fighters with confidential counseling, support, or assistance in dealing with a physical, financial, emotional, or substance abuse problem.
- As a driver/operator, you have a duty to educate other crew members on their roles and responsibilities to support your function. The driver/operator is a teacher, a mentor, a vital crew member, and a safety advocate. You must lead by example—especially in regard to safety.
- Compliance with standard operating procedures or guidelines is essential. Always follow these procedures, and promote compliance among your crew members.
- All fire apparatus are operated in two basic ways: driving operations and on-scene operations. The driver is responsible for the safe and efficient operation of the vehicle in both settings.
- NFPA 1002 identifies the minimum requirements for a driver/operator.
- NFPA 1451 identifies the requirements for a fire department's driver training program.

KEY TERMS

assessment center A series of simulation exercises for a promotional examination.

blind spots Areas around the fire apparatus that are not visible to the driver/operator.

Code of Federal Regulations (CFR) A collection of permanent rules published in the *Federal Register* by the executive departments and agencies of the U.S. federal government. Its 50 titles represent broad areas of interest that are governed by federal regulation. Each volume of the CFR is updated annually and issued on a quarterly basis.

commercial driver's license (CDL) A government-issued license that ensures the driver has met the requirements to operate certain types of commercial vehicles depending on the weight of the vehicle, the number of passengers, and the presence (or not) of any hazardous materials.

critical incident stress debriefing (CISD) A postincident meeting designed to assist rescue personnel in dealing with psychological trauma as the result of an emergency. (NFPA 1006)

critical incident stress management (CISM) A program designed to reduce acute and chronic effects of stress related to job functions. (NFPA 450)

driver/operator A person who has satisfactorily completed the requirements of driver/operator as specified in NFPA 1002, *Standard for Fire Apparatus Driver/Operator Professional Qualifications*, and who is authorized by the authority having jurisdiction to drive, operate, or both drive and operate fire department vehicles. (NFPA 1451)

due regard The care exercised by a reasonably prudent person under the same circumstances.

employee assistance programs (EAPs) An employee-sponsored service designed for personal or family problems, including mental health, substance abuse, various addictions, marital problems, parenting problems, emotional problems, or financial or legal concerns. (NFPA 450)

fire department vehicle Any vehicle, including fire apparatus, operated by a fire department.

freelancing The dangerous practice of acting independently of command instructions.

job aids A tool, device, or system used to assist a person with executing specific tasks.

Occupational Safety and Health Administration (OSHA) The U.S. federal agency that regulates worker safety and, in some cases, responder safety. OSHA is part of the U.S. Department of Labor.

stressors Conditions that create excessive physical and mental pressures on a person's body; any type of stimulus that causes stress.

tactical benchmarks Objectives that are required to be completed during the operational phase of an incident.

vehicle dynamics Vehicle construction and mechanical design characteristics that directly affect the handling, stability, maneuverability, functionality, and safety of a vehicle.

vehicle intercom system A communication system that is permanently mounted inside the cab of the fire apparatus and allows fire fighters to communicate more effectively.

REFERENCES

American Cancer Society. Alcohol Use and Cancer. 2017. https://www.cancer.org/cancer/cancer-causes/diet-physical-activity/alcohol-use-and-cancer.html. Accessed August 22, 2017.

Centers for Disease Control and Prevention. Findings from a Study of Cancer Among U.S. Fire Fighters. July 2016. https://www.cdc.gov/niosh/pgms/worknotify/pdfs/ff-cancer-factsheet-final.pdf. Accessed August 21, 2017.

Firefighter Behavioral Health Alliance. www.ffbha.org. Accessed August 22, 2017.

Fire Fighter Cancer Support Network. Who We Are. https://firefightercancersupport.org/%20Who%20We%20Are/. Accessed August 21, 2017.

National Fallen Firefighters Association. Everyone Goes Home. Confronting Suicide in the Fire Service. https://www.everyonegoeshome.com/2014/12/02/suicides-preventable-reaching-vulnerable/. Accessed August 22, 2017.

National Fire Protection Association. Firefighter Fatalities in the United States—2016, Figure 2. June 2017. http://www.nfpa.org/news-and-research/fire-statistics-and-reports/fire-statistics/the-fire-service/fatalities-and-injuries/firefighter-fatalities-in-the-united-states. Accessed August 22, 2017.

National Fire Protection Association (NFPA) 1001, *Standard for Fire Fighter Professional Qualifications*. 2013. https://www.nfpa.org/codes-and-standards/all-codes-and-standards/list-of-codes-and-standards/detail?code=1001. Accessed January 29, 2018.

National Fire Protection Association (NFPA) 1002, *Standard for Fire Apparatus Driver/Operator Professional Qualifications*. 2017. https://www.nfpa.org/codes-and-standards/all-codes-and-standards/list-of-codes-and-standards/detail?code=1002. Accessed January 29, 2018.

National Fire Protection Association (NFPA) 1451, *Standard for a Fire and Emergency Service Vehicle Operations Training Program*. 2018. https://www.nfpa.org/codes-and-standards/all-codes-and-standards/list-of-codes-and-standards/detail?code=1451. Accessed January 29, 2018.

National Fire Protection Association (NFPA) 1500, *Standard on Fire Department Occupational Safety and Health Program*. 2018. https://www.nfpa.org/codes-and-standards/all-codes-and-standards/list-of-codes-and-standards/detail?code=1500. Accessed January 29, 2018.

National Fire Protection Association (NFPA) 1582, *Standard on Comprehensive Occupational Medical Program for Fire Departments*. 2018. https://www.nfpa.org/codes-and-standards/all-codes-and-standards/list-of-codes-and-standards/detail?code=1582. Accessed January 29, 2018.

Smith, Denise, PhD. Can SMARTER Technology Reduce Fire Fighter Injuries and Fatalities? http://horizons.globeturnoutgear.com/can-smarter-technology-reduce-firefighter-injuries-and-fatalities/. Accessed August 21, 2017.

On Scene

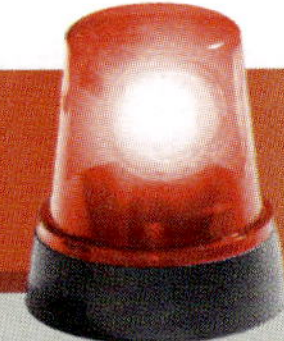

While studying for the promotional exam, you and several other candidates form a study group. The group decides that each candidate should make up several questions and bring the questions to the next study group session. All of the questions will then be compiled, and each of you will have a practice test to take before the promotional examination. Here are some of the questions that your study group created.

1. Which NFPA standard identifies the requirements of a driver/operator?

A. NFPA 1001
B. NFPA 1002
C. NFPA 1003
D. NFPA 1004

2. NFPA 1451 requires that fire departments evaluate the effectiveness of the vehicle training program once every _____ year(s).

A. 1
B. 3
C. 5
D. 10

(continued)

On Scene Continued

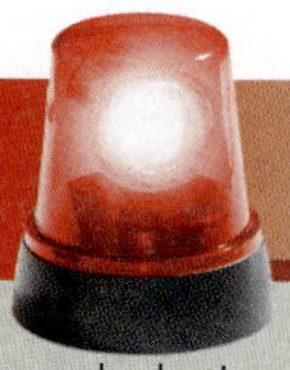

3. What is the acronym to remember the correct sequence to start power units?

   A. FCSP (fuel, choke, switch, pull)

   B. FSPC (fuel, switch, pull, choke)

   C. SCFP (switch, choke, fuel, pull)

   D. CFSP (choke, fuel, switch, pull)

4. At the fire scene, the driver is usually responsible for all of the following EXCEPT:

   A. safely operating equipment to support operations.

   B. placement of the apparatus at the scene.

   C. securing equipment before leaving the scene.

   D. repairing the apparatus if it is broken.

5. How much water should be consumed to maintain proper hydration for each 5 to 10 minutes of physical exertion?

   A. 4 to 6 ounces (0.1 to 0.17 liter)

   B. 8 to 10 ounces (0.2 to 0.3 liter)

   C. 12 to 16 ounces (0.35 to 0.4 liter)

   D. 20 to 24 ounces (0.6 to 0.7 liter)

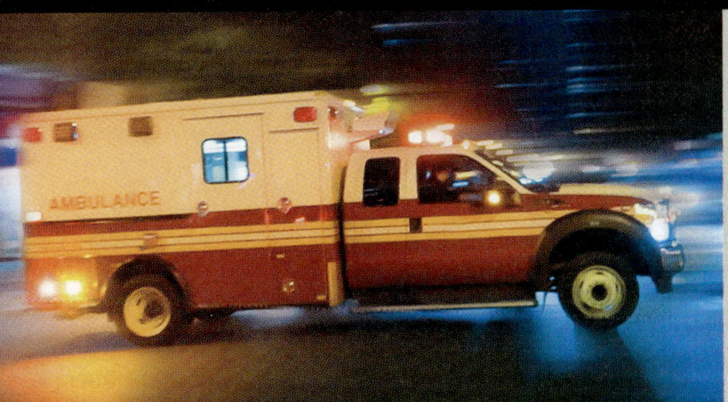

CHAPTER 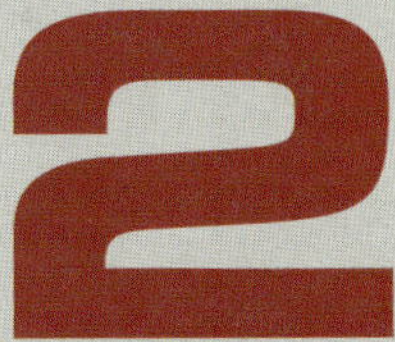

Making Safety a Priority

OBJECTIVES

2.1 Discuss the importance of safety in any emergency response.

2.2 Discuss the importance of ensuring mental preparedness by avoiding or managing sleep deprivation, excessive emotion, stress, and any physical ailments that may inhibit decision making.

2.3 Discuss the importance of developing a "safety-first" attitude.

2.4 Discuss the importance of proper seatbelt placement, airbags, headrest positioning, mirror position, the use of a spotter, and equipment restraint.

2.5 Explain how to secure a patient to the stretcher.

2.6 Demonstrate how to safely transport adult and child patients and passengers.

2.7 Demonstrate how to establish a safe work zone in the event of a roadway incident.

2.8 Outline the appropriate steps to respond safely to mechanical failure.

SCENARIO

On July 13, 2001, a 27-year-old female EMT died when the ambulance she was working in struck a support column for an elevated train track. The EMT had been riding unrestrained in the patient compartment while attending to a patient during a nonemergency medical transport. Since the transport was a nonemergency it is not clear whether being unrestrained was necessary to patient care.

Leading up to the collision, the crew departed the hospital with the patient at 11:56 AM. The patient had been placed supine on the cot, secured with lap-belt-type leg and hip restraints and loaded into the ambulance. The ambulance was traveling southbound without lights and siren on a two-lane city street. At approximately 12:15 PM, 1.5 miles from the hospital, the driver drifted through the northbound lane toward oncoming traffic and struck an elevated train track support column at an estimated speed of 26 mph **FIGURE 2-1** and **FIGURE 2-2**. At approximately 12:20 PM, the EMT/driver called the office of the ambulance service to report the incident. At about the same time, witnesses called 9-1-1.

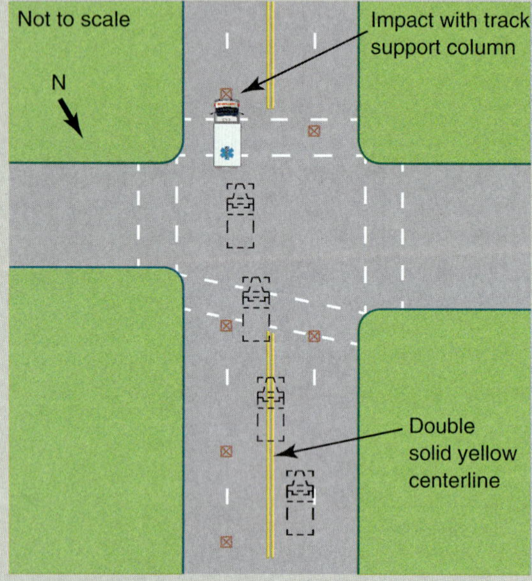

Figure 2-1 Overhead view of the crash scene.

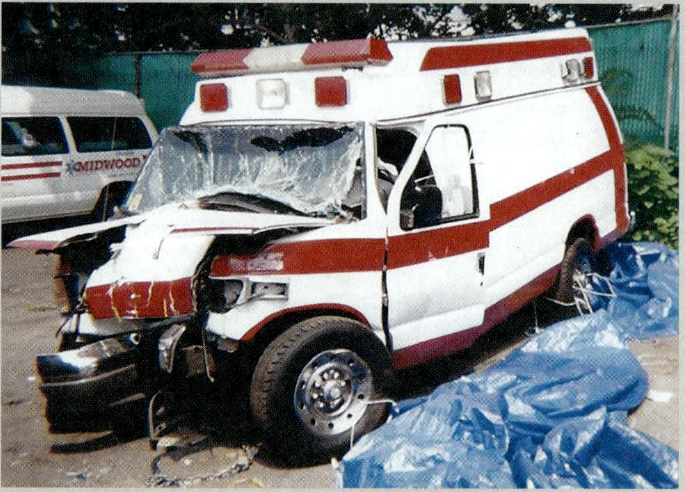

Figure 2-2 The front/driver's side view of the damage that resulted from the ambulance striking the track support column ("El" pillar).
Courtesy of Rob Raheb.

During the collision, the patient was partially ejected from the cot restraints and struck the rear-facing captain's seat at the front of the patient compartment. The EMT/driver, who was riding unrestrained, contacted the vehicle's dash and the inflating airbag. The EMT attending to the patient impacted and broke a handrail at the end of the squad bench and struck a cabinet at the front of the patient compartment.

The EMT/driver, EMT, and patient were transported by ambulance to a hospital. The EMT from the patient compartment was pronounced dead as a result of injuries, including a thoracic spine cord laceration, complete cord syndrome with dislocation, bilateral lung contusions, and cerebellum subarachnoid hemorrhage.

A conclusive determination could not be made as to why the ambulance veered left across traffic and struck the support column. However, the National Automotive Sampling System (NASS) case file for this incident indicated that no avoidance maneuvers had been attempted and listed "inattentive or distracted, sleepy or fell asleep" under the category for distraction. Witnesses interviewed said that the driver admitted having no recollection of the crash.

1. Have you ever caught yourself drifting off while driving your personal vehicle or the ambulance?
2. How often do you use all available restraints for yourself and your patient?
3. Have you ever had a close call because you were not focused while driving?

Sources: Centers for Disease Control and Prevention. (2003). Ambulance crash-related injuries among emergency medical services workers—United States, 1991–2002. *Morbidity and Mortality Weekly Report, 52*(8), 154–156. Retrieved from http://www.cdc.gov/mmwr/preview/mmwrhtml/mm5208a3.htm; Centers for Disease Control and Prevention. (2004). Emergency medical technician dies in ambulance crash—New York. Fatality Assessment and Control Evaluation (FACE) Program. *National Institute for Occupational Safety and Health (NIOSH) In-house FACE Report*. Retrieved from http://www.cdc.gov/niosh/face/In-house/full200112.html.

Introduction

An EMS provider's abilities, skills, and knowledge of emergency vehicle operation contribute to every EMS response. Every year there are millions of EMS responses that place the EMS provider and the general public at risk. The priority for every EMS provider is to ensure his or her own safety and the safety of his or her partner, the patient, and any passengers. Your own personal safety must be placed ahead of everyone else's. Ensuring your own safety includes being mentally and physically prepared, fastening your seatbelt, and making sure the unit is safe to operate.

You play a key role in keeping your partner safe by ensuring the proper use of seatbelts, in both the front and the patient compartments of the ambulance. Proper safety belts are also important for patient safety, including all of the gurney shoulder straps provided by the manufacturer. The best patient care can be provided only by enforcing a "safety-first" attitude and ensuring that everyone around does the same. The right thing to do may feel uncomfortable, such as telling your partner to put on a seatbelt before you move the vehicle or asking the driver to slow down. However, vehicle collisions continue to be the main cause of death for EMS providers (aeromedical excluded), and it is important to do the right thing: Practice safety first, all the time.

Personal Preparedness

As the operator of an emergency vehicle, you are responsible for safe vehicle operation, including the safety of the public and those in the vehicle. Emergency vehicle operators must be both mentally and physically prepared to perform their jobs. Mental preparation includes an awareness and management of **sleep deprivation**, emotions, and stress while maintaining physical awareness and a safety-first attitude.

Sleep Deprivation

Sleep deprivation is a common cause of driver error. Most adults require 7 to 9 hours of sleep per night. Being well rested improves concentration, reaction times, and physical capabilities. Drowsy driving occurs when a person does not get the proper amount of sleep. Common signs of drowsy driving include:

- Difficulty focusing, frequent blinking, or heavy eyelids
- Daydreaming; wandering or disconnected thoughts
- Microsleeping
- Trouble remembering the last few miles driven; missing exits or traffic signs
- Yawning repeatedly or rubbing your eyes
- Trouble keeping your head up
- Drifting from your lane, tailgating, or hitting a shoulder rumble strip
- Feeling restless and irritable

It is your personal responsibility to ensure that you are well rested for your shift and are not a danger to yourself or others.

According to the National Sleep Foundation's (NSF) 2009 Sleep in America poll, 54% of respondents indicated that they had driven a vehicle within the past year while feeling drowsy; 28% of those who drive reported having actually fallen asleep at the wheel. The National Highway Traffic Safety Administration (NHTSA) estimates that about 100,000 police-reported crashes are the direct result of driver fatigue annually. International estimates fault drowsy driving for 10% to 30% of all automobile crashes. The NHTSA and the Centers for Disease Control and Prevention report that 2.5% of all fatal crashes are a result of drowsy driving, which results in an estimated 1,550 deaths each year. Drowsy driving annually results in an estimated 2% of all injury crashes or 71,000 injuries. These large numbers result in an estimated $12.5 billion in monetary losses annually. Unfortunately, these figures are believed to be low estimates and may not capture the true prevalence of drowsy driving-rated incidents, since without a way to test for it, it is difficult to attribute crashes to sleepiness.

According to the NSF's 2001 Sleep in America poll, a number of the nearly three-quarters of U.S. adults (71%) who drive a car to and from work are drowsy drivers. More than one-quarter of those surveyed (27%) reported they had driven drowsy to or from work at least a few days a month, 12% said they drove drowsy a few days a week, and 4% reported they drove drowsy every day or almost every day. Drowsy drivers are more likely to have lapses of attention while on the road.

Sleep deprivation and fatigue may also affect behaviors that can lead to crashes, such as speeding. According to the NSF's 2000 Sleep in America poll, when asked about their behavior while driving drowsy, 42% of respondents said they become stressed, 32% said they get impatient, and 12% reported that they tend to drive faster.

The NSF also notes several trends about drivers who fall asleep at the wheel. Drivers are more likely to fall asleep on high-speed, long, boring, rural highways. However, those who live in urban areas are more likely to doze off while driving compared to rural or suburban counterparts (24% vs. 17%). Crashes or near misses most commonly occur between the hours of 4:00 AM and 6:00 AM, 12:00 AM and 2:00 AM, or 2:00 PM and 4:00 PM. According to the NSF's 2005 Sleep in America poll, of the approximately one-third of drivers who reported having ever fallen asleep, or microslept, while driving, 13% reported having done so at least once a month. Nearly one-quarter of adults say they know someone personally who has crashed due to falling asleep at the wheel.

Drowsy driving has been compared to another extremely dangerous and illegal practice: driving under the influence of alcohol. In the United States, 0.08% blood alcohol concentration is considered impaired and illegal. There are studies that show that being awake for 18 consecutive hours is impairment equal to a blood alcohol concentration of 0.05%. Being awake for a full 24 hours produced impairment similar to a 0.096% blood alcohol concentration, which is legally intoxicated in all 50 states.

Wrecks from drowsy driving can result in high personal and economic costs. Several drowsy driving incidents have resulted in jail sentences for the driver. These crashes have resulted in multimillion-dollar settlements against drivers and their companies. These costs do not include the damage to reputation and accompanying losses that a company will have due to news of the crash.

As an emergency vehicle operator, you are ultimately responsible for the safe operation of the vehicle. However, companies should take precautions and create policies that ensure providers have the opportunity to rest before shifts. This should include mandating time off between shifts and setting maximum consecutive hours of work to prevent impairment. EMS is currently one of the very few transportation-related fields that is not regulated with mandatory time off and rest periods.

SAFETY POINTER

It is your responsibility as an EMS provider to ensure you are well rested, having received a recommended 7–9 hours of sleep, and fit for duty prior to the start of your shift.

Emotions

Although emotions can be difficult to manage, EMS providers have a responsibility to be emotionally prepared for their shifts by not bringing personal distractions to work or allowing professional challenges to affect decision-making abilities. Some common emotions that can affect your ability to make decisions are anger, love, hate, fear, grief, and happiness.

Loss of control of emotions can interfere with the ability to think and focus. This lack of focus and inability to concentrate create an environment in which a driver can be distracted, affecting the ability to process information and increasing risk-taking behavior. As part of your personal preparedness, it is your responsibility to ensure that you are emotionally capable of operating an emergency vehicle. The type of run, the patient, the behavior of other drivers, and many other factors can be triggers for cumulative stress reactions. The emergency vehicle operator needs to be able to recognize and control those reactions when driving.

Stress

EMS providers are constantly placed in high-stress environments. You must be able to properly manage your stress level and prevent it from interfering with your decision-making abilities. Stress associated with an EMS response can occur frequently and affects each individual differently. For example, your stress may increase when a call involves a pediatric patient, while another person's stress may increase when the call involves an Alzheimer's patient. These responses may be delayed or cumulative, manifesting in reaction to other situations.

As stress levels increase, so do levels of adrenaline and cortisone, as the body prepares for a fight-or-flight response. The increase in these stress hormones affects the vehicle operator by increasing pulse rate and elevating blood pressure. Adrenaline also causes the pupils to dilate and take in more light, increasing the field of vision. However, as blood is redistributed from certain areas of the brain to the muscles and internal organs, peripheral vision is decreased (tunnel vision), which consequently narrows the visual field. Increased levels of stress hormones may also result in increased risky behavior and more emotional reactions, such as frustration or anger. In addition to the physical effects of adrenaline and cortisone, stress may also affect a person physically, causing gastrointestinal discomfort, headaches, or back pain. Longer-term and consistent exposure to stress can lead to memory and concentration problems, which are the enemy of the emergency vehicle operator.

At one time or another, all EMS providers will be adversely affected by job-related stress. It is imperative that EMS providers recognize stress and change their behaviors to compensate for its adverse effects. An excellent way to combat the effects of stress is to practice safe driving habits every day. During stressful events, people who have reinforced good habits with education and training are able to make better decisions. By practicing safe vehicle operations every day, you will reduce your risk during a stressful event. The key is to stay focused, understand that other drivers will react to the presence of your emergency vehicle in a variety of ways, and remain prepared and in control when other drivers undertake crazy maneuvers. Maintaining self-control involves not internalizing others' actions and creating a new stressor.

Physical Awareness

Your state of health, both physical and mental, can affect your ability to operate an emergency vehicle. Therefore, physical awareness is an important part of ensuring your preparedness and safety. Physical awareness includes being sensitive to any health problems. It is also important to remember that over-the-counter (OTC) treatments can affect physical awareness and the ability to react and respond to emergencies. The following are some examples of physical disruptions that could affect your performance:

- A leg sprain or strain may cause difficulty in moving your foot from the accelerator to the brake, thus delaying reaction time.
- Gastrointestinal distress may cause you to become less focused and attentive to detail or to rush your actions.
- A cold or flu may be associated with distracting symptoms such as a runny nose, which can lead to loss of focus; the use of OTC medications can impair your ability to operate the vehicle safely.
- Headaches, especially migraine headaches, may cause changes in vision and hearing, which can severely diminish your ability to operate an emergency vehicle.

Attitude

A person's attitude is a key component of mental preparedness for emergency vehicle operation. Many people feel empowered and confident when they use lights and sirens as the driver of an emergency vehicle. These feelings of empowerment and confidence may lead to angry and aggressive driving, which can lead vehicle operators to take chances that they would not otherwise take, jeopardizing providers and patients. Aggressive driving can lead to serious injury or even death. There is no excuse for aggressive driving, even when other drivers are not reacting to your approach as legally required. As a professional, it is your job to focus on your driving, be cautious, and refuse to allow emotions to guide you behind the wheel.

A related issue concerns those vehicle operators who feel that because they already know how to drive, there is nothing to teach them that they do not already know. This type of attitude is misguided, as it is critical that vehicle operators know and understand the unique hazards inherent in operating an emergency vehicle. Avoiding aggressive driving and having a safety-first attitude are central to safe vehicle operation.

Safety Equipment

Emergency vehicles are equipped with safety equipment, such as seatbelts and airbags. Proper use of this equipment is essential to ensure the safety of vehicle operators, technicians, EMS providers, and the patients they transport.

Seatbelts

Seatbelts are an extremely effective method of reducing injuries and deaths from vehicle collisions. Over 15,000 lives are saved each year by proper use of seatbelts, and most EMS organizations have polices requiring the use of seatbelts in emergency vehicles.

For seatbelts to be effective, they must be worn properly. The lap belt needs to be placed snugly over the hips. The shoulder belt should be placed over the shoulder and diagonally across the torso away from the neck **FIGURE 2-3**. The shoulder belt should never be placed under the arm. Shorter or taller individuals may need to adjust the seatbelt restraint system or the position of the seat to ensure that the seatbelt fits properly. In older vehicles with separate lap and shoulder restraints, both systems must be used. Wearing a safety belt improperly may increase the risk of injury to a level similar to that of not wearing a seatbelt at all.

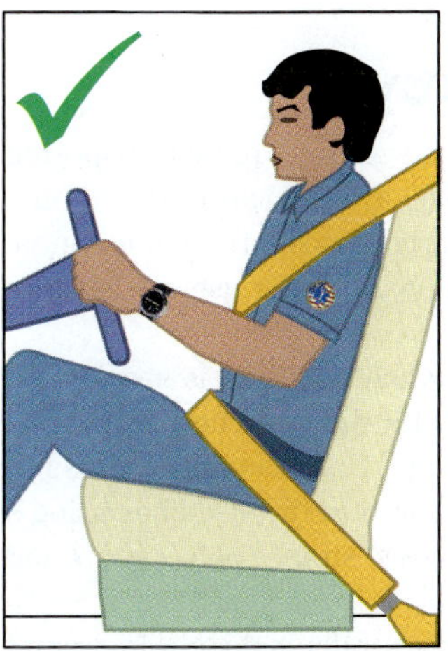

Correct

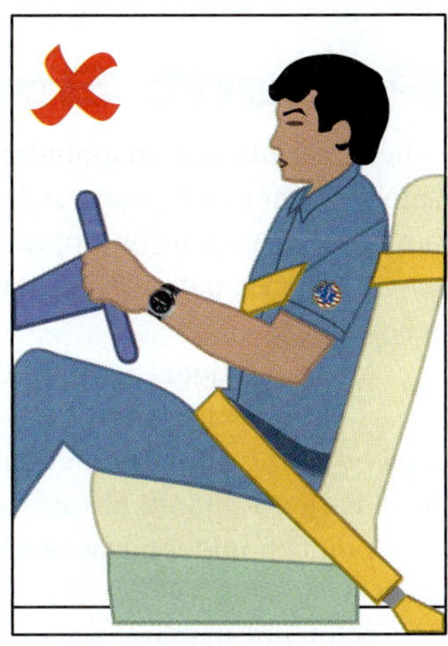

Incorrect

Figure 2-3 Proper seatbelt use.

Although the evidence is overwhelming that seatbelts save lives, many people still do not wear them, including people working in EMS. Providers may think it is acceptable to stand or move around unrestrained in the patient compartment when the vehicle is in motion. Even those who have witnessed the often tragic consequences of not wearing a seatbelt may rationalize this practice, but unrestrained providers providing patient care are at significant risk for injury and death in the event of a collision.

As the emergency vehicle operator, you are responsible for ensuring that everyone is wearing a seatbelt properly before moving the vehicle. This includes providers in the patient compartment. Unrestrained or improperly restrained EMS providers die or are seriously injured each year in motor vehicle collisions. Even though it is legal, it is not safe practice for EMS providers to be unrestrained, even when providing patient care.

SAFETY POINTER

The single most important factor in seatbelt use is personal commitment. Make a commitment to ensure your safety first.

It may be more difficult or inconvenient to provide patient care while wearing a seatbelt, but this is no excuse to not wear one. Research is under way to develop a more ergonomic work space that will allow providers to tend to patients while being restrained. Regardless of the system in place, the vehicle operator must be properly restrained and ensure that all crew members are wearing seatbelts. This simple step can mean the difference between a minor injury and death in the event of a motor vehicle collision.

SAFETY POINTER

Seatbelts save lives. There is no excuse for not using seatbelts in the front compartment. Moreover, they should be used in the patient compartment.

Airbags

Airbags are important safety features that help to reduce **morbidity** and **mortality** in the event of a collision. Frontal airbags in emergency vehicles are usually located in the steering wheel or the dash and are designed to protect the occupant from hitting the steering wheel, dash, and windshield. Newer ambulances may include other types of airbags such as side curtain airbags, rollover airbags, knee bolsters, carpet airbags, and/or anti-slide airbags.

Vehicle occupants should be a safe distance from the airbag (at least 10 inches). No objects, including mobile data terminals or other devices, should obstruct the path between the occupant and the airbag. Objects located in this path during airbag deployment could interfere with the release of the airbag or become projectiles and cause further injury. It is important to remember that airbags are only part of the occupant safety system and that proper seatbelt use is required.

Headrests or Head Restraints

Head restraints, more commonly called headrests, in emergency vehicles vary depending on the make, model, and year of the vehicle. When available, they may help to reduce neck injuries in the event of a rear-end collision. Many drivers have improperly adjusted head restraints. The most common error is head restraints that are adjusted too low. A head restraint should be positioned no more than 2 inches behind the driver's head, with the center of the headrest at approximately ear level. When adjusted properly, the driver's head should contact the head restraint before the neck does. Properly positioning the head restraint may reduce whiplash and other neck injuries in the event of a rear-end collision.

Mirrors

Properly adjusted mirrors are important to safe vehicle operation. It is the emergency vehicle operator's responsibility to ensure the mirrors are positioned to maximize the operator's field of vision and limit blind spots. Mirrors may need to be adjusted multiple times during a shift in situations where drivers change frequently.

It is important to remember that even when you have properly maximized your field of vision, blind spots are still present behind the vehicle. To back the vehicle safely, use a spotter to provide directions. Services should have strict policies requiring use of a spotter when backing a vehicle.

SAFETY POINTER

Being safe is a personal commitment and is a *must* for every emergency vehicle operator. Be committed to your safety and the safety of others.

Helmets

When an ambulance is involved in a collision or evasive maneuver, unrestrained providers may fall and strike their heads. Unrestrained equipment such as oxygen gauges or suction unit bottles may become airborne and strike providers, and sharp corners or edges may cause injuries. Thus, some safety experts advocate the use of safety helmets for EMS personnel during patient transport.

Dr. Nadine Levick, CEO of Objective Safety and Research Director of EMS Safety Foundation, reports that 74% of EMS fatalities are the result of vehicle collisions and that 64% of those deaths are the result of serious head injuries. It is logical to presume that helmets could help reduce morbidity and mortality in these situations. Specially designed helmets for protecting EMS personnel have yet to be developed, and traditional fire helmets would not be effective for this purpose. The use of helmets, however, would not reduce the need to improve ambulance design and testing for greater safety. Routine helmet use will require further education, training, positive reinforcement, and practical policies implemented by visionary leaders who are committed to safety and research.

Equipment Security

Properly securing equipment is essential to prevent it from becoming a projectile during a collision or sudden stop. Unsecured equipment such as first-in bags (jump kits), oxygen caddies, defibrillators, or monitors may become deadly projectiles and have been documented to cause provider and patient injury. Equipment should always be secured in cabinets or in specifically designed locations. One method of securing gear is to attach carabineers to the bag and clip it to a specified location in the box. Properly securing equipment takes only a few seconds; there is simply no justifiable reason to leave equipment unsecured. Ambulances should be properly equipped with monitor locks and computer docking stations to secure equipment in a usable position.

SAFETY POINTER

Gear should always be secured in a compartment or specified location.

Patient Safety

When patients call an ambulance, they expect to be transported safely. Remember rule number one: Do no harm. You should never put a patient in jeopardy during transport. One essential way to ensure patient safety is through proper use of stretcher restraints.

Many providers assume that when a patient is secured on the stretcher with three lap belts and the stretcher is properly latched to the floor, the patient is safe. Unfortunately, this is not true. Patients should always be secured to the stretcher using a four-point shoulder harness with a chest strap, a pelvis strap, and a leg strap FIGURE 2-4.

Stretcher manufacturers now generally include a four-point shoulder harness as part of their standard equipment. Many providers believe that the shoulder harnesses are optional, but in fact, they are critical for ensuring that the patient does not

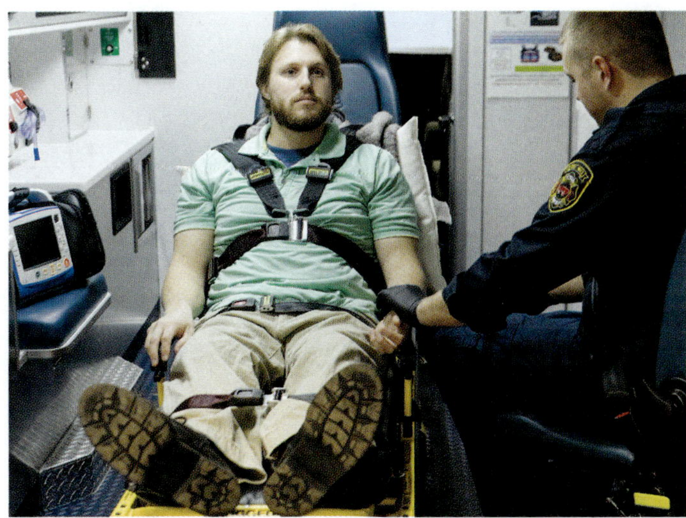

Figure 2-4 Proper patient restraints.

slide out of the stretcher straps during a collision. It is imperative that providers use the manufacturer's specifications for securing patients; failure to do so could result in increased liability for injuries in the case of a collision. The scenario at the beginning of this chapter is a good example of this happening. When the shoulder harnesses are properly secured in accordance with the manufacturer's recommendations, they should not interfere with your ability to provide patient care, including a 12-lead ECG or other monitoring.

SAFETY POINTER

You have the responsibility to ensure that your patients are properly secured. In many instances, patients who were improperly secured without the use of the provided shoulder harnesses have been killed or severely injured following a vehicle collision. Your patient's safety is your responsibility.

The stretcher should be secured to the floor during transport. Slightly raise the head end to help prevent the patient from hitting the captain's seat or bulkhead in the event of a frontal impact crash. Note, however, that even when properly secured, ambulance crash tests have revealed that stretchers can detach from the mounts and become projectiles in the event of a collision. It is interesting to note that in the United States, the locking system of the most commonly used stretchers and mounting systems is designed to withstand only 2,200 foot-pounds of force—roughly equivalent to only 74 pounds moving at 30 mph. In addition, stretchers are secured at only a single point of contact on a rack that prevents the wheels from rolling too far forward. This design is significantly inferior to stretchers used in Europe. In Europe, stretchers and their mounting systems are able to endure loads 10 times the force of gravity over a crash impulse window of less than 100 milliseconds without failure. Further, stretchers are secured to the floor at three points of contact, each of which restrains motion on at least two axes.

Passenger Safety

Family members and friends often want to accompany patients in the ambulance. Your company should have a policy for this case, and you should be familiar with the policy to ensure that this is an approved practice.

An adult passenger should be transported in the front passenger seat and wear a seatbelt. The emergency vehicle operator should assist the passenger into the front seat and ensure that the seatbelt is properly attached. The emergency vehicle operator should also assist the passenger out of the vehicle upon arrival at the destination. Any passenger who refuses to wear a seatbelt should not be permitted to ride in the ambulance. Small folding stools may be useful to help passengers into and out of the passenger seat. These stools may be stored behind the passenger seat of the ambulance.

EMS providers should not allow themselves to become distracted by conversing with accompanying family members or friends. The primary objective is getting to the hospital safely, and this may require the operator's full attention. It is not discourteous to inform passengers that you are unable to talk while driving to ensure that everyone arrives safely at their destination.

While in general, passengers should be seated in the front compartment, there are certain circumstances in which it may be advantageous for a passenger to ride in the patient compartment. For example, it may be beneficial for a parent to ride in the patient compartment to provide support to a pediatric patient. In this event, the child must be properly restrained in accordance with his or her age and size and with local laws. Children should never be transported on the parent's lap, even if the parent is secured to the stretcher. Parents in the patient compartment must also be properly restrained.

Prior to allowing the parent to ride with the patient, a member of the crew should explain any necessary interventions so that the parent knows what to expect during transport. Parents who are overly emotional or unable to control themselves should not be permitted to ride in the patient compartment. Family members or friends should never be transported in the patient

SAFETY POINTER

EMS providers should never sit on the end of the stretcher to provide patient care during transport. This practice places the patient at risk of being injured by the provider should a vehicle collision occur.

compartment when the patient is in respiratory or cardiac arrest or when other critical conditions exist.

In special situations, children may need to be transported as passengers when their parent is a patient. This practice should be limited to situations in which no other options exist. Children who are eligible to ride in the passenger seat according to your state law should ride in the passenger seat with proper restraints. Children who require a safety seat must be transported in a child safety seat or booster seat. Safety seats may not be placed on side-facing seats. Children who are not required to use a child safety seat of any kind may ride in the captain's seat (rear-facing seat) with a seatbelt, based on your department's policy.

When necessary, additional emergency responders may be transported as passengers. It is the responsibility of the emergency vehicle operator to ensure that they are properly restrained the same as any other crew member. Remember that the number of occupants should never exceed the number of seatbelts in the vehicle.

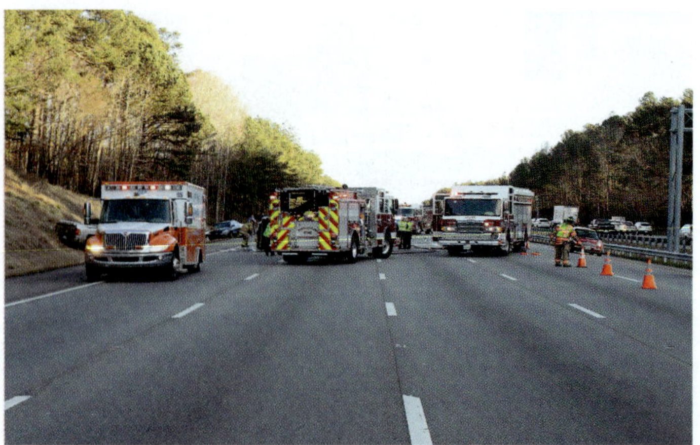

Figure 2-5 Proper traffic blocking techniques and high-visibility gear will help to keep you safe.

Roadside Safety

Many emergency incidents occur on interstates, highways, and other roadways. An emergency scene on the roadway presents unique hazards to the emergency vehicle operator. Every year, many EMS providers are injured or killed at roadway incidents.

Motorists may be distracted by the scene and not paying attention to their driving. When drivers see the lights on an accident scene, they are likely to drive toward it because our hands follow our eyes. The safest place for an emergency vehicle responding to a highway incident is off of the roadway and away from traffic. Emergency vehicle operators need to ensure they are seen by other motorists and have been given the right of way. Whenever possible, you should avoid working on a roadway or highway or at least aim to limit the amount of time you spend on the roadway as much as possible, even if it means delaying patient care until you can move to a safe location. When it is necessary to work on a roadway, you should take proper precautions:

- Establish a safe work zone by having the police or fire department block traffic and using traffic-control devices **FIGURE 2-5**.
- Position the vehicle properly ("downstream" of the collision).
- Consider the use of warning lights.
- Wear high-visibility apparel.

Safe Work Zone

Emergency vehicles can be positioned to establish a safe work zone by blocking traffic and providing protection for personnel operating at the emergency scene. Ideally, fire apparatus should be used to block traffic. Cones and traffic warning devices should be used to warn unsuspecting motorists at extended incidents whenever possible. The key is having the first-arriving unit block traffic from the scene. It is not ideal for the ambulance to perform this function, but it is needed to secure the scene and warn oncoming drivers. The preferred placement of the ambulance is in front (downstream) of the collision, which limits exposure to moving traffic during patient loading. It is also the best position for egress once it is time to transport the patient.

If an ambulance is being used to block traffic, angle the vehicle so that it is aimed away from the scene, with the rear doors not directly facing on-coming traffic. Keep the rear doors closed so that the vehicle's lights are visible. This positioning provides additional protection so that providers can access equipment. In addition, turn the vehicle's wheels away from the work zone so that in the event it is struck by a motorist from behind, it will not directly collide with the scene. Note that the patient should not be loaded into the vehicle until it is moved around the incident and positioned such that the collision scene serves as a protective barrier.

At high-risk incidents and incident locations, it may be necessary to request assistance from additional responders (e.g., police, fire, EMS, and highway services) to ensure scene safety. The Traffic Incident Management (TIM) system can help responders coordinate their efforts when more than one response vehicle is necessary at an incident to avoid placing the ambulance in an area that may be blocked by other emergency vehicles.

The TIM system comprises several components that both allow traffic to move safely and smoothly around an emergency scene and allow the first responders to work in a relatively safe environment **FIGURE 2-6**. The system is made up of the following:

- *Advanced warning area.* This area gives motorists ample warning of an incident ahead and is usually marked with a *pink* diamond-shaped warning sign placed by the first unit arriving on scene.
- *Transition area.* This area begins the flare or cone pattern, which is used to taper the number of lanes and move traffic away from the incident.
- *Buffer space.* This area starts to slow traffic and funnel it away from the incident.

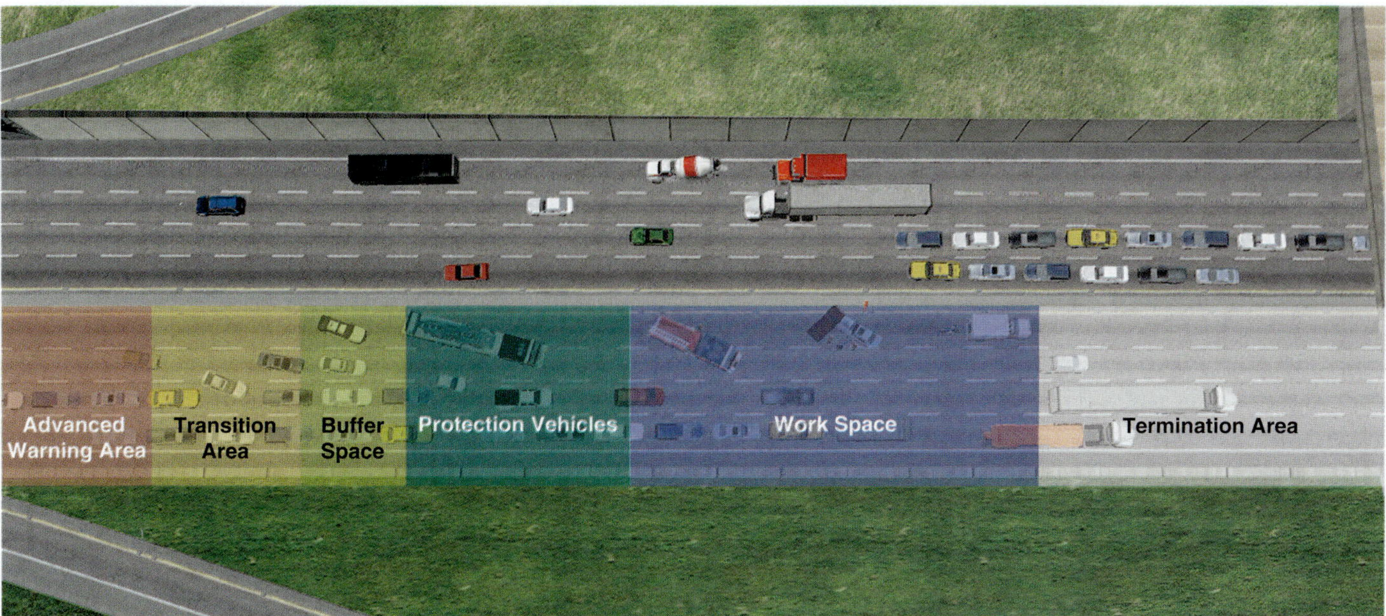

Figure 2-6 The traffic incident management system.
Courtesy of FAAC, Inc. Based on original figure by Emergency Responder Safety Institute.

- *Protection vehicles.* This area is directly "upstream" from the incident. Vehicles positioned here are primarily used for blocking and secondarily used as resource vehicles. "Lane + 1 blocking" affords a good work space for rescuers and a "shadow" area that limits drivers' ability to rubberneck. Position vehicles to both block and direct traffic.
- *Work space.* This is the area of the incident, and it must remain as open and as safe as possible. Protection vehicles may have to be repositioned as the operation progresses to maintain a high level of safety while allowing traffic to flow with as little impediment as possible.
- *Termination area.* This is the area immediately downstream of the incident that allows traffic to continue to move in a controlled manner. This area should be avoided by rescuers at all times and at all costs. If the incident dictates that rescuers enter into the termination area, then the work space should be extended and the termination area moved further downstream. This area can be used for staging of tow trucks, medical examiner vehicles, and other ancillary vehicles that are not actively engaged in the rescue process.

SAFETY POINTER

Become familiar with the Traffic Incident Management (TIM) system. If you have any questions about vehicle placement, consult with the incident commander who has overall responsibility for scene safety and comprehensive knowledge about the operations.

For more in-depth information regarding the TIM system, visit the Emergency Responder Safety Institute website.

Vehicle Positioning

It is important to position the emergency vehicle properly at an emergency scene to ensure the safety of motorists, patients, and providers. Consider the location of the incident and unique hazards, such as inclement weather and poor visibility, when determining the safest places to position the vehicle. For example, vehicles should not be placed on corners, at the crest of hills, or in blind spots. Providers need to be aware of the unique hazards within their response district.

When staging the vehicle at a scene, several issues may need to be taken into account in the placement of the vehicle, not only for safe scene operations but also for easy egress once scene management is complete. Examples include placing vehicles uphill from spilled liquids and vapors, downwind from fumes and smoke, upstream when first on scene, and downstream when on scene with other units and loading patients. Vigilance should be used when positioning the ambulance so as not to get blocked in by additional emergency vehicles, prohibiting rapid transport from the scene.

A majority of emergency responses occur at a residence or other locations where there is a driveway. In these instances, the driveway is usually the safest place to park the ambulance. When arriving at the incident location, depending on the situation and priority of the assignment, your partner should exit the vehicle wearing high-visibility apparel and serve as a spotter to help you back into the driveway. In some situations, it may be necessary to park at the curb in front of the residence. Either way, once the vehicle is parked, the emergency lights

VEHICLE OPERATOR INCIDENT

In southwestern Colorado in March 2007, several teenagers were killed due to improper parking and misuse of warning equipment by an emergency provider at the scene. A deputy investigating a car off the road drove past a collision on a curve and parked without using emergency lights, leaving his headlights on. The deputy parked to the right of the travel lanes and left of the disabled vehicle. This created an optical illusion with the stopped car, creating the appearance that the oncoming lane was further right than it really was. As a result, the fatigued driver of an oncoming utility truck drove into the scene on the shoulder, striking the teenagers inside of and around the disabled vehicle. The truck driver saw the deputy's headlights and mistakenly thought the deputy was in the approaching lane. Had the deputy used his emergency lights, turned off the headlights, or lit the scene properly, this incident may have been avoided.

and headlights should be turned off if they might interfere with the normal flow of traffic in any way.

Warning Lights

It may seem counterintuitive, but emergency lights may actually be a safety hazard. It is not uncommon for motorists to crash into parked emergency vehicles that have warning lights operating. The flashing lights attract the drivers' attention, which may lead them to steer toward the emergency vehicle. When possible, warning lights should be limited to amber lights in an alternating pattern on the vehicle's corners. When this lighting option is not available, the vehicle's hazard lights should be used. Drivers are accustomed to seeing yellow or hazard lights and recognize that they need to slow down and proceed with caution. Most drivers are not accustomed to emergency lighting and may be distracted by the lights and unsure how to respond. Today, most states require blue lights on the rear portion of all emergency vehicles. Provided your specific state does not prohibit the use of a blue light, this is a helpful recommendation.

The use of warning lights for blocking vehicles is discussed in detail in NFPA 1451, *Standard for a Fire and Emergency Service Vehicle Operations Training Program.*

High-Visibility Apparel

High-visibility apparel increases the provider's visibility when working along a roadway. Federal law requires all workers within the right of way along a federal highway to wear an ANSI 107 (2004) Class 2 or 3 high-visibility vest. This law applies to all first responders, though exceptions do exist for police personnel based on tactical need. The use of high-visibility vests increases personnel visibility and reduces the risk of severe injury or death FIGURE 2-7. These vests are also required to come with a five-point breakaway feature for safety. However, it is important to understand that the use of high-visibility apparel alone does not make you safe.

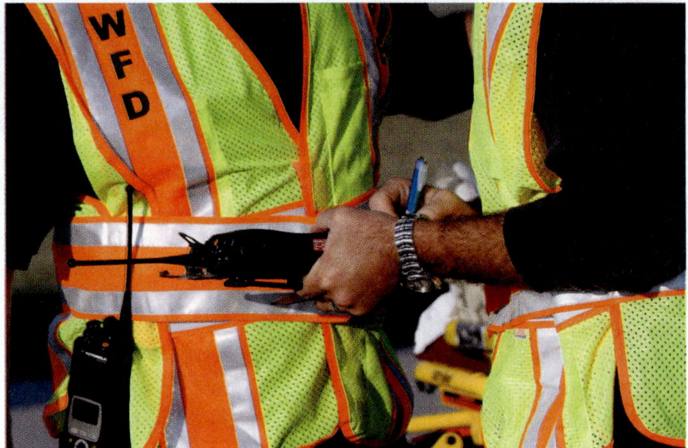

Figure 2-7 Agencies should obtain high-visibility vests (ANSI-107 [2004] Class 2 or 3 garments or ANSI-207 [2006]-compliant garments) for their personnel. Ensure that vests are sized to fit when worn on top of full turnout gear, such as in cold-weather situations, responses to motor vehicle crashes where there is no fire, or where otherwise appropriate.

SAFETY POINTER

Place approved high-visibility apparel in an easily accessible location. Use positive reinforcement and lead by example so that wearing high-visibility apparel becomes the norm.

Mechanical Problems

As an emergency vehicle operator, you may encounter situations that involve safety hazards such as a mechanical problem or vehicle fire. In these situations, the overriding concern should be your personal safety and the safety of your partner, patient, and passengers.

Common mechanical problems such as engine failure, transmission failure, an overheating vehicle, or a flat tire can create an unexpected and hazardous situation. When a mechanical problem occurs, every attempt should be made to move the vehicle away from traffic. If your vehicle is blocking traffic in any way, immediately turn on your hazard lights to warn oncoming motorists. Do not use your emergency lights, as this may confuse drivers who associate the emergency lights with an incident such as a motor vehicle collision. After turning on your hazard lights, you should request assistance to control the traffic hazard in accordance with your agency's policies. Remember to request an additional unit to transport your patient, if necessary.

SAFETY POINTER

Take precautions to protect yourself in the event of mechanical difficulties:

- Move the vehicle away from traffic.
- Put on the vehicle's hazard lights.
- Call for assistance.
- Safely exit the vehicle.
- Use traffic-control devices.

Once assistance has been requested, you should don high-visibility apparel and exit the vehicle. To provide additional protection and warn oncoming traffic, you should set up flares, warning triangles, or other traffic-control devices. Whenever possible, place warning devices at least 300 feet from the vehicle in equal increments to direct traffic away from the disabled vehicle. Roadside repairs should never be attempted by nonqualified personnel; always defer to local policies. Keep in mind that flares may create additional danger if there are leaking fluids on the ground.

Although rare, vehicle fires can occur in an emergency medical vehicle. Emergency medical units carry oxygen, which is an accelerant and can be extremely dangerous in the event of a fire. If a vehicle fire occurs, you must rapidly assess the situation and take actions to maximize safety. The priority should be removing the patient from the vehicle. If the vehicle is on fire, you should not take time to remove equipment. Since the oxygen system on board could result in an explosion, your main concern is to move yourself and the patient a safe distance away from the vehicle.

SAFETY POINTER

Safety is the number one priority during an unexpected or hazardous situation.

WRAP-UP

SUMMARY

- The priority for EMS providers is to ensure their own safety and the safety of their partner, patients, and passengers.
- Having a safety-first attitude is a critical component of safe vehicle operation.
- Safety is a habit and a culture that relies on personal responsibility and commitment to excellence.
- Mental and physical preparedness includes efforts to reduce or avoid sleep deprivation, stress, extreme emotions, or physical ailments, which may inhibit decision making.
- To be effective, a seatbelt must be placed properly, with the lap belt snug over the hips and the shoulder belt over the shoulder and diagonally across the torso.
- Care providers must always be properly restrained during transport, even when they are providing care to the patient in the patient compartment.
- Emergency vehicle airbags located in the steering wheel or dash are designed to protect the driver and front passenger in the event of a collision.
- Properly positioned headrests can reduce the risk of neck injuries.
- Correct mirror positioning and use of spotters when backing are important safety precautions.
- It is necessary to secure all equipment to avoid projectiles if the vehicle stops suddenly.
- Patients should always be secured to the stretcher using a four-point shoulder harness with chest strap, pelvis strap, and leg strap.

- Adult passengers should ride in the front passenger seat with a seatbelt.
- Children should always be properly restrained according to their age, size, and weight in accordance with state guidelines.
- To establish a safe work zone in the event of a roadway incident, position the vehicle properly, consider the use of warning lights, and wear high-visibility apparel.
- In the event of a mechanical failure, move the vehicle away from traffic, use hazard lights, call for assistance, safely exit the vehicle, and use traffic-control devices.

GLOSSARY

morbidity Illness or harm; a diseased state.

mortality Death; the quality of being mortal.

sleep deprivation The state of having insufficient sleep.

ADDITIONAL RESOURCES

Emergency Responder Safety Institute, http://www.respondersafety.com

National Highway Traffic Safety Administration, http://www.nhtsa.gov

National Safety Council, http://www.nsc.org

U.S. Department of Labor: Occupational Safety and Health Administration (OSHA), http://www.osha.gov

REFERENCES

McCallion, T. (2012). Consider the dangers of shift work: It's important to have a fatigue management plan in place. *Journal of Emergency Medical Services*. Retrieved from http://www.jems.com/article/emsinsider/consider-dangers-shift-work

National Fire Protection Association. (2013). *NFPA 1451: Standard for a fire and emergency services vehicle operations training program*. Quincy, MA: Author, 2013.

National Sleep Foundation. (2005). *2005 sleep in America poll: Summary of findings*. Retrieved from https://sleepfoundation.org/sites/default/files/2005_summary_of_findings.pdf

National Sleep Foundation. (2009). *2009 sleep in America poll: Summary of findings*. Retrieved from https://sleepfoundation.org/sites/default/files/2009%20SLEEP%20IN%20AMERICA%20SOF%20EMBARGOED_0.PDF

National Sleep Foundation. (2015). *Facts and stats: Drowsy driving – Stay alert, arrive alive*. Retrieved from http://drowsydriving.org/about/facts-and-stats/

Proudfoot, S. L. (2005). Ambulance crashes: Fatality factors for EMS workers. *EMS World*. Retrieved from http://www.emsworld.com/article/10323905/ambulance-crashes-fatality-factors-for-ems-workers

U.S. Department of Homeland Security Science and Technology Directorate, First Responders Group. (2015). *Ambulance patient compartment human factors design guidebook*. Retri-eved from http://www.firstresponder.gov/TechnologyDocuments/Ambulance%20Patient%20Compartment%20Human%20Factors%20Design%20Guidebook.pdf

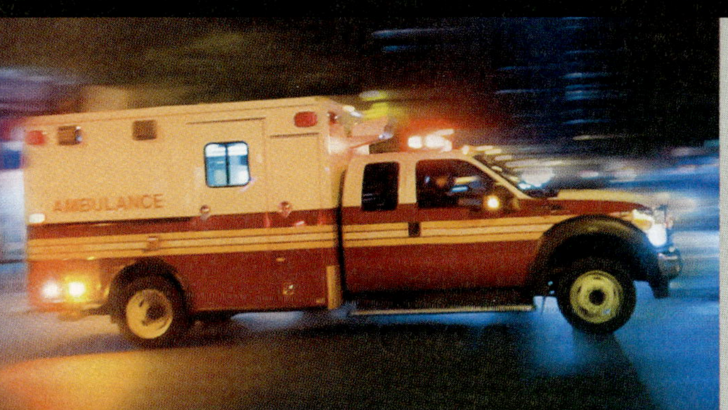

CHAPTER 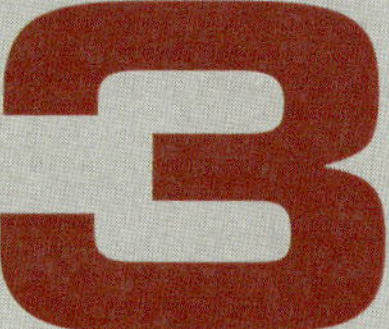

Mental, Emotional, and Physical Preparedness

OBJECTIVES

3.1 Explain the importance of mental, emotional, and physical preparedness.

3.2 Discuss how avoiding distractions is a key component of safe vehicle operation.

3.3 Discuss how paying attention to detail helps ensure safe vehicle operation.

3.4 Outline the key elements of a safety-first attitude.

3.5 Discuss steps the emergency vehicle operator can take to ensure emotional preparedness, reducing the effects of stress and emotion.

3.6 Explain the importance of physical preparedness in emergency vehicle operation, including hearing and vision testing and hazards related to physical ailments, sleep deprivation, and medication and substance use.

SCENARIO

On Sunday, September 23, 2007, in Cranberry Township, Pennsylvania, the fog was so thick that it created virtual "white-out" conditions, making it nearly impossible to see the cars in front of one's vehicle or the headlights of oncoming traffic. An ambulance was transporting a 90-year-old patient for heart problems when it approached a standing red light. The emergency vehicle operator proceeded through the intersection with lights flashing, not engaging the siren until just 2 seconds before the ambulance broadsided a Chevy Cavalier with two occupants.

The patient, emergency vehicle operator, and medic in the ambulance all suffered minor injuries, while both the driver and passenger in the car were killed. The patient eventually died of a heart condition several days later, but it was not considered related to the collision. The roadway was shut down for 9 hours while police investigated the crash. Initial reports stated that the police did not know if speed played a part in the crash, but after additional investigation, they discovered that the emergency vehicle operator had been driving 70 mph in a 40-mph zone and had been under the influence of alcohol. The prosecutor stated that the patient's condition did not require the driver to exceed the speed limit. The emergency vehicle operator was charged with two counts of homicide by vehicle and two counts of homicide by vehicle while driving under the influence. She faced up to 14 years and 9 months behind bars but will spend 1 to 2 years in the county jail as part of her plea agreement.

1. What would you do if you suspected a coworker of being unfit for duty?
2. What conditions require emergency transport to the hospital?
3. What happens to your visibility and the visibility of emergency lighting in the fog?

Sources: WPXI.com. (2007). Two Killed in Pennsylvania Ambulance Crash. Retrieved from http://www.emsworld.com/news/10339925/2-killed-in-pennsylvania-ambulance-crash; Kane, K. (2007). Ambulance driver charged in fatal crash will be fired under zero tolerance policy. *Pittsburgh Post-Gazette*. Retrieved from http://www.post-gazette.com/local/north/2007/11/11/Ambulance-driver-charged-in-fatal-crash-will-be-fired-under-zero-tolerance-policy/stories/200711110225.

Introduction

Every operator of an emergency vehicle is responsible for the safe operation of their vehicle as well as for the safety of the passengers, patients, and general public who might be affected by their vehicle's operation. Emergency vehicle operators must be mentally, emotionally, and physically prepared every time they get behind the wheel. Mental preparedness means having a safety-first attitude and concentrating on the details of driving. Emotional preparedness includes managing stress, anxiety, and other emotions. Physical preparedness includes avoiding driving when affected by illness or injury, undergoing regular hearing and vision testing, and maintaining adequate sleep. Obviously the use of any substance that can alter your body's ability to react quickly to an emergency should be avoided as well.

SAFETY POINTER

Emergency vehicle operators must ensure that they are mentally, physically, and emotionally prepared to focus on the high stress environment of vehicle operations.

Education, training, and experience are all important aspects of being a safe emergency vehicle operator; however, the most important aspect of being a safe operator is a personal commitment to safety and excellence. The concepts discussed in this chapter do not exist simply for the sake of creating company policy or guidelines. They must be embraced by the individual emergency vehicle operator. They play an integral part in ensuring the safe operation of an organization's vehicles and limiting the organization's risk.

Mental Preparedness

As an emergency vehicle operator, you must stay focused solely on the task of safely operating the emergency vehicle. The key to focus is avoiding distractions such as thoughts about what is going on in your personal life or technological distractions like cell phones or mobile data terminals. Many times the emergency vehicle operator is doing something in addition to driving. He or she is receiving urgent radio traffic or transmitting on the radio while navigating an intersection. At the same time, the vehicle operator and his or her partner are discussing the nature of the call based on dispatch information, and what equipment and potential additional resources they need. All things considered, the emergency vehicle operator is on scene mentally, but the vehicle has not even finished clearing the intersection.

One of the most prevalent mental distractions is mentally placing oneself at the scene while still responding. It is extremely dangerous and the emergency vehicle operator must instead refocus his or her attention on the present and the driving tasks at hand. Considering questions such as, "What equipment do I need?" and "What will we find?" can help responders mentally prepare but should not take precedence over the task of arriving at the scene safely. Failure to focus on vehicle operations can have deadly consequences.

Even during "routine" assignments, emergency vehicle operators must be mindful that simple conversations about "Where should I go for dinner?" or "What are you doing after work?" can lead to collisions. In the airline industry, pilots are required to have a "sterile" cockpit during critical phases of operation. This means that during critical phases of a flight such as ground operations, departure, or arrival, pilots are permitted to discuss only issues directly related to the task being performed. This approach increases awareness and decreases errors caused by inattention due to distraction. Research has demonstrated the effectiveness of the sterile cockpit, which can be adapted for use in a variety of settings, including EMS vehicle operation. The sterile cockpit is an important concept that should be embraced to help you perform your duties safely and effectively. Complacency is one of the EMS service's worst enemies. Remember, the smallest mistakes usually lead to the most horrific crashes.

Avoid Technological Distractions

Cellular phones, radios, and other technological devices are a major source of potential distraction. Many EMS systems rely on cell phones as the primary form of communication between the responding vehicle and receiving hospitals. However, cell phone and radio use distracts drivers and causes them to lose focus, leading to thousands of injuries and fatalities each year. When talking on a cell phone, the driver can be distracted mentally, emotionally, and physically, leading to tragic consequences. The use of cell phones by emergency vehicle operators in any form while driving is neither a safe nor an accepted practice. Some local municipalities and states have created laws prohibiting cell phone use while driving, and emergency vehicle operators need to be aware of and follow such laws. These laws can include prohibiting calls from supervisors, who should avoid calling crews while they are on calls *unless an absolute emergency*. If an emergency vehicle operator does use a cell phone during a response, the passenger should be the one to hold the phone to limit the likelihood of the driver becoming distracted.

The practice of texting while driving is especially unsafe and irresponsible. There is no way in which the operator of any vehicle can maintain constant visual contact with the road while texting FIGURE 3-1. Even if you only take your eyes off the road for a fraction of a second, your vehicle is continuing to travel. At a speed of 55 mph, it will go 60 feet in just three-quarters of a second. Studies show that texting while operating an emergency vehicle increases the likelihood of a collision by a factor of 23 because it takes the hands, eyes, and mind off of driving. Distracted driving increases the amount of time it takes the vehicle operator to react and is a leading cause of collisions FIGURE 3-2. There is simply no excuse for it. As an emergency vehicle operator, you must possess a safe and positive attitude and not engage in dangerous activities. You must aim to eliminate distractions and focus on the task of operating your vehicle safely.

Mobile data terminals (MDTs), which are becoming common in EMS vehicles, are intended to be used only by the occupant of the passenger seat or when the vehicle is safely stopped. Use of an MDT by an emergency vehicle operator while the

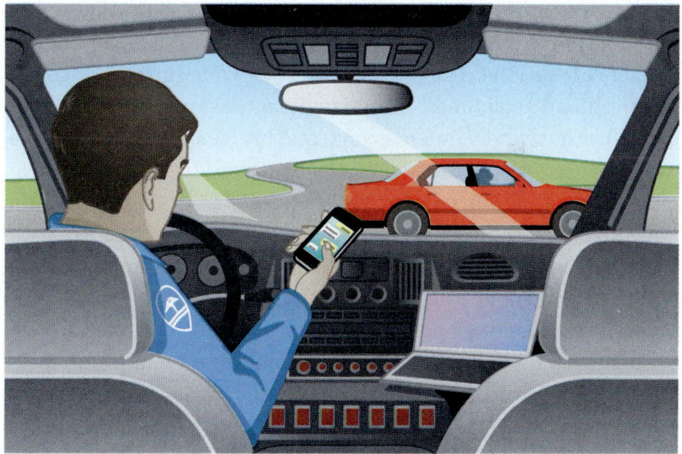

Figure 3-1 Texting while driving puts everyone at risk.
© Jones & Bartlett Learning.

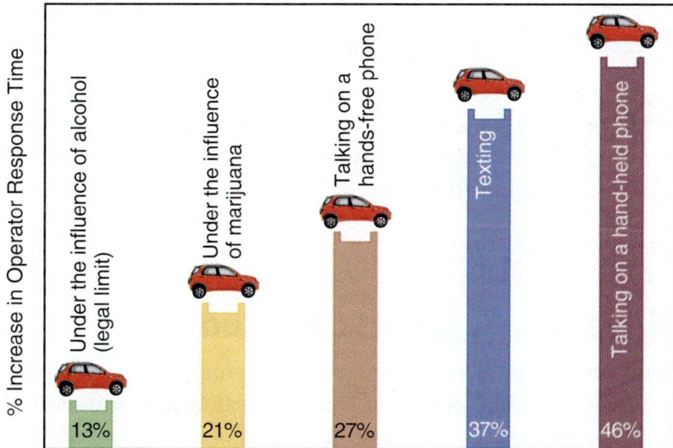

Figure 3-2 Driving distractions and their respective percentage increase on the operator's response time.
Data from Reed, N., and R. Robbins. "The Effect Of Text Messaging On Driver Behaviour: A Simulator Study." RAC Foundation. Transport Research Laboratory, 1 Sept. 2008. http://www.racfoundation.org

vehicle is in motion is a dangerous distraction. Operation of this type of device requires the driver to remove one hand from the steering wheel and to divert his or her attention from the road. Focus on the screen and/or keyboard of the device takes the driver's attention completely away from what is happening in front of and around the vehicle. It only takes a second of distraction for a collision to occur. For this reason, use of MDTs should be restricted by department policy as well as the individual driver's conscience. Coworkers in the passenger seat should be using mapping functions and using the MDT whenever possible. Drivers should plan their route before leaving a scene so they won't need to look at the map while driving, unless the vehicle is stopped.

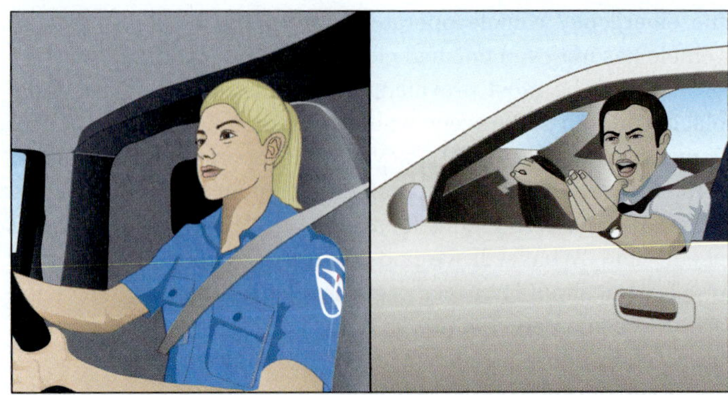

Figure 3-3 Do not respond to aggressive drivers or let your emotions get the best of you.

Pay Attention to Detail

Paying attention to detail is a way of ensuring everyone's safety. As an emergency vehicle operator, you must ensure that everyone is properly restrained prior to moving the vehicle and during vehicle operations. You must be aware of your surroundings and environment at all times. Attend to the roadway environment and any hazards present, such as one-lane bridges, low underpasses, weight restrictions, narrow roads, or hazardous locations. Also pay close attention to your vehicle, constantly monitoring the dash, console, gauges, and warning lights. Lack of attention can create dangerous and unprofessional situations, such as driving with compartment doors unintentionally left open or partially open bay doors, leaving the garage with the shoreline still connected, driving with items or equipment left on rear bumpers or the hood, or overlooking hazards such as low wires, tree limbs, or overhangs. A quick walk around the vehicle prior to leaving is a good habit to avoid issues with open compartments and equipment misplacement.

SAFETY POINTER

Adverse weather conditions can make it more difficult to identify potential hazards. When operating in adverse weather conditions, you must pay close attention to details and remain aware of your surroundings.

Have a Safety-First Attitude

Your attitude is a key component of mental preparedness for emergency vehicle operation. Having a safety-first attitude can help you be mentally prepared. Examples of this type of attitude include remaining calm at all times, making sure the vehicle is in safe operating condition before moving it, and constantly evaluating your driving to make sure you are doing things the safest way possible under the circumstances. Allowing yourself to be lulled into a false sense of confidence when driving with your lights and siren on can result in mistakes that can lead to a collision.

Another risky behavior is aggressive driving, which can stem from knowing that the patient is in urgent need of hospital care. Aggressive driving is not justified even in the most serious patient situations, since the time saved in transport is small, especially when compared to the increased risk of being involved in a collision. Remember that the driver needs to keep a clear mind and focus on driving, not on patient care. Without a smooth transport, patient care can suffer. Keeping a safety-first attitude will engender good defensive driving and help combat the urge to become aggressive **FIGURE 3-3**.

SAFETY POINTER

Your personal attitude toward safe vehicle operations is the single most important element in reducing emergency vehicle collisions. Your ability to recognize emotional responses and maintain a mature attitude in dealing with these temporary visceral reactions can save your life, and the lives of your partner, patients, and the public.

Having the right attitude also means not responding to other drivers who are showing signs of **road rage**. Road rage is thought to be responsible for thousands of collisions, resulting in injury or death each year. As an emergency vehicle operator, you are held to a higher standard and should not let your emotions control your actions. Do not respond to aggressors; always be courteous and remember that the vehicle you are operating is a billboard for your organization and profession. *Consider that everything you do is being filmed and could be on the Internet 2 minutes later.* Do not take other drivers' actions personally. For example, a driver who fails to yield the right-of-way may have a vehicle with a quiet cab or may freeze when approached by an emergency vehicle. The person's inappropriate response was purely accidental and did not reflect any disrespect for you or your profession.

Emotional Preparedness

Another important factor in emergency vehicle operation is emotion. Our emotions affect us strongly and can result in dangerous behavior if not properly controlled. Anger and hate can lead to aggressive driving, while love, grief, fear, and happiness can be dangerous if we allow them to distract us while driving. A lack of concentration due to these very strong emotions can easily lead to a collision in which people could be hurt or even killed. Controlling emotions is a very difficult task, but it is essential to maintaining focus on the primary duty of operating your vehicle safely.

Stress can also interfere with your ability to focus. EMS by definition is stressful, so knowing how to prevent stress from affecting your driving is critical. Every person deals with stress differently, and no one technique will work for everyone. In addition, different types of calls affect responders differently. Most of us are stressed when the patient is a child, but we may just as easily be overstressed if the patient reminds us of a loved one, such as a grandparent. The important point is to recognize when you are stressed and take action to prevent it from affecting your vehicle operation. Remember, that without a smooth and safe ride, very little care will happen during transport. Furthermore, if the ambulance does not make it to the scene and then hospital, no one will be helped.

Stress can cause physical symptoms such as headaches, increased blood pressure, back pain, or gastrointestinal distress. These physical symptoms of stress will also complicate vehicle operation. To deal with stress, you must first recognize it, and physical symptoms are sometimes the best clues. Other signs that you are stressed include rapid breathing, nervousness or shaking, and a strong urge to do everything as fast as possible. Probably the most effective way of dealing with stress for most people is to attempt conscious acts of relaxation. Deep breathing or slowly counting to 10 (or higher) before leaving the scene may allow you to reduce the stress that you may be experiencing from dealing with the patient's condition, which can help prevent the stress from affecting your driving. This technique may be needed before the run starts as well. Emergency vehicle operators must be able to leave whatever emotions they were experiencing before the run at the station.

When responding to what sounds like a serious call, it is easy to get excited and allow your adrenaline to push you to take risks, reasoning that you have to get there as fast as possible. You and your partner should remember that many calls are not as serious as they sound when dispatched. In addition, you should remember that risky behavior while responding to a scene will possibly save a minute or two, while exposing you to a greater chance of collision, which will then take even longer to get help to the patient and possibly cause injury to others. Managing stress is one of the most important things you can do to maintain your focus on driving and reach your destination safely.

Physical Preparedness

Physical preparedness is essential to the operation of an emergency vehicle. To be prepared physically, you must start by having regular physical exams, including hearing and vision tests. You must also be aware of any physical ailments you might have that could affect your driving and must make sure you are getting an adequate amount of sleep. Finally, avoiding any substances, especially drugs (even over-the-counter ones) and alcohol, which can affect your body's ability to function, is critical. The emergency vehicle operator needs to be in sufficient physical shape to operate the vehicle and keep the crew safe at all times. Remember, your job is one of the most important. Every person in the ambulance depends on you. Their lives are in your hands.

Hearing Testing

People often take their sense of hearing for granted and do things that can diminish their ability to hear such as listening to loud music. However, as an emergency vehicle operator, hearing is essential to ensuring your safety on the job. Your hearing can be compromised by colds, sinus problems, headaches, and exposure to loud noises, such as sirens and air horns. You need to recognize and be honest with yourself when these types of issues are affecting your ability to hear well.

Hearing loss is usually gradual and often difficult for people to recognize until it becomes severe. You should have your hearing checked annually to ensure that you have not unknowingly sustained hearing damage FIGURE 3-4. As mentioned, exposure to noises such as sirens can result in hearing loss, especially when the exposure occurs over a long course of time, as is sure to be the case for EMS professionals. Noise levels within the cab of an ambulance are of particular concern to emergency vehicle operators. Headsets may be needed to help keep noise exposure within Occupational Safety and Health Administration (OSHA) recommendations, which can be found in OSHA's General Industry Standards, Occupational Noise Exposure guideline (29 CFR 1910.95). The emergency vehicle operator needs to ensure that noise levels and use of headsets do not interfere with their ability to hear other emergency vehicles or outside warning devices and should consider a hearing conservation program as outlined in OSHA 29 CFR 1910.95(c).

If an emergency vehicle operator has hearing loss, hearing aids may provide great assistance. Hearing aids must be worn correctly, with the volume properly adjusted.

SAFETY POINTER

EMS leaders and personnel should ensure systems are in place to prevent hearing loss. The siren speaker should not be mounted directly over the front cab, and vehicle windows should be closed to minimize siren noise in the cab. Some services have also considered the use of ear protection.

SAFETY POINTER

Use of the siren and other audible warning devices may affect the emergency vehicle operator's hearing over time, thereby increasing the risk of vehicle collisions. Undergo regular hearing tests and take steps to protect your hearing.

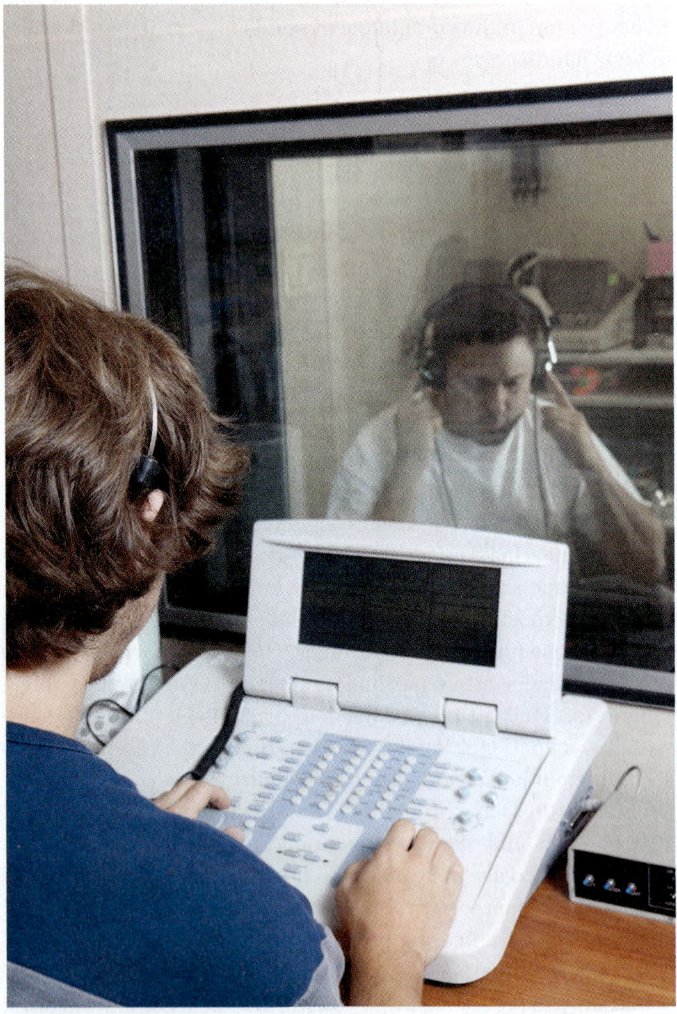

Figure 3-4 Annual hearing tests are essential to ensure your ability to perform your job safely.

Vision Testing

While it may seem obvious that a person should have good vision to safely operate an emergency vehicle, there are many people who drive every day with serious visual impairments. There are many conditions that affect a person's vision, including the following:

- Color blindness
- Night blindness
- Farsightedness (hyperopia)
- Nearsightedness (myopia)
- Eye irritation
- Age
- Medical conditions (e.g., colds or allergies)
- Incorrect eyeglass prescriptions
- Self-tinting eyeglass lenses
- Failure to get annual eye exams

It is important to recognize that vision changes. Annual eye exams are necessary to pick up on any changes in vision FIGURE 3-5. Some insurance policies cover the cost of annual eye exams, but they are necessary even if not covered by insurance. In addition, age plays a major role in your vision. It is quite common for a person to have a change in vision around 40 years of age. It is not adequate to rely solely on the eye exam given every several years to renew your driver's license as proof that your vision is acceptable. It is important to remember that if your

SAFETY POINTER

Some emergency vehicle operators wear contact lenses during the day and resort to glasses for calls during the night. This is fine, as long as they have the most up-to-date prescription.

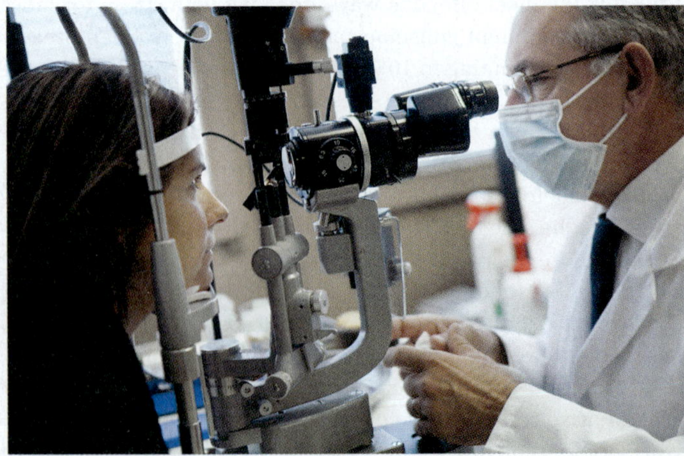

Figure 3-5 You should get your vision checked every year.

driver's license says you are to wear corrective lenses, then they are required while operating the ambulance.

Physical Ailments

You must be aware of your body and sensitive to any health problems, injuries, or illnesses. While many people do not think that muscle strains affect their ability to operate a vehicle, these simple physical injuries can have a major impact on your ability to function. A muscle strain can significantly reduce your ability to move your feet, legs, hands, and arms, thus increasing the time it takes you to make sudden motions. In many cases, you will not realize how much your reaction time has been affected, and when an incident occurs that requires your quick reaction, you may not be able to react to avoid a collision.

In addition to muscle injuries, a person can be injured in a manner such that they are required to wear a walking cast or a joint immobilizer. These devices are designed to help a person heal by reducing the function of the injured area. The subsequent reduction in function places the individual in an unfit, and therefore unsafe, state to operate an emergency vehicle. When a person is required to wear any type of immobilizing device, he or she should not operate an emergency vehicle.

Illnesses such as colds, flu, gastrointestinal distress, or headaches can also affect your ability to operate an emergency vehicle. While you may think you are not affected by a cold or a minor case of the flu, symptoms of these conditions such as runny nose, sneezing, or coughing will definitely affect your ability to drive a vehicle safely. Thinking about these illnesses or discomforts can cause a mental distraction for the operator. In addition, medications to control the associated symptoms will often make you drowsy. *If a medicine has a warning that says do not operate machinery, it would be inappropriate to take the medicine while working as the emergency vehicle operator.* Gastrointestinal distress can be serious as well, since having a sudden bout of vomiting or diarrhea while driving could easily lead to a collision by taking the driver's mind and eyes off the road. Even something as seemingly minor as a headache can be serious if it suddenly becomes worse while you are driving, especially if you are experiencing sensitivity to light.

During any illness, you may be distracted mentally and more likely to react negatively or aggressively toward other drivers. Whenever you are suffering from an illness, you must ensure that it is not severe enough to impact your ability to operate an emergency vehicle. Failure to recognize when your ability to drive the ambulance is impaired can greatly increase your risk.

Tired Driving

Sleep deprivation can be a common cause of driver error **FIGURE 3-6**. Since EMS providers often work long shifts, including through the night, they often do not get the 7 to 9 hours of sleep that most adults require. While the excitement of an emergency call may make us think we are alert, many symptoms of sleep deprivation can occur even in these situations. Symptoms of sleep deprivation include:

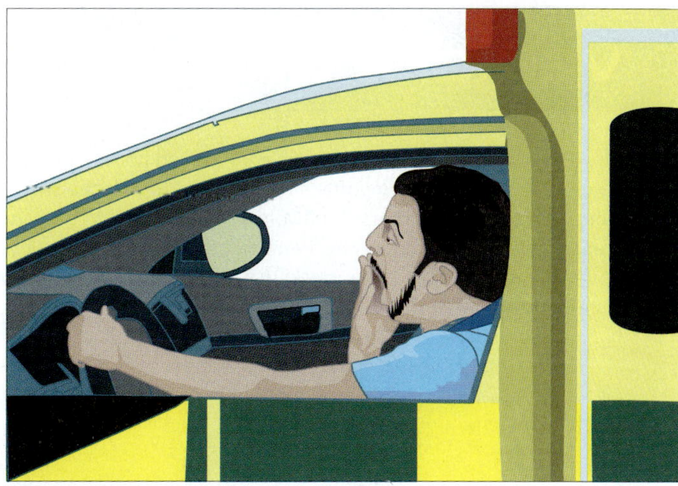

Figure 3-6 Safe driving practices involve never driving while drowsy.

- Confusion or difficulty focusing
- Yawning or rubbing of the eyes
- Weaving within one's lane of traffic or even crossing into another lane
- Impaired reaction time, judgment, and vision
- Decreased performance, vigilance, and motivation
- Increased moodiness and aggressive behaviors
- Problems with information processing and short-term memory

Long transfers of nonemergency patients can also lead to drowsiness for the emergency vehicle operator and even episodes of microsleeping.

Mircosleeping is basically a brief lapse of consciousness or awareness that occurs when someone momentarily enters a state of sleep. A person experiencing episodes of microsleep will experience head nodding, heavy eyelids, and periods of long blinks or seconds of the eyes being closed. Generally, microsleeping is thought to be the result of sleep deprivation, though microsleeping has been seen in non-sleep-deprived individuals during monotonous or boring tasks. There is little agreement on the best ways to identify and classify microsleep. In situations that demand constant alertness, such as driving a motor vehicle or working with heavy machinery, microsleeping can lead to critical mistakes—a problem that is worsened by the fact that people who experience microsleeping usually remain unaware of it.

Since the emergency vehicle operator is required to function with the safety of all in mind, it is essential to never drive when drowsy. Taking turns driving with your partner may be helpful, as may carrying on a conversation with your partner when you are both in the cab at the same time. If you feel you are operating the vehicle while drowsy, you should notify your

VEHICLE OPERATOR INCIDENT

All providers have their own circadian rhythms and hormones that physiologically regulate their sleep and wake cycles. EMS offers several styles of shifts, and it is important for providers to find the shift that best accommodates their lifestyle. For example, one provider was working the day shift from 7:00 AM to 7:00 PM but did not want to get up in the morning and had trouble getting to work and being prepared for calls without several cups of coffee. The same employee moved to nightshift, which was from 7:00 PM to 7:00 AM and woke up regularly without an alarm clock, was active prior to going to work, and arrived at work ready to take calls. Even when the activities were similar after work and this person stayed up until 11:00 AM on nights and 11:00 PM on days, the employee functioned better on nights than on days.

Emergency vehicle operators should attempt to find shifts that fit their personal rhythms and needs. In many cases, maintaining an ideal sleep schedule is not easy or possible, but doing so will help ensure that the emergency vehicle operator has the necessary energy to function properly.

partner and switch roles, if possible. If both you and your partner are extremely sleep deprived, you should consider notifying dispatch and asking about taking your unit out of service. It is much better to deal with the ramifications of this request than to be involved in a vehicle collision caused by drowsy driving. The bottom line is that you are responsible for having enough sleep before coming to work that you will be able to complete your shift without encountering problems relating to sleep. Studies show that being awake for 18 consecutive hours results in impairment equal to a blood alcohol concentration of 0.05%. Being awake for a full 24 hours produces impairment similar to a 0.096% blood alcohol concentration, which is legally drunk in all 50 states.

SAFETY POINTER

It is extremely important that EMS providers ensure the safety of themselves, partners, patients, passengers, and the public by being aware of the signs of sleep deprivation.

Medication or Substance Use

Occasionally, EMS providers will get sick, and it may be necessary to take medications that can affect their ability to perform their jobs. Before you take any over-the-counter medications, read the labels to ensure they will not compromise your ability to function, and never take any medication that warns of drowsiness and advises against operating machinery or motor vehicles. You should be aware of any potential synergistic effects with other medications or caffeine. Be sure to read and understand all warning labels and package inserts before taking any medication FIGURE 3-7. Be especially cautious with cold, allergy, pain, diet, or sleep medications.

SAFETY POINTER

Always read medication labels carefully and seek advice from your pharmacist prior to taking a new medication.

Sleep aids are available over the counter and come in many forms. Studies indicate that sleep aids can cause effects more severe than alcohol, hours after being taken. There are documented cases of what is known as "sleep driving" in which a person gets out of bed and drives without any memory of the event. EMS providers should never take any form of sleep aid while at work or prior to a shift. If you are prescribed a sleep aid, you should consult your physician to determine what the time frame is between using the medication and reporting for work.

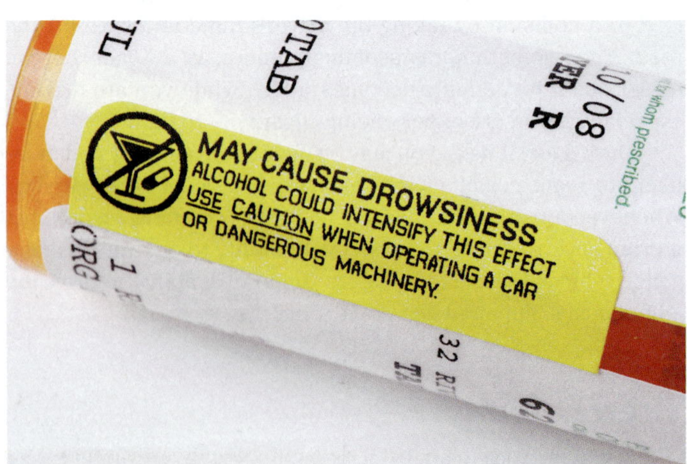

Figure 3-7 Read labels carefully and avoid medications that can cause drowsiness.

Although the use of alcohol prior to or during a shift seems ludicrous to many EMS providers, there are some EMS providers who use alcohol and then operate emergency vehicles and provide patient care. Although this may seem more likely to be a problem with volunteer services, it occurs in paid EMS services as well. This behavior is unprofessional and dangerous to everyone involved. The federal blood alcohol limit for commercial drivers is 0.04%, but emergency vehicle operators follow local and state-specific regulations and are not subject to the federal transportation rules of other commercial transportation workers. Even before this level, alcohol can slow reaction time, impair vision, cause drowsiness, increase confidence, and impair a person's ability to function.

It is also important that employees are aware of, and employers have, policies that prohibit alcohol consumption for at least 8 hours prior to shift. These policies will help emergency vehicle operators be cognizant that alcohol takes time to be fully eliminated from the body before the start of the shift. Remember, conditions such as a hangover can decrease concentration, reaction time, and the ability to safely operate an emergency vehicle.

The use of illegal street or other recreational drugs is unacceptable in all forms and at all times by EMS providers. Drugs can greatly reduce your ability to think, react, and function. In some instances, EMS providers involved in incidents that resulted in patient and provider fatalities and criminal prosecutions were found to have used recreational drugs before or during their shift. Any attitude that promotes rationalizing this type of activity is unhealthy and unprofessional. The only attitude to have regarding any type of recreational drug use is an attitude of zero tolerance. With states starting to make recreational marijuana use legal, it is important that employees and employers have clear policies addressing the use of this drug FIGURE 3-8.

It is your responsibility to be mentally, physically, and emotionally prepared every time you get behind the wheel of an emergency vehicle. You owe it to yourself, your partner, and the public.

Recreational and Medical Marijuana

Applicants for employment and volunteer opportunities should be aware of the City of Colorado Springs' current policies concerning the use of drugs or alcohol.

These policies have not been altered by Amendment 64 as it was not intended to require employers to permit marijuana use and it specifically states: "Nothing in this section is intended to require an employer to permit or accommodate the use, consumption, possession, transfer, display, transportation, sale or growing of marijuana in the workplace or to affect the ability of employers to have policies restricting the use of marijuana by employees." Colo. Const. art. XVIII, § 16(6)(a).

This language mirrors the Colorado Constitutional provision allowing medical marijuana which states: "Nothing in this section shall require any employer to accommodate the medical use of marijuana in any work place." Colo. Const. art. XVIII, § 14(10)(b).

Civilian Policy (Civilian PPM #39), Sworn Policy (Sworn PPM #35) and the Drug/Alcohol Procedures Manual outline the City's policies and remain in effect. Specifically, Drug/Alcohol

Procedures Manual, Section II, includes:

- An employee is prohibited from the unlawful manufacture, distribution, dispensing, possession or use of a Controlled Substance in the workplace or on City property.
- An employee who reports to work under the influence of or whose performance is Impaired through the use of alcohol or drugs is subject to corrective action in accordance with City policies and procedures, up to and including termination.
- Marijuana is a prohibited drug in Schedule I of the Controlled Substances Act and it remains a violation of City policy for any employee to use marijuana.

Marijuana, whether it is used medically or recreationally, remains a violation of the Federal Controlled Substances Act, 21 U.S.C. §§ 801 et seq.

Figure 3-8 An example of a marijuana-use policy, from the Colorado Springs, Colorado, Fire Department.

WRAP-UP

SUMMARY

- It is your responsibility to ensure you are mentally, emotionally, and physically prepared to complete all aspects of emergency vehicle operations.
- Mental preparedness includes a commitment to avoid distractions, pay attention to details, and put safety first.
- Distracted drivers pose a significant risk to other motorists.
- Emotional preparedness includes reducing stress and emotional distractions.
- The emergency vehicle operator must be physically capable of operating an emergency vehicle at all times.
- An individual's physical capabilities can be affected by a variety of issues, such as illness, injury, sleep deprivation, medication, or substance use.

GLOSSARY

microsleeping A brief break with consciousness in which a person loses awareness of his or her surroundings and momentarily enters a state of sleep.

road rage Aggressive or angry behavior by a driver of a motor vehicle that may include rude gestures, verbal insults or threats, or unsafe driving.

sleep deprivation The state of having an insufficient amount of sleep.

REFERENCES

McCallion, T. (2012). *Consider the dangers of shift work: It's important to have a fatigue management plan in place. Journal of Emergency Medical Services.* Retrieved from http://www.jems.com/article/emsinsider/consider-dangers-shift-work

U.S. Department of Transportation. (2009). *Driver distraction in commercial vehicle operations*. Retrieved from http://www.distraction.gov/downloads/pdfs/driver-distraction-commercial-vehicle-operations.pdf

CHAPTER 4

Emergency Vehicle Operation and the Law

OBJECTIVES

4.1 Define the types of laws that affect EMS vehicle operation.

4.2 Explain the legal terms related to EMS vehicle operation.

4.3 Describe the appropriate use of lights and sirens.

4.4 Discuss safety considerations for responding to an emergency scene.

4.5 Outline the types of preventable collisions most common to emergency vehicle operations.

4.6 Discuss the assessment of liability and how liability affects the emergency vehicle operator.

4.7 Explain steps the emergency vehicle operator can take to avoid legal entanglements.

4.8 Describe how to respond appropriately in the event of a collision.

SCENARIO

You and your partner are at the daily meeting in the center of town when a Priority 1 response is dispatched for your zone. As you drive past the airport, with your lights and siren on, you approach a red traffic light. There is no traffic to the left and a few vehicles to your right. Though they have a green light, they are stopped at the intersection. You slow down slightly and proceed through the intersection. Suddenly, almost out of nowhere, a BMW pulls directly in front of your ambulance from the right. You react quickly and hit the brakes, but your vehicle hits the driver's side door.

You are unharmed. You quickly check on your partner; he says he is okay but that his sternum is sore. Next, you get out to check on the driver of the other vehicle. She is conscious, alert, and oriented. Her left leg appears to be broken. She also appears to be trapped in the vehicle and will require extrication.

You notify dispatch to assign another ambulance to the original call and request that police, fire rescue, an ambulance, and a supervisor come to your crash scene. An additional ambulance arrives to take both you and your partner to the hospital, but you are both discharged after a few hours with only minor bruising. The front end of the ambulance has significant damage and will be out of service until it can be repaired. Local media picks up the story and your name appears in the newspaper. You are interviewed by the town's police traffic safety unit, which will be investigating the incident. According to your service's policy, all crashes are investigated by police traffic safety, and they ultimately issue a report if there was fault or a need for education or retraining. Witnesses report that the driver of the BMW was talking on her cell phone prior to the collision. The police department will not be issuing a report, but the town attorney's office is notified that the driver has brought a $7 million lawsuit against your service. You must hire an attorney because you are personally named in the suit. Eventually, all parties agree to a settlement after a long and difficult legal battle.

1. How often do you review and have trainings on local driving laws?
2. What are your standard operating procedures, protocols, and/or responsibilities when you witness or are involved in a collision?

Introduction

This chapter introduces the legal considerations for emergency vehicle operators. Service policy makers and their driver trainers should outline very clearly what your responsibilities are for operating the emergency vehicle. They should also provide high-quality training to you to prepare you for your job. Department leadership should also remain current with all laws and policies that pertain to driving emergency vehicles in your jurisdiction. However, it is ultimately your responsibility to properly perform your job and know the laws that govern your actions. If you are involved in a crash in which someone is seriously injured or killed and you broke traffic laws, violated department standard operating procedures (SOPs), or acted without due regard to others (a subject discussed later), you could face legal consequences, possibly even manslaughter or negligent homicide charges in the case of a fatality.

SAFETY POINTER

The vehicle operator should be familiar with the state traffic laws, specific municipality ordinances, and all department rules related to emergency vehicle operation.

Criminal and Civil Law

The U.S. judicial system is divided into two primary types of law, criminal and civil.

Criminal law involves determining whether a statute has been violated and, if so, assessing an appropriate punishment, whether that be a fine, jail or prison incarceration, or both. For a minor criminal offense, such as illegally parking your ambulance when not on an emergency call, a police officer could issue a citation requiring you to appear in front of a judge, who would most likely impose a fine. For a more serious criminal offense, such as striking and killing a pedestrian, the vehicle operator could be arrested and placed in jail and would need to arrange for legal representation in the ensuing criminal proceedings.

Motor vehicle laws involve the criminal justice system. If you violate a traffic law, such as exceeding the speed limit in your personal vehicle, you have committed a criminal offense. While emergency vehicles are given a certain amount of latitude with regard to following all motor vehicle laws, emergency vehicle operators may still be ticketed or fined if they disregard these laws and put the public at risk.

Civil law is much broader and more often invoked against a vehicle operator in cases of vehicle collisions (even when the incident does not lead to criminal charges). In a civil action, an injured person files a lawsuit naming the vehicle operator as the **defendant**. The **plaintiff** (person suing) asks for monetary compensation for his or her physical, emotional, and psychological injuries as well as other damages, such as loss of employability or other financial harm.

In criminal cases, the state (or prosecution) must prove to a jury that the accused is guilty of the crime beyond a **reasonable doubt**, meaning that a reasonable person would not doubt the accused party's guilt. In civil cases, however, the plaintiff must prove his or her case based on only a **preponderance of the evidence**, meaning there is slightly more evidence of guilt than of innocence. In a civil case, the jury may choose to award the plaintiff compensation from the defendant at the requested amount or at a higher or lower amount, based on the jury's determination of the defendant's level of guilt.

Legal Terms

The most common cause of legal trouble for a vehicle operator is a collision. In a vehicle collision there may be criminal charges brought against the operator, but much more likely there will be a civil suit naming the operator as a defendant. In civil suits involving collisions, the primary goal is to establish **liability**, which is the determination of who is primarily at fault for the collision. In civil cases involving emergency vehicles, the primary determination of liability is based on a term called **negligence**, which indicates that the vehicle operator did not perform his or her responsibilities correctly. To prove negligence in a vehicle collision, the plaintiff must prove that the defendant had a responsibility to act in a certain way and that he or she failed to do so, resulting in a collision that caused injury to the plaintiff.

Gross negligence is a more serious form of negligence, and implies reckless conduct and a blatant disregard for the safety and lives of others. Consider, for example, a vehicle operator driving under the influence of alcohol who collides with a vehicle that is stopped at an intersection and kills the vehicle's driver upon impact. To prove gross negligence, the plaintiff would need to prove that the defendant's conduct was deliberately reckless and without concern for other drivers' safety. The line between negligence and gross negligence can be unclear and may need to be determined by a court.

In the event of a collision involving an EMS vehicle, a court primarily bases its judgment on these two questions:

1. Did the emergency vehicle operator have reasonable grounds to believe he or she was responding to a *true emergency*?
2. Did the emergency vehicle operator exercise *due regard* for the safety of others?

A **true emergency** is a situation in which there is a high probability of death or serious injury to an individual or of significant property loss, and the actions of the responders can mitigate the situation. **Due regard** refers to taking appropriate considerations in a given situation. The determination of "appropriate" is based on what a reasonably careful person could be expected to do if he or she were performing similar duties under similar circumstances. Thus, "due regard for the safety of others" means taking precautions that a reasonably prudent person would take to safeguard the public in a similar situation.

VEHICLE OPERATOR INCIDENT

The following comparisons are loosely based on incidents that tragically occur somewhere almost every day. Note how differently the incident appears to the public when it involves an ambulance.

In a small suburban neighborhood, there was a tragic crash that involved a preschool-aged child on a big wheel, who rolled down his driveway and entered the street. A pine tree at the foot of the driveway was a potential obstruction to the view of the oncoming traffic. Two middle-aged couples were in a car traveling through this suburban neighborhood on their way to dinner. They were traveling at the posted speed limit. The child suddenly darted out in front of them, and they did not see the child before striking and fatally injuring him. While EMS was attempting to resuscitate the child, police took statements from witnesses, did a field sobriety test, and checked for skid marks as a part of their investigation. In the end, there was no ticket issued because it was determined that the vehicle could not have avoided hitting the child.

In another collision a few months later in a different small community, an ambulance was responding to a call on a residential street. They were exceeding the posted speed limit but not by more than the 10 mph that their company policy allows. A school-aged child rode his bicycle into the side of the ambulance. He was not wearing a helmet and he too was fatally injured. The EMS crew tried to revive the child, but they were unsuccessful. The police again interviewed witnesses, measured skid marks, and did a field sobriety test. In this case, although no evidence appeared to indicate that the EMS crew was at fault and no tickets were issued, the case was turned over to the grand jury for further investigation. The media attacked the EMS service and published the name and address of the emergency vehicle operator. In the end, the grand jury determined that the crash could not have been avoided and the emergency vehicle operator was not at fault, but the service's and operator's reputations were deeply damaged.

As you can see from these two similar cases, the due regard provision sets a higher standard for EMS providers. Always make every effort to take due regard for the safety of others while operating an EMS vehicle.

The law gives a tremendous amount of responsibility to emergency vehicle operators when a call is classified as a true emergency; however, operators must still show due regard for the safety of all others. To show due regard, the emergency vehicle operator must give sufficient notice of the vehicle's approach (e.g., lights and sirens) to allow other motorists and pedestrians to clear a path and protect themselves. If you do not give notice of your approach until a collision is unavoidable, you have not satisfied the principle of due regard for the safety of others.

SAFETY POINTER

The emergency vehicle operator is held to a higher standard than all other drivers on the road.

Use of Lights and Siren

Lights and sirens are used to alert motorists and pedestrians of the approach of an emergency vehicle. State laws mandate that the emergency vehicle operator use emergency warning devices such as lights and/or siren, when reasonably necessary, especially when taking advantage of any traffic law exemptions FIGURE 4-1. However, the use of signaling equipment does not guarantee that motorists and pedestrians are aware of the presence of the vehicle, nor do they protect the vehicle operator from civil or criminal liability if a collision occurs.

SAFETY POINTER

Legally your emergency warning devices require traffic to yield the right of way. However, you have no guarantee that you will receive it. Motorists or pedestrians who do not give you the right of way are breaking the law, but you are still required to give them due regard!

The use of emergency lights must comply with state and local laws, state and local EMS rules and regulations, and your company's policy. The lights do not provide as much protection or warning as you may think. Furthermore, in parking at the scene of an emergency, the use of the warning lights may actually make the scene unsafe and draw other motorists' vehicles toward your location. It is important to remember that low sun, glare, fog, and tinted windows in other vehicles can reduce the effectiveness of warning lights. At night, red warning lights may blend in with other red lights in traffic or the neon light along the side of the streets. Warning lights mounted on top of a vehicle may not be visible in the rearview mirror of vehicles in front of the emergency vehicle.

There are similar concerns with the effectiveness of the siren. In general, sirens can be heard only to a distance of 230 feet ahead of the vehicle. At speeds greater than 40 mph, you can completely outrun the effectiveness of your siren. Even

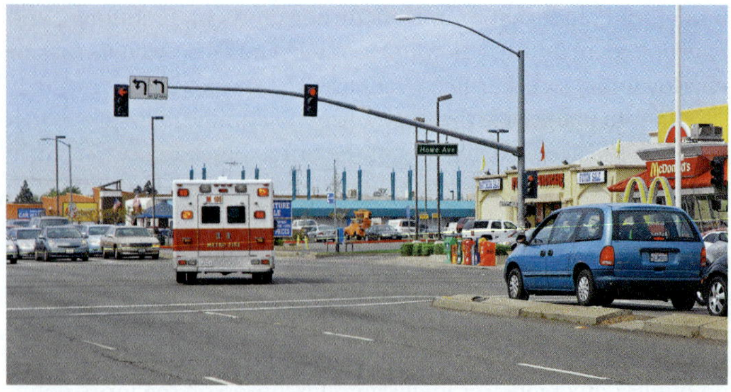

Figure 4-1 Emergency warning devices should be used when taking any exemptions to vehicle and traffic laws.

at close range, the siren may not be heard by a motorist who has the vehicle's windows closed and is using the air conditioning or radio. Newer cars even advertise how much outside noise the car blocks, and this includes emergency vehicle's sirens.

SAFETY POINTER

Do not overestimate the reach of your emergency warning devices.

Responding Safely

When responding to an incident, emergency vehicle operators should be made aware if they are being dispatched on a potential emergency. Dispatch should obtain information from the caller to determine how the vehicle operator should respond (i.e., emergency or non-emergency) by using an emergency medical dispatch system. EMS system directors may be liable if they do not have a policy regarding what information responders should receive when they are dispatched.

Nonemergency responses include incidents involving chronic illness (without life-threatening complications), minor injuries, and stable patients. True emergencies include cardiac or respiratory complications, major trauma, or other complaints based on your system's 9-1-1 dispatch categories. In EMS systems, the emergency vehicle operator should initiate a high-priority response to a presumed, true emergency that includes the use of emergency warning devices. The response mode may change or downgrade if a first responder reports that the call does not involve a life-threatening situation.

The decision about routine or emergency transport should be made by asking the following questions:

- Will the time saved make a significant difference in the patient's outcome?
- Will emergency transport create an unnecessarily unsafe situation for the public, myself and my partner(s), and the patient?
- What effect will the emergency warning devices have on the surrounding public, patient, driver, and crew?

It is important to note that in situations in which it is necessary to respond to the station or emergency scene in your own private vehicle, you must adhere to all applicable motor vehicle laws. Privately owned nonemergency vehicles are not granted any exemptions or special privileges by most states and must obey all state vehicle and traffic laws, even when states allow the use of emergency warning devices. State rules and department policies vary greatly in what they consider an authorized emergency vehicle. Regardless, if you are responding in a nonemergency vehicle, you should be careful not to let the excitement affect your driving and should make a special effort to drive in a safe manner. As with emergency vehicles, you should pay close attention to speed limits, road and weather conditions, intersections, and maneuvering your vehicle around the emergency scene.

If your private vehicle has an emergency identification light, you must comply with the applicable emergency motor vehicle rules and regulations that cover size, type, color, and candle power of the light. You must also recognize that you are representing your emergency response organization and drawing attention to yourself when you respond with a light on your private vehicle. You might consider shutting off the light when you are stopped at traffic lights or stop signs to avoid distracting motorists and pedestrians FIGURE 4-2 . Always follow the SOPs of your organization and any state laws concerning the use of colored lights on personal vehicles.

SAFETY POINTER

You can be held both criminally and civilly liable if a collision occurs while you are on duty as an emergency responder. The agency for which you work can also be brought into a lawsuit if the case can be made that you were improperly or inadequately instructed or that no effort was made to control unsafe or reckless vehicle operation.

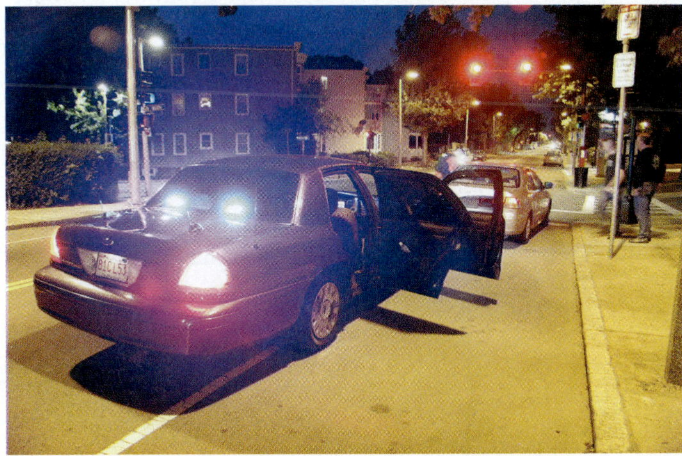

Figure 4-2 Private vehicles may be issued emergency warning devices for emergency response.

Types of Collisions

One of the most common causes of legal issues for an emergency vehicle operator is a collision involving the emergency vehicle he or she is driving. There are many types of collisions common to emergency vehicle operations. The ones most likely to involve legal trouble for the operator are preventable collisions.

A **preventable collision** is one in which the driver failed to do everything reasonable to prevent its occurrence. Note that the word *reasonable*, rather than *possible*, is used in this definition. There is always something possible that could have been done to prevent a collision (such as not responding to the call or taking another street). Reasonable preventive measures include knowing, understanding, and obeying traffic laws; adjusting speed to existing conditions; scanning ahead to anticipate stops; and anticipating the reactions of other drivers and pedestrians to your emergency vehicle.

There are many different types of preventable collisions:

- Parking collisions may result from double-parking, failure to warn traffic of your parked position, and parking in an unconventional location, to name a few examples.
- Intersection collisions are those that happen at stop lights, stop signs, or other intersections, where different directions of traffic must cross paths.
- Backing collisions occur while the vehicle is in reverse gear.
- In rear-end collisions, the emergency vehicle impacts a vehicle in front of it; these incidents are commonly caused by not maintaining a safe following distance, not looking ahead to anticipate the need to stop, or not controlling vehicle speed.
- Pedestrian collisions are always considered preventable, even though children and adults may perform sudden, unexpected maneuvers.
- Mechanical failure collisions are often the result of lack of attention during the vehicle inspection, reckless or abusive vehicle handling, or operating the vehicle beyond its mechanical limits (e.g., over the gross vehicle weight rating).
- Adverse weather collisions may be caused by failure to drive according to the existing conditions, failure to postpone nonemergency calls, failure to use snow chains, or driving in adverse weather conditions.
- Traffic lane encroachment collisions may be the result of using improper passing techniques, weaving through or merging with traffic at unsafe times, or changing lanes in an unsafe manner.
- Collisions with fixed objects such as low overheads, buildings, poles, parked cars, and trees or collisions resulting from running off the roadway or overturning the vehicle may be caused by unsafe evasive action on the part of the emergency vehicle operator FIGURE 4-3 .

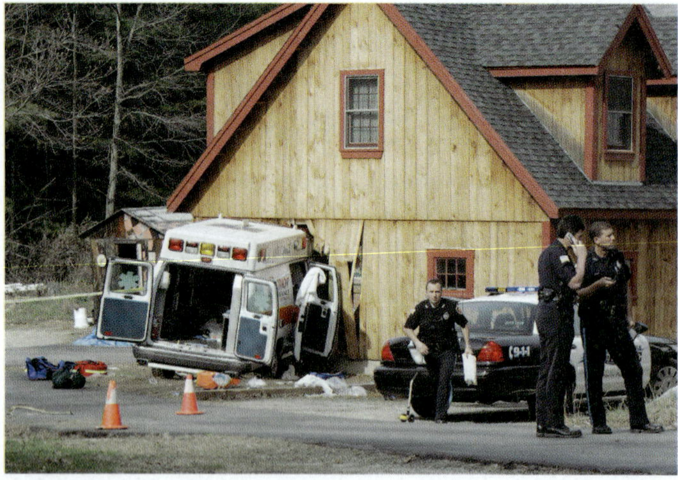

Figure 4-3 Collisions into stationary objects are considered preventable collisions.
© Jon Hill/The Lowell Sun/AP Photo.

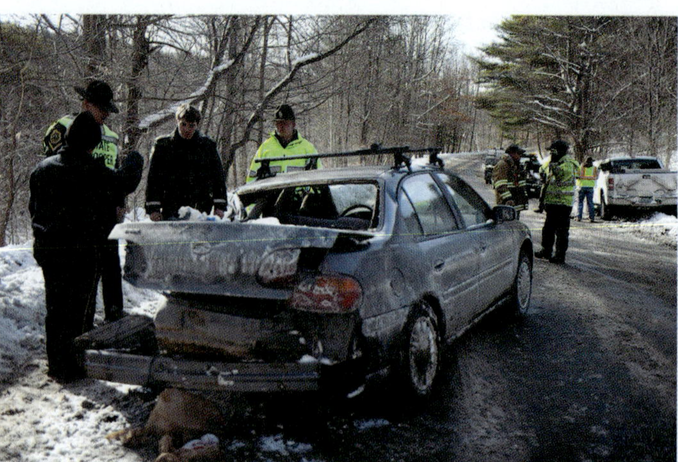

Figure 4-4 Always cooperate with a crash scene investigation.
© Valley News, photographer: Jennifer Hauck.

Criminal and Civil Law

Liability in Cases of Collisions

As mentioned earlier, liability is the determination of who is primarily at fault in the event of a collision. In addition to evaluating whether the emergency vehicle was responding to a true emergency with due regard for the safety of others, the judge or jury may ask the following questions:

- Are there any state, national, or department standards for emergency vehicle operation that may apply? If so, did the specific emergency operator comply with them?
- Do any state statutes regarding emergency vehicle exemptions apply?
- Was the emergency vehicle operator properly trained and supervised per accepted standards, and did the operator follow the SOPs of the agency?
- Was the vehicle properly equipped, was the equipment being properly operated, and are there records of relevant repairs and preventive maintenance?
- Were the manufacturer's ratings exceeded?
- Did the emergency vehicle have seatbelts, and if so, were they properly utilized?

A finding of liability in a vehicle collision involving an ambulance will likely result in monetary damages being assessed to the vehicle operator, as well as the EMS service he or she represents. It is in everyone's best interest for the emergency vehicle operator to avoid any action that might result in a collision for which he or she might be liable.

SAFETY POINTER

The greatest likelihood of a legal entanglement in the EMS profession is associated with collisions that occur while responding to calls for service and during transport.

Avoiding Legal Entanglements

Ultimately, it is your responsibility to know and obey the laws of your state and the SOPs of your organization as they relate to driving an emergency vehicle. State laws may vary regarding the maximum speed at which emergency vehicles can drive during an emergency operation and which traffic law exemptions emergency vehicles have, but in all states, emergency vehicle operators must drive with due regard for the safety of others. The best way to stay out of legal entanglements is to be attentive and practice safe driving.

If you do become involved in a collision, stay calm, follow your agency's SOP, and notify the police. Care for any injured persons immediately and always remain courteous and polite. You should not make any statements to the media but should cooperate with any investigations or police documentation FIGURE 4-4.

WRAP-UP

SUMMARY

- Criminal law involves determining whether a statute has been violated and, if so, assessing an appropriate punishment, whether that be a fine, jail or prison incarceration, or both.
- Civil law is much broader and more often invoked against a vehicle operator in cases of vehicle collisions (even when the incident does not lead to criminal charges).
- In criminal cases, the state (or prosecution) must prove to a jury that the accused is guilty of the crime beyond a reasonable doubt, meaning that a reasonable person would not doubt the accused party's guilt.
- In civil cases, the plaintiff must prove his or her case based on only a preponderance of the evidence, meaning there is slightly more evidence of guilt than of innocence.
- A true emergency is a situation in which there is a high probability of death or serious injury to an individual or of significant property loss, and the actions of the responders can mitigate the situation.
- Due regard is taking appropriate considerations in a given situation. The determination of "appropriate" is based on what a reasonably careful person could be expected to do if he or she were performing similar duties under similar circumstances.
- Lights and sirens are used to alert motorists and pedestrians of the approach of an emergency vehicle. State laws mandate that the emergency vehicle operator use emergency warning devices such as lights and/or siren, when reasonably necessary, especially when taking advantage of any traffic law exemptions.
- A preventable collision is one in which the driver failed to do everything reasonable to prevent its occurrence. Note that the word *reasonable*, rather than *possible*, is used in this definition.
- The best way to stay out of legal entanglements is to be attentive and practice safe driving.

GLOSSARY

civil law The type of law that pertains to determining responsibility for a wrongful act and imposing monetary penalties (with or without criminal charges) if the defendant is found guilty.

criminal law The type of law that pertains to determining whether a statute has been violated and, if so, imposing a punishment (fine and/or imprisonment) on the guilty party.

defendant The person or party in a lawsuit who is charged with breaking the law and harming the plaintiff.

due regard Appropriate consideration and responsibility shown for the safety of others.

gross negligence A more serious form of negligence that implies reckless conduct and a blatant disregard for the safety and lives of others. The line between negligence and gross negligence may need to be determined by a court.

liability Legal accountability or obligation.

negligence Failure to exercise due caution.

plaintiff The person or party who files a complaint in a lawsuit claiming to have been harmed by the defendant.

preponderance of the evidence A requirement in determining the guilt of a defendant that the majority of evidence presented in a case favor the plaintiff's argument.

preventable collision A collision in which the driver failed to do everything reasonable to prevent its occurrence.

reasonable doubt The lack of certainty that a person may justifiably feel based on the evidence at hand regarding the alleged guilt of a defendant.

true emergency A situation in which there is a high probability of death or serious injury to an individual or of significant property loss.

REFERENCES

Auerbach, P. S., Morris, J. A., Phillips, J. B., Jr., et al. (1998). An analysis of ambulance accidents in Tennessee. *Journal of the American Medical Association, 258*, 1487–1490.

Clawson, J. J. (1991). Running "hot" and the case of Sharon Rose. *Journal of Emergency Medical Services, 16*(7), 11–13.

Colwell, J. J., Pons, P., Blanchet, J. H., et al. (1999). Claims against a paramedic ambulance service: A ten-year experience. *Journal of Emergency Medicine, 17*, 999–1002.

DeLorenzo, P. A., & Eilers, M. A. (1995). Lights and siren: A review of emergency vehicle warning systems. *Annals of Emergency Medicine, 20*(12), 1331–1335.

Elling, R. (1989). Dispelling myths on ambulance accidents. *Journal of Emergency Medical Services, 14*(7), 60–64.

Emergency Medical Response Task Force, for the National Association of EMS Physicians and the National Association of State EMS Directors. (1994). Use of warning lights and siren in emergency medical vehicle response and patient transport. *Prehospital Disaster Medicine, 9*, 133–136.

Garza, M. (1998). Ohio paramedic jailed in deaths from ambulance crash. *Journal of Emergency Medical Services, 21*(12), 21.

George, J. E., & Quattrone, M. S. (1991). Above all do no harm. *Emergency Medical Technician Legal Bulletin, 15*(4).

Hunt, R. C., Brown, L. H., Cabinum, E. S., et al. (1995). Is ambulance transport time with lights and sirens faster than without? *Annals of Emergency Medicine, 25*(4), 507–511.

NAEMSP. (1994). Use of warning lights and siren in emergency medical vehicle response and patient transport (Position Paper). *Prehospital and Disaster Medicine, 9*(2).

Pirrallo, R. G. (1994). Characteristics of fatal ambulance crashes during emergency and non-emergency operations. *EVS Monitor, 3*(4).

Slattery, D. E., & Silver, A. (2009). The hazards of providing care in emergency vehicles: An opportunity for reform. *Prehospital Emergency Care, 13*, 388–397.

CHAPTER 5

Vehicle Inspection and Maintenance

OBJECTIVES

5.1 Explain the importance of vehicle inspection and preventive maintenance. (**NFPA 1002, 4.2.1**)

5.2 Demonstrate how to perform a complete vehicle inspection of the exterior and interior. (**NFPA 1002, 4.2.1, 4.2.2**)

5.3 Explain the function, inspection, and maintenance procedures for the various mechanical components and systems of your emergency vehicle.

5.4 Explain how to respond appropriately to vehicle problems.

5.5 Discuss the value of road testing for vehicle performance. (**NFPA 1002, 4.3.1**)

5.6 Describe relevant standards and certification programs for vehicle inspection and maintenance.

SCENARIO

Kelsey moved the ambulance out of the bay for the morning checkout and noticed a pool of fluid on the bay floor. She noted the presence of fluid on her checkout sheet and reported the problem to her supervisor. The supervisor asked what color the fluid was, but Kelsey did not know. She returned to the bay area to look, but someone had already mopped the bay and cleaned up the fluid.

The supervisor explained that color is an important clue to determine what type of fluid is leaking. For example, motor oil is typically golden to black in color, antifreeze is typically green and watery, and transmission fluid is red with an oil-like consistency. By noting the color of the fluid, Kelsey would have been able to make an educated guess about potential vehicle problems.

1. Do you have a clear list of reasons for when and how an ambulance can be marked out for mechanical problems?
2. What are your standard operating procedures (SOPs) and training for checking the mechanical elements of the ambulance?
3. As an operator, what liability do you hold for the mechanical function of the ambulance?

Introduction

As the emergency vehicle operator, you are responsible for the proper mechanical operation of your vehicle. This does not mean that you need to be a mechanic, but you should have at least enough understanding of how the vehicle operates to identify potential problems before they occur. It is also important to understand your role and responsibility based on your department's policy. Each department will have different standards for which the emergency vehicle operator will be responsible.

Vehicle Inspection

Most emergency services require daily inspections of vehicles and equipment. Daily checks can help manage any known or developing problems with the vehicle by identifying trends as well as finding anything unexpected. Most services have a mandatory checklist that is completed on a routine basis FIGURE 5-1. Never complete a vehicle inspection checklist without verifying each element on it. You should complete a thorough inspection of the entire vehicle prior to each shift to ensure there is no damage to the vehicle or any safety hazards that could affect the vehicle's performance. This inspection includes the vehicle's exterior, interior compartments, and the functional systems and mechanical components. As the operator of an emergency vehicle, it is your responsibility to be aware of the function, conduct an inspection, and perform maintenance of the various components of the vehicle for which you are responsible.

SAFETY TIP

Vehicle inspection checklists are legal documents that can be subpoenaed, so take your documentation seriously.

SAFETY TIP

During the vehicle inspection, emergency personnel should review the location and confirm the presence of all emergency equipment.

Exterior Inspection

All services want to present a professional appearance, and many people base opinions about a service simply on the appearance of the vehicle. Therefore, during the inspection, you should check that the vehicle body is clean and free of damage, noting any new damage that may not have been reported. Next, examine the tires to ensure they are in good condition and have adequate tread, with no bulges along the sidewall. Any uneven wear should be noted, and the spare tire (if present) should also be examined. The air pressure in the tires should be checked to make sure they are properly inflated. Remember that the proper inflation is determined by the vehicle manufacturer and not the tire manufacturer. Variations in tire inflation, such as a reduction of 3–4 psi (10%) can alter handling and fuel economy.

All external lights should be checked for proper operation, including emergency lights in responding and traffic-blocking modes. Check for signs of internal moisture and for rusted reflectors inside the lights, and also make sure the lights are securely fastened. To safely check emergency lights in the responding mode, it is necessary for the engine to be running with the transmission in park and the parking brake depressed. This will activate the high idle, which supports the power drain of the emergency lights. Next, put the transmission into drive with the parking brake engaged, and while one person has a foot on the brake, have another person walk around the vehicle to check for proper operation of each light, including turn signals.

Daily Ambulance Inspection Checklist

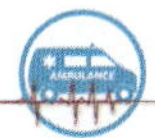

AMBULANCE OPERATION

Ambulance Equipment

- Plugged in (electrical)............................ ___
- Radio (operational)................................ ___
- Telephone (operational).......................... ___
- Emergency lights (operational).............. ___
- Fuel (above ½ tank)............................... ___
- Key (starts unit)...................................... ___
- Tires (proper inflation, tread depth)........ ___
- Inspection sticker (up to date)................ ___
- Insurance card.. ___
- IV warmer working (seasonal)................ ___
- Windows clean.. ___
- Unit clean (outside)................................ ___

Driver's Compartment

- 1–Hand light (6–12V)................................ ___
- 1–Spotlight (working)............................... ___
- 2–Protective gear (bunker coat, pants)...... ___
- 1–Emergency Response Guidebook......... ___
- Driver's log book (mileage recorded)...... ___
- Map/information book............................. ___
- Garage door opener................................ ___
- Hospital map book.................................. ___
- Keys/gas card... ___
- Clean/trash removed............................... ___
- Trip sheets box (with extra trip sheets)... ___
- Completed patient paperwork/turned in.. ___
- Accountability ring.................................. ___

DRIVER-SIDE COMPARTMENTS

DA Compartment (Oxygen)

- 1–Oxygen cylinder M (500 psi)................. ___
- 1–Regulator (2,500–2,550 psi)................. ___
- 2–Padded board splints (54")................... ___
- 2–Padded board splints (36")................... ___
- 2–Padded board splints (15")................... ___
- Reeves stretcher..................................... ___
- Scoop stretcher....................................... ___
- 1–Fire extinguisher (2A:10BC, charged).... ___
- 1–Folding litter.. ___

DB Compartment (Tool)

- Bag buster... ___
- 2–Bunker helmets (hard hats).................. ___
- 2–Clear eye protection............................ ___
- 4–Disposable blankets (yellow)................ ___

Access Equipment Toolbox ...... # ☐

DC Compartment (Drawer)

- 2–Leather work gloves............................. ___
- 3–Flares (30 min.).................................... ___
- Tow strap... ___
- Battery jumper cables .... ___
- Wheel simulator wrench......................... ___
- 2–Goggles.. ___

DD Compartment (VacuSplint)

- 1–SCBA/face mask (pressurized)............. ___
- 1–Vacu-splint mattress, with pump (child). ___
- 1–Vacu-splint mattress, with pump (child). ___
- Vacu-splint kit (L, M, & S and pump)...... ___
- Air-splint kit (6 pieces)........................... ___
- 1–Hand light (6–12V)................................ ___

Primary Trauma Bag................. # ☐

PASSENGER-SIDE COMPARTMENTS

PD Compartment (Backboard)

- 2–Long backboards (straps)..................... ___
- 1–KED (adult)... ___
- 1–Pediatric immobilization board............. ___
- 1–Stair chair... ___

PC Compartment (C-Collar)

- 2–CID blocks (with straps)....................... ___

Cervical Collar Bag

- 1–C-spine collar (infant)........................... ___
- 2–C-spine collars (pediatric)..................... ___
- 2–C-spine collars (no-neck)...................... ___
- 2–C-spine collars (short).......................... ___
- 1–C-spine collar (regular)......................... ___
- 1–C-spine collar (tall)................................ ___

– OR –

- 3–C-spine collars (adjustable).................. ___

PB Compartment (Side Door)

- 2–Oxygen cylinder D (> 500 psi).............. ___
- 1–Oxygen cylinder D (on cot).................... ___
- 2–Flowmeter (1–25 lpm) with guard.......... ___
- 1–Wrench (as required)............................ ___
- 1–Folding litter/cot................................... ___
- Unit clean/tidy (inside)........................... ___

PA Compartment (Drug Box)

- 1–Portable suction unit (& water)............. ___
- 1–Suction tubing....................................... ___
- 1–Rigid suction catheter........................... ___
- 1–French suction catheter......................... ___
- MAST with pump (adult)........................ ___
- MAST with pump (child)......................... ___

Pediatric Kit.............................. # ☐

Auto Vent Kit............................ # ☐

Drug Box (locked)..................... # ☐

Jonesville VFC Ambulance • 111 Main Street • P.O. Box 978 • Jonesville, MA 01803 • (888) 555-1234

Figure 5-1 The emergency vehicle operator needs to document that the vehicle and all its systems are in proper operating condition. Here is a sample page from a form used for this purpose.

Once the walk-around is complete, turn off all emergency lights, put the vehicle in park, and turn the engine off. Check that all doors open, close, and lock properly, including door locks on the patient compartment. Examine the windows; they should be clean and free of cracks and should open properly if designed to do so. The external antennas should be intact and secure. The exhaust system should be intact and directed toward the side or rear of the vehicle, as appropriate. The windshield should be clean and free of cracks and debris. The windshield wipers should include pliable wiping material that cleans the windshield without leaving any streaks. To check the windshield washer level, look at the reservoir inside the engine compartment. If the level appears low, add washer fluid to fill the reservoir according to company policy.

SAFETY TIP

Antennas frequently strike overhead objects, so pay particular attention to their condition during the vehicle inspection.

Finally, as part of the exterior inspection, it is useful to check that all auxiliary equipment stored on the exterior of the vehicle is present and fully functional. Some outside compartment doors may not fully protect equipment from the elements, so steps must be taken to ensure cleanliness and regular maintenance of this equipment.

Interior Compartments

The operator compartment (or cab) should be clean and neat. Electrical loads should be switched off, and all radios, audible warning devices (e.g., public address systems and sirens), and other necessary equipment should be present, functional, and accessible. For example, you should check that fire extinguishers are placed appropriately in both the driver and patient compartments and that their expiration date and gauge levels are appropriate, that the nozzles or hoses are intact and free of obstructions, that there is no rust or physical damage, and that the pins are intact and secure. It is essential for all equipment to be properly secured before the vehicle is in motion, as any unsecured equipment is likely to become a projectile and injure the patient or providers.

SAFETY TIP

Equipment for basic maintenance, such as a tool set and jumper cables, should be kept on the vehicle. A basic set of tools may be used for basic repairs to the vehicle and may allow you to help someone else in need. Know your state guidelines regarding which hand tools are required to be on the unit.

Next, check that the seatbelt and restraints operate correctly without binding. All belt webbing should be intact with no cuts, and buckles should easily release when activated and close securely. Many emergency vehicles are equipped with air ride seats, which are adjustable for height, position, and angle. These seats should be adjusted for optimal comfort and vehicle control.

All mirrors should be properly adjusted for the maximum field of vision so that the vehicle operator can see down the length of the vehicle. Convex mirrors should be adjusted so the inside of the mirrors has the edge of the emergency vehicle as a reference. If the mirrors have a heat control, the operator should be familiar with this function. Examine the lights in the interior to ensure they are functional, and check for signs of internal moisture.

SAFETY TIP

When mounting equipment, such as the mobile data computer inside the front compartment, be sure it will not block the operator's vision yet is within sight as needed.

The vehicle operator should also examine all gauges and meters to ensure they are fully functional and within an acceptable range for safe vehicle operation. The gauges and meters that should be checked are described as follows:

- The *fuel gauge* shows the amount of fuel in the tank. The vehicle should have an adequate level of fuel to respond to a call. If the vehicle has dual tanks, note which tank the gauge is reading and switch to the other tank to check the level in it as well. Experience with a particular vehicle will provide the operator with functional knowledge of its fuel range.
- The *oil pressure gauge* indicates the delivery pressure of lubricating oil to the engine.
- The *air pressure gauge* shows the amount of air in the air brake system. Typically, these systems have multiple tanks with safety valves installed to prevent catastrophic loss of air. Many systems will have two different-colored indicator needles for front and rear pressure systems installed in a single gauge or multiple gauges.
- The *coolant temperature gauge* indicates the temperature of the engine coolant.
- The *speedometer* indicates the speed of the vehicle when moving.
- The *odometer* records miles traveled.
- The *hour meter* registers the number of hours the engine has been running.
- The *tachometer* registers the speed of the engine in rpm.
- The *voltmeter* (or ammeter) indicates battery voltage and shows if the alternator is charging the system.

Any warnings that are indicated should be reported as required by your company policy.

Mechanical Components and Systems

Your ambulance is a machine that is designed to perform specific functions. As with any other machine, it can be more efficiently operated and maintained if you understand its various mechanical components and systems. Ambulances have many of the same mechanical components as your personal vehicle plus some extras.

Engine

The power for operating the vehicle is provided by the **engine**, which in most cases runs on either gasoline or diesel. The engine creates power by combusting fuel in cylinders that are within the block (inner core) of the engine. This combustion process pushes pistons in each cylinder that are attached to a rotating crankshaft. The pressure of the combustion on the top of the piston pushes it down and the combination of all of the pistons moving in synchronization causes the crankshaft to rotate. Most ambulances have a tachometer gauge that tells the operator how many revolutions per minute (rpm) the crankshaft is turning—usually between about 500 and 3,000, depending on the vehicle.

The engine must have lubrication between the pistons and the cylinder walls to allow the pistons to move smoothly inside the cylinder. The engine oil, which is held in a pan at the bottom of the engine and is pumped through the engine as it is running, provides this lubrication. If the amount of engine oil gets too low, friction will build up between the pistons and the cylinder walls and may cause a piston to lock up inside the cylinder, ruining the engine.

The exhaust gases from the internal combustion are removed from each cylinder by the revolution of the crankshaft pushing the piston back up and the gases above the piston out through the open exhaust valve. These gases are routed through pipes located on the sides of the engine to the exhaust system underneath the vehicle. The exhaust system also includes catalytic converters that reduce the pollutants in the exhaust gases and mufflers that reduce the noise caused by the escaping gases. The exhaust system gets very hot during operation and remains hot for quite a while after the engine is turned off. The engine exhaust gases contain carbon monoxide, which is a very deadly odorless gas when inhaled, so the vehicle should never be left running inside an enclosed area without adequate ventilation.

The internal combustion of the engine produces a significant amount of heat, which can also damage the engine. To avoid overheating, the engine has a cooling system that uses engine coolant to circulate around the outsides of the cylinders (within the engine block) absorbing the heat of the engine. This coolant is pumped through the engine and then through hoses to the radiator located in front of the engine. As the coolant flows through tubes inside the radiator, the air passing across the radiator around these tubes removes the heat it has absorbed from the engine. Once the heat has been removed, the coolant is again circulated through the engine to repeat the process. The coolant, which in most cases is a combination of water and other chemicals such as ethylene glycol, is very efficient at removing heat without freezing inside the engine if the outside temperature gets too cold and the engine is not running. The coolant often reaches temperatures in excess of 200°F during operation and creates pressures of around 15 to 20 pounds per square inch (psi) inside the cooling system. Most ambulances will have a gauge that indicates the temperature of the coolant. If the coolant temperature gets too high, the vehicle should be stopped and the engine turned off to prevent permanent engine damage due to overheating.

On the front of the engine, there are often several devices mounted that have pulleys on them. One or more rubber belts to the crankshaft of the engine attach these pulleys. This arrangement allows the rotation of the engine to drive these devices, such as an alternator for producing electricity for the vehicle, a power steering pump that provides hydraulic assistance for the steering of the vehicle, and an air-conditioning compressor that allows cool air to circulate through the unit in hot weather. In addition, on some units there may be an air compressor that provides compressed air if the vehicle is equipped with an air brake system. As you can imagine, if these belts break, the devices they operate will stop functioning, putting the unit out of service.

The engine compartment should be clean FIGURE 5-2. A clean compartment allows for the detection of new leaks or problems and helps the engine stay cool. Any belts should be intact and snug, with no cracks, cuts, or damage. Hoses should be properly attached and show no signs of leakage.

In the engine compartment, you should check the levels of oil and coolant.

To check the oil level, first ensure that the engine has been turned off for at least 5 minutes so that the oil reading will be accurate (oil distributes throughout the engine when it is running and then drains back into the oil pan). Next, locate the dipstick and remove it, wipe it off, and reinsert it. Completely reseat the dipstick and then remove it again and read the oil level in relation to the markings on the stick FIGURE 5-3. The engine dipstick typically has marking indicating whether the oil level is sufficient or additional oil needs to be added. Depending on the engine, anywhere from 1 quart to 1 gallon may be required to bring the level from low to full. When adding oil, ensure that it is the proper type and viscosity required for the engine of your specific vehicle per the owner's manual. This information is also found on the oil fill cap of most new engines. If oil is leaking, you may notice pools of fluid under the engine in the color of the oil, which is typically golden or black. Conduct these checks and refill oil only if it is within your company's policy.

SAFETY TIP

Be knowledgeable about the engine of your vehicle and follow the manufacturer's recommendations for inspection and maintenance. This information can be found in the vehicle owner's manual.

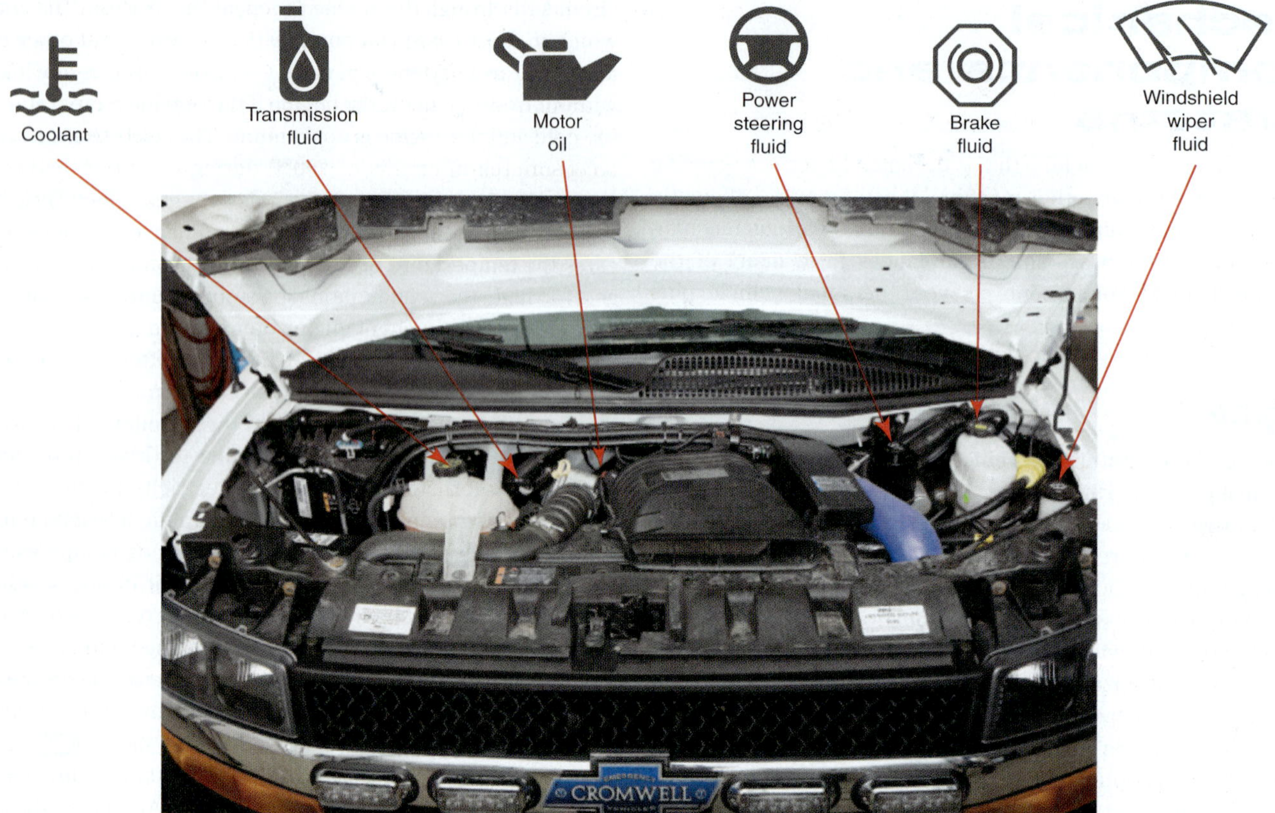

Figure 5-2 The symbols for coolant, transmission fluid, motor oil, power steering fluid, brake fluid, and windshield wiper fluid, and their respective locations in a typical ambulance engine compartment.

Photo: © Jones & Bartlett Learning. Brake Fluid Icon: © A Aleksii/Shutterstock. Motor Oil Icon: © Liudmyla Marykon/Shutterstock. Transmission, Power Steering, Windshield Wiper Fluid Icons: © Alexandr III/Shutterstock.

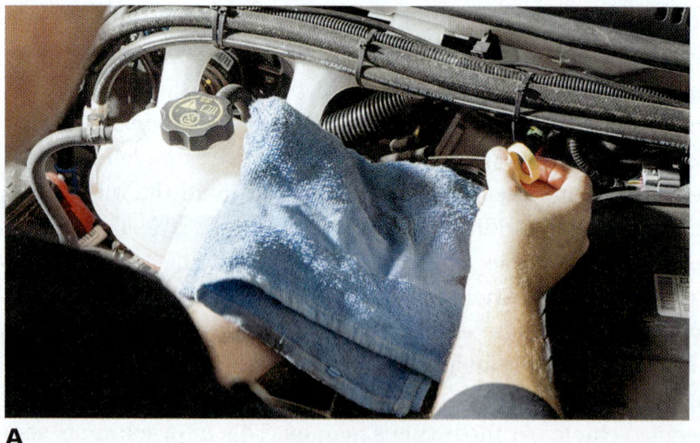
A

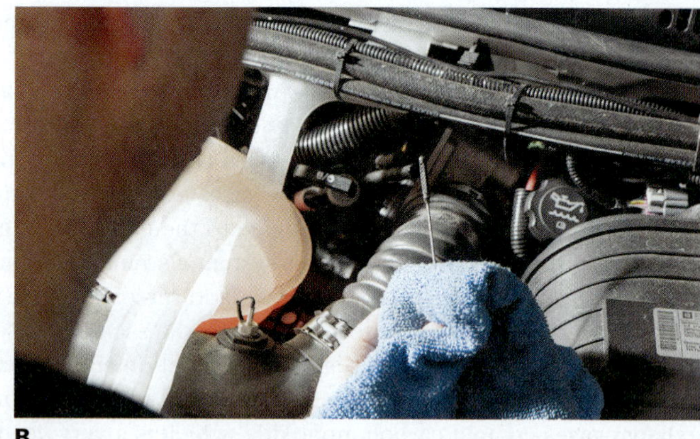
B

Figure 5-3 When performing an oil check, you must first wipe off and fully reseat the dipstick. You then **A.** remove it a second time and **B.** check the oil level.

© Jones & Bartlett Learning.

To check the coolant, ensure that the engine has been turned off for at least 5 minutes for safety. Removing the radiator cap when the engine is hot can easily release coolant as steam and cause a boilover of the coolant and possible injury. Most newer vehicles have see-through coolant reservoirs with hot and cold markings, making it easy to visualize coolant levels and unnecessary to remove the radiator cap.

Electrical System

The **electrical system** provides all electrical energy for vehicle operation and takes on heavy demands in the modern emergency vehicle. Although efforts have been made through the federal specifications to limit the electrical demands of emergency vehicles, they are still heavy. There are several key components of the electrical system:

- **Alternators** produce current for the electrical system and are powered by an engine-driven belt.
- **Batteries** store electrical energy to help start the vehicle and provide a backup power source should the alternator fail; they typically provide only a few minutes of power under these circumstances.
- **Inverters** convert direct current (DC) power from the vehicle's electrical system to alternating current (AC) power—the same as household current—to enable the operation of hospital-type equipment, such as suction units, during transport or the ability to use an AC-powered accessory charger for charging cell phones in the ambulance.

Emergency vehicles typically have a high electrical demand and can occasionally suffer from electrical problems. Jumper cables may be useful to "jump-start" a vehicle when the battery has died. Care should be taken to clearly understand the procedure for jump-starting a vehicle, and eye protection should be worn when performing this task. Since jump-starting a vehicle can result in electrical spikes to the system, all electronic devices on the emergency vehicle should be turned off when performing the procedure. Always follow your service's SOPs, since some agencies do not allow crew members to perform any mechanical procedures on the vehicles.

Drivetrain

The drivetrain is the entire system of components that provide power to the wheels, including the transmission, transfer case, driveshafts, and differential.

The engine is connected to a **transmission** that is located behind the engine and that uses internal gears to convert the revolutions of the engine to slower revolutions that are required by the vehicle wheels as it is accelerating. As the speed of the vehicle increases or decreases, the transmission allows the revolutions of the wheels to change within the normal range of rpm of the engine by applying different gears. At slow speeds, a lower gear is used, and higher gears are applied as the vehicle reaches higher speeds. The transmission must have constant lubrication for the gears as well as for the internal hydraulics, which shift the gears when appropriate. Transmission fluid is a special type of hydraulic fluid. It is usually dark red in color and rarely causes problems unless a seal at one end of the transmission fails, allowing the fluid to leak out.

Most ambulances have automatic transmissions. New technology has allowed for the design of automatic transmissions to handle the heavier weight of emergency vehicles. These transmissions are hydraulic systems, which require proper levels of fluid to function properly. Additionally, they are usually electronic, requiring a properly functioning electrical system to select the proper shift patterns.

Newer transmissions are being designed to utilize computer programming to prevent damage to the unit. For example, if the vehicle is rolling forward, the computer would ensure that the transmission would not shift into reverse before the vehicle was brought to a complete stop. Designs have also been developed to ensure that the vehicle cannot be placed into drive unless the vehicle is idling.

The transmission revolutions are transmitted to the wheels through a driveshaft and a rear-end gear that changes the direction of rotation and causes the wheels to turn. There are rarely any problems with this part of the drivetrain, but fluid leaking from the rear-end gear would be cause for concern. The rear-end gear is located in the middle of the rear axle (the shaft going from side to side between the rear wheels). If you find fluid (usually dark gray to black) leaking from this area, the unit should be put out of service for repair.

Routine preventive maintenance for the drivetrain includes checking transmission and power steering fluid levels. The transmission is a hydraulic system, and the dipstick is commonly marked with hot and cold notations. Some vehicles require checks with the transmission in neutral, and some in park, but almost always with the engine running. Make sure the parking brake is applied if the engine is in neutral. The procedure for checking the power steering fluid is the same as for the engine oil (just using a different dipstick and with the engine running). The power steering is also a hydraulic system. It is commonly checked with a dipstick installed on the cap and marked with hot and cold notations. The power steering fluid level should be checked with the engine off. Many power steering units simply use automatic transmission fluid, but make sure to follow the manufacturer's recommendations, found in the owner's manual and company policy.

Braking System

Historically, the **braking system** has been one of the most abused systems on an ambulance. Since most ambulances have a greater gross vehicle weight rating than a typical passenger car, these heavier vehicles are outfitted to handle additional stress and strain. Some vehicles are also equipped with auxiliary braking devices, which slow the vehicle by acting on the driveshaft, transmission, or engine. These devices normally act on the rear wheels and can be set to varying degrees of deceleration. However, caution should be used when using these devices on slick roads where they may cause the rear of the vehicle to skid.

There are several different types of brakes used in emergency vehicles. **Drum brakes** have a circular wheel hub with two semicircular brake shoes FIGURE 5-4. When the brake pedal is pressed, a piston spreads the brake shoes outward against the drum, using friction to slow the vehicle. Release of the brake pedal allows springs to return the brake shoes to their resting position. **Disc brakes** are designed with a disc and a brake caliper, with brake pads on the inside of the caliper FIGURE 5-5. The caliper is installed over the disc. Pressing on the brake pedal causes the caliper to compress the brake pads against the rotating disc, slowing the vehicle.

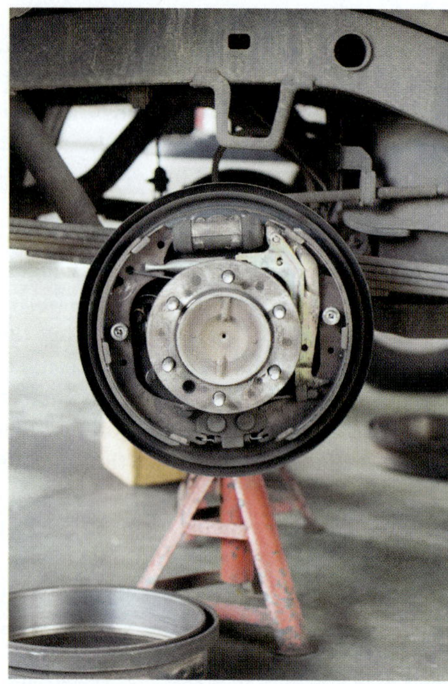

Figure 5-4 Drum brakes.
© Toa55/iStock/Getty.

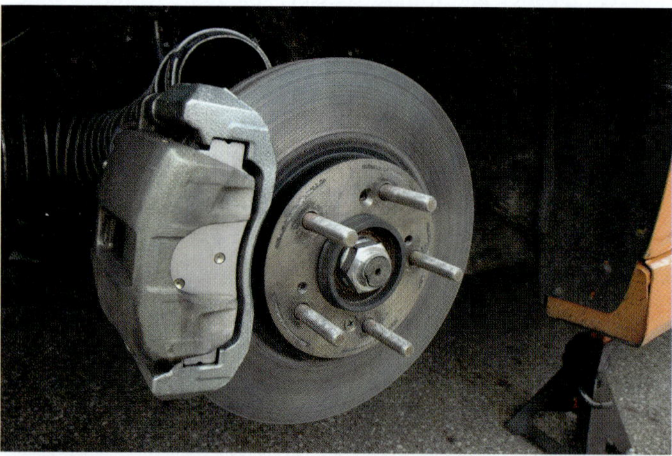

Figure 5-5 Disc brakes.
© schlol/iStock/Getty.

Hydraulic brakes use fluid to charge and activate the brakes. When you step on the brake pedal, fluid is compressed through the system and the pressure is applied to the brake pads or shoes, forcing them out against the rotor or drum. If fluid is lost due to a leak or other means, the system cannot pressurize and the result is complete brake failure.

Air brakes have the same task as hydraulic systems but function differently and require different maintenance. In a triple-valve air brake system, the air holds the brake pads away from the wheel, allowing it to turn freely. Depressing the brake pedal releases air from a chamber to activate the brake system instead of fluid pushing against the system. The parking system on air brakes also works differently from a hydraulic system. The park position on air brakes allows a mechanical spring to activate the brakes and holds the vehicle in place. This design enables a vehicle with common noncritical slow leaks in the air system to be parked for an indefinite amount of time. A certain amount of air pressure, typically about 60 psi, is required to deactivate the spring system on the brakes. Their deactivation allows the parking brake to be released so the vehicle can roll. It is important to note that at any time while operating this type of vehicle, if the air pressure becomes lower than the spring pressure, the springs will take over, locking the brakes and causing the vehicle to skid to a stop.

Antilock brakes are a type of brake system that uses a computer system to detect wheel lockup and briefly reduce braking action to that particular wheel, allowing rotation and directional control to be maintained. Antilock brakes do not necessarily decrease stopping distance, but they protect the wheels from locking up and prevent the turning of the vehicle. Antilock brakes are especially useful on slippery surfaces. Caution should be exercised when using an antilock braking system on uneven roads, such as cobblestone or gravel, since braking distance can be increased.

Since inspection of the mechanical brake components requires the removal of the wheels, this process is not included in daily routine vehicle inspection. Brake systems should, however, be checked by qualified mechanics on a regular schedule. If the vehicle has hydraulic brakes, the brake fluid should be checked routinely. Most new vehicles are equipped with a see-through reservoir where the level of this fluid can be visualized. If the brake fluid level appears low, notify a supervisor. Low brake fluid usually indicates worn brakes, which will require the unit to be out of service for maintenance. Low brake fluid may also be caused by leaks, so make sure to check underneath the reservoir as well as behind each wheel for puddles of brake fluid. If you discover brake fluid leaks, this should also be reason to put the unit out of service. Never simply add fluid and continue driving the vehicle; doing so could lead to catastrophic brake failure. Some newer brake fluids are hydroscopic (absorb moisture), so opening the reservoir daily simply introduces unwanted moisture into the system. This problem can be avoided by simply looking through the reservoir to gauge the level of the brake fluid.

Air brakes should be tested daily by performing the ALSAPS method:

- *Air brake leakage test.* Depress the brake pedal and hold it. There should be an immediate reduction of air, but not more than 10 psi. Continue to depress the pedal for 1 minute. The system should not lose more than 2 psi in that time.
- *Low air warning test.* Turn on the power supply, but do not start the vehicle. Begin fanning (rapidly pressing and releasing) the brakes until pressure drops and the warning light and buzzer activate. Note that pressure on the gauge should be around 70 psi.
- *Spring brake test.* With the vehicle on level ground, push the parking brake in. Begin fanning the brake

pedal until the parking brake "pops" out. Note that pressure on the gauge should be around 40 psi.

- *Air compressor cutoff test.* Start the engine and monitor the air compressor gauge. The air compressor should cut off around 125 psi. This process should be completed in under 2 minutes.
- *Parking brake test.* With the vehicle still running and the parking brake on, shift into gear and gently step on the accelerator, checking that the parking brake is holding.
- *Service brake test.* With the vehicle in drive and your foot on the brake, depress the parking brake and allow the vehicle to roll slowly 15 to 50 feet. Depress the brake and stop the vehicle. The service brake is functional.

If the brakes are used heavily during a trip, you may notice a burning smell coming from the area of the wheels. This odor is caused by the brake pad material overheating and is a sign that the brakes have been pushed to their limit. Occasionally under extremely heavy use, brakes can fail, resulting in an inability to stop the vehicle. This true emergency can often be avoided by limiting heavy use of the brakes through reasonable and careful driving.

Tires

Tires on the ambulance are expected to be durable and perform well at high speeds. They should be inspected at the beginning of each shift, and examined for proper inflation, adequate tread, and any signs of damage such as cuts, cracks, or uneven wear. You will need to check the tire inflation pressure to ensure that it falls within the manufacturer's recommendations for the specific vehicle type. These recommendations are normally located on a sticker inside the driver's door, the door jam, or the glove box door FIGURE 5-6. Because the manufacturer recommendations for tire pressures are based on the gross vehicle weight rating, they may vary from the maximum pressure listed on the tire. It is important to follow the vehicle manufacturer's guidelines, while not exceeding the tire manufacturer's stated limits.

To check the tire pressure, you will need a high-quality tire pressure gauge. Tire pressure gauges come with different measurement ranges. Typical car gauges measure pressure up to only 50 psi, but commercial vehicle gauges may have a range of greater than 100 psi. Make sure your gauge is appropriate for the task at hand. It is important to note that tire pressure increases when the tires are hot, so it is best to check tire pressure after the vehicle has been idle for at least 3 hours. To check the tire pressure, first remove the protective cap from the air valve, then firmly press the gauge inlet against the **valve stem** to prevent air loss FIGURE 5-7. Read the measurement on the gauge and adjust air pressure as needed by adding air with an air compressor hose and nozzle or releasing excess air by compressing the needle inside the valve stem to remove air from the tire. Do *not* let air out of a tire that has just been driven or is hot; doing so can cause the tire to be underinflated when it cools. Note, it should not usually be necessary to reduce the air pressure unless someone has previously overinflated the tire. Make sure all tires are inflated equally. Unequal inflation will lead to poor vehicle handling as well as a higher likelihood of tire failure. Just remember that changes in weather and barometric pressure can change the pressure of a tire.

Wear bars are small portions of rubber that lie underneath the tire's surface and perpendicular to the tread FIGURE 5-8. As the tread slowly wears away, the wear bars become more prominent until they become level with the tire's tread. When this occurs, it is mandatory to change the tire since the sipes are not deep enough to channel away water. Actual tread depth

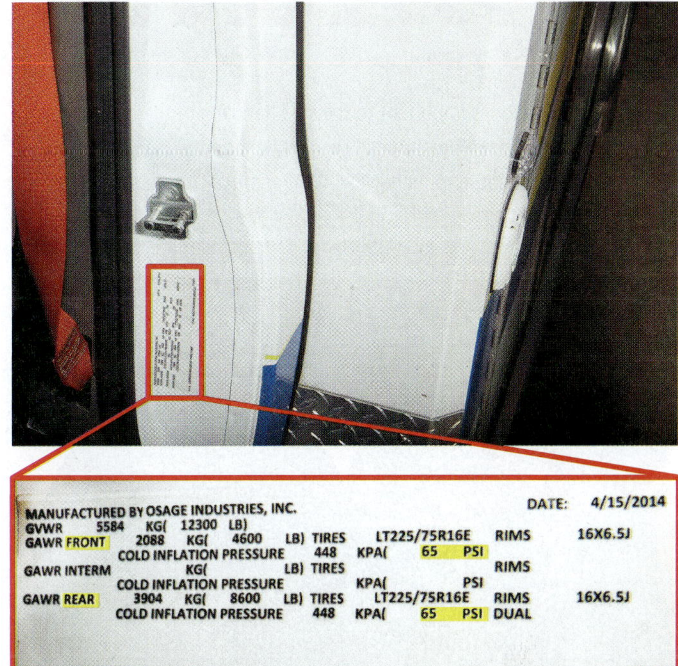

Figure 5-6 The tire pressure tag (inset) is typically found on the inside of the driver's door.

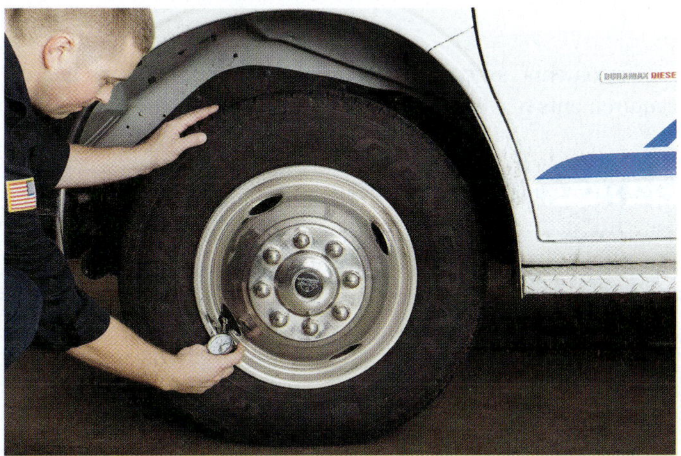

Figure 5-7 Check tire pressure regularly.

SAFETY TIP

Proper tire inflation is important to the safe handling of the emergency vehicle. Automatic tire pressure gauges will be included in those ambulances built or updated to meet NFPA 1917, *Standard for Automotive Ambulances*.

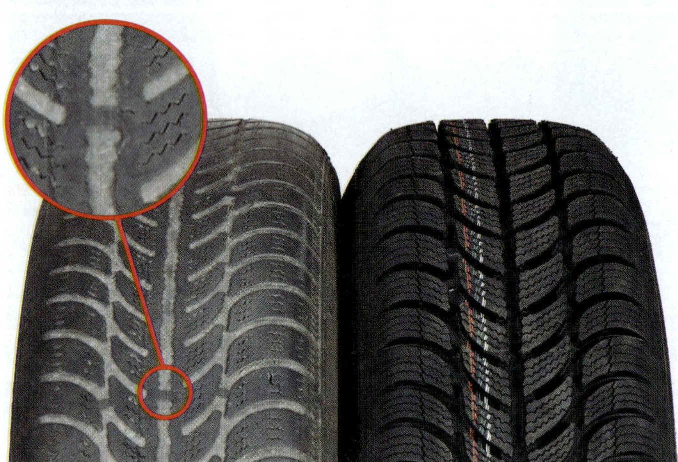

Figure 5-8 Prominent wear bars (inset) indicate that the tread is worn and that the tire must be replaced.

measurements are tire specific, but commercial driver's license requirements of $^{2}\!/_{32}$ inch can be used as a guideline.

Suspension System

The **suspension system** is what supports the vehicle above the drivetrain. Most ambulances are equipped with heavy-duty suspension systems to withstand the rigors of emergency use. Suspension systems have improved greatly in recent years, and many newer vehicles have air suspension systems that provide a smooth and comfortable ride. The suspension system in newer vehicles may also lower the rear of the vehicle to make it easier to get in and out of the patient compartment. Combined with stabilization systems, which reduce vehicle body roll (a tendency for the top of the vehicle to lean outward) in curves, improved suspension systems have made the vehicles much more comfortable and safer to use. Since the suspension system is all located under the vehicle, it should be inspected by qualified mechanics on a regular schedule.

Heating and Air-Conditioning System

In accordance with federal guidelines, all ambulances used to transport patients must have adequate heating and cooling systems to maintain a temperature of 68–78°F in the patient compartment. Most emergency vehicle heating systems work off of the vehicle coolant system. A series of hoses channel hot coolant to the patient module where a fan and radiator arrangement introduces heated air into the patient compartment. Electronic or mechanical valves controlled by a thermostat system regulate the temperature. Some vehicles are also equipped with electrical or mechanical valves under the hood that may cut off the flow of coolant to the patient module when it is not needed due to warm external temperatures. Most ambulance air-conditioning systems have one compressor and condenser to cool the cab and a secondary compressor and condenser system to cool the patient compartment.

SAFETY TIP

While not required, it is a good idea to maintain a temperature of 68–78°F in the patient compartment so the area is at the proper temperature when the need to transport a patient arises.

Exhaust System

The **exhaust system** of the vehicle should be intact and functional, channeling all exhaust gases safely out the side or the rear of the vehicle. It is important to note where the exhaust exits the vehicle and to avoid aligning the exhaust output with the area of injured patients at a scene. Remember that the carbon monoxide in exhaust gases is colorless and odorless and can cause serious problems if it leaks into the ambulance. To avoid this situation, some ambulances are equipped with carbon monoxide detectors in the patient module. A qualified mechanic should regularly inspect the exhaust system, which is located underneath the unit.

Preventive Maintenance

Most EMS services require a daily inspection of the vehicle. This inspection is important to maintain the vehicle, helping it to last longer and perform more efficiently, and also to reduce potential liability from a failed vehicle due to a defective or damaged component. **Preventive maintenance**, regularly inspecting and servicing the vehicle, helps reduce equipment downtime and repair costs. It is more economical to schedule servicing and replacement at regular intervals than to pay for unexpected repairs. Preventive maintenance may be performed at intervals determined by the vehicle's mileage or a certain amount of time. For example, engine oil changes are not dependent on the vehicle's mileage as in personal vehicles, since emergency vehicles typically spend more time in idle (i.e., the engine is running, but this engine work is not registered by the odometer); however, tire inspection and maintenance should be based on the vehicle's mileage rather than a designated amount of time.

VEHICLE OPERATOR INCIDENT

During the morning checkout, Danny was behind schedule and completed the inspection sheet in a hurry. Later that day, another EMT, Carl, was responding to a call and was unable to contact anyone on the radio. He had to resort to the unit's cell phone to get in touch with the hospital. After wheeling the patient into the hospital on the stretcher, he returned to the vehicle, but the engine would not start. He tried to turn the unit's headlights on to determine if there was a problem with the battery and discovered that the headlights weren't working either. He opened the hood of the unit and noticed the alternator belt lying beneath the radiator. The alternator belt could have been easily replaced if only Danny had done a thorough vehicle inspection.

Maintenance schedules may vary based on the severity of the problem. Any problems that affect the safety of the vehicle (e.g., a cut in a tire or brake issues) should be addressed immediately. Less critical problems (e.g., a nonoperative clearance light) may be repaired during scheduled routine maintenance.

Road Performance

Some EMS systems include vehicle road performance in their required routine inspections, since certain problems can be detected only by driving the vehicle. If your service requires this test, you should check the following:

- The steering wheel should be properly aligned and should turn smoothly, accurately directing the vehicle with little play.
- There should be no unexpected noises. For example, a high-pitched squealing noise may indicate a worn or loose power steering belt.
- The brake pedal should be firm, and the vehicle should slow in proportion to pedal pressure.
- The brakes should stop the vehicle evenly without pulling to the left or right and should perform consistently, even during repeated stops.
- The vehicle should accelerate with smooth engine operation and no skipping.

Relevant Guidelines and Organizations

Several standards and organizations provide useful guidelines and resources for emergency vehicle inspection and maintenance. Vehicle operators should be familiar with NFPA 1071, *Standard for Emergency Vehicle Technician Professional Qualifications*. This standard outlines the minimum job performance requirements for a person qualified as an emergency vehicle technician who is engaged in the inspection, diagnosis, maintenance, repair, and testing of an emergency vehicle. While this standard is intended for the fire service, it does have some useful information that can be applied to all providers of emergency services. In addition, NFPA 1911, *Standard for the Inspection, Maintenance, Testing, and Retirement of In-Service Automotive Fire Apparatus*, provides minimum requirements for a preventive maintenance program for fire apparatus and sets a standard for many emergency providers and agency SOPs.

NFPA 1917, *Standard for Automotive Ambulances*, is becoming the new standard for ambulance design and construction and is steadily replacing the KKK specifications for ambulances built on or after January 1, 2013.

The Emergency Vehicle Technician (EVT) Certification Commission, Inc., is a nonprofit corporation that seeks to improve the quality of emergency vehicle service and repair. This organization offers a certification program for vehicle operators recognizing the training and experience they have in the service and repair of emergency vehicles. Automotive Service Excellence (ASE) is another nonprofit certification agency that tests professionals' vehicle repair and service abilities.

When your inspection or use of your emergency vehicle reveals a problem, you should report the problem in accordance with your chain of command and the SOPs within your agency. You should not drive a vehicle that you feel is unsafe. Remember that as the emergency vehicle operator, you will be held responsible for any collisions or injuries that occur. It is the employer's responsibility, in accordance with the Occupational Safety and Health Act, to provide a safe work environment, free of any hazards that may cause injury to the employee. States may have additional standards and different enforcement policies. NFPA 1911 allows the authority having jurisdiction to define defects considered unsafe for vehicle operation and outlines the responsibility to remove the vehicle from service.

WRAP-UP

SUMMARY

- As the emergency vehicle operator, you are generally charged with making sure your unit is mechanically ready prior to your initial operation of the vehicle.
- You should be generally familiar with the mechanical operation of your vehicle and potential problems that might routinely occur.
- You should be very familiar with the daily inspection checklist for your vehicle and complete it in a thorough and responsible manner on every shift.
- You should be able to determine which maintenance you can reliably perform and which maintenance needs to be referred to a qualified mechanic, based on your company's policies.
- You should be able to road test a vehicle and handle any performance issues, including reporting them to the proper person.
- The emergency vehicle operator should mark out of service any unit he or she believes to be unsafe, pending repair.

GLOSSARY

air brakes A braking system that uses air as a medium for applying the brakes.

alternator An electromechanical device that converts mechanical energy to electrical energy in the form of alternating current; automotive alternators use a set of rectifiers to convert alternating current to direct current to charge the vehicle batteries.

antilock brakes A computerized braking system that prevents wheel lockup, helping the vehicle maintain directional control.

battery A device that chemically stores electrical energy; it is generally used for starting the vehicle and short-term electrical use.

braking system The entire system that allows the vehicle operator to stop the vehicle by applying pressure to the vehicle's brake pedal.

disc brakes A braking system designed with a disc and a brake caliper installed over the disc.

drum brakes A braking system that has a circular wheel hub with two semicircular brake shoes installed inside.

electrical system The system that generates and maintains electrical energy required for vehicle operation as well as for patient care activities.

engine A device that provides the mechanical motive force for propelling a vehicle and powering its subsystems.

exhaust system The system for removing dangerous exhaust gases from the engine.

hydraulic brakes A braking system that uses fluid to charge and activate the brakes.

inverter An electrical device that converts direct current to alternating current; it provides 110-volt current.

preventive maintenance Scheduled servicing, inspection, or replacement of specific items in the vehicle to reduce potential problems.

suspension system The system that supports the vehicle and allows it to absorb the impact from bumpy roads without affecting the ride inside the cab and patient compartment.

transmission A device that provides speed and torque conversions from the engine to the wheels using gear ratios; it reduces the higher engine speed to the slower wheel speed, increasing torque in the process.

valve stem An opening to the valve that admits air to a tire and automatically closes to seal in pressure.

ADDITIONAL RESOURCES

Automotive Service Excellence, http://www.ase.com

Emergency Vehicle Technician Certification Commission, http://www.evtcc.org

REFERENCE

U.S. Fire Administration, Federal Emergency Management Agency. (2014). *Emergency vehicle safety initiative.* FEMA FA-336. Retrieved from https://www.usfa.fema.gov/downloads/pdf/publications/fa_336.pdf

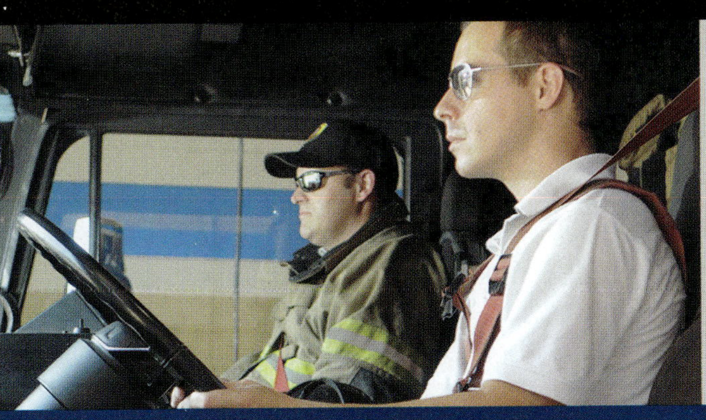

CHAPTER 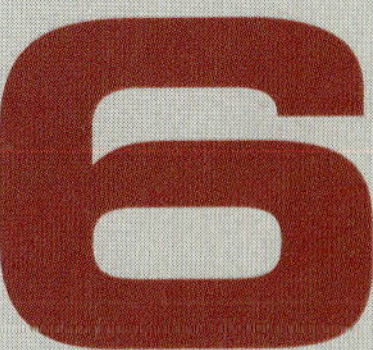

Driving Emergency Vehicle Apparatus

KNOWLEDGE OBJECTIVES

After studying this chapter, you will be able to:

- Describe the 360-degree inspection.
- Describe the process to start the apparatus, get it under way, and shut it down. (**NFPA 1002, 4.3, 4.3.1, 4.3.1(A)**)
- Describe the seat belt requirements of NFPA 1500. (**NFPA 1002, 4.3.1(A)**)
- Describe the various driver-training exercises required by NFPA 1002. (**NFPA 1002, 4.3.1, 4.3.1(A), 4.3.2, 4.3.2(A), 4.3.3, 4.3.3(A), 4.3.4, 4.3.4(A), 4.3.5, 4.3.5(A)**)
- Describe the procedure to back up the apparatus. (**NFPA 1002, 4.3.2, 4.3.2(A)**)

SKILLS OBJECTIVES

After studying this chapter, you will be able to:

- Perform a 360-degree inspection.
- Start the fire apparatus. (**NFPA 1002, 4.3.1, 4.3.1(B)**)
- Perform the serpentine exercise. (**NFPA 1002, 4.3.3, 4.3.3(B)**)
- Perform a confined-space turnaround. (**NFPA 1002, 4.3.4, 4.3.4(B)**)
- Perform a diminishing clearance exercise. (**NFPA 1002, 4.3.5, 4.3.5(B)**)
- Back a fire apparatus into a fire station bay. (**NFPA 1002, 4.3.2, 4.3.2(B)**)
- Shut down and secure a fire apparatus. (**NFPA 1002, 4.3.1, 4.3.1(B)**)

Additional NFPA Standards

- **NFPA 1500**, *Standard on Fire Department Occupational Safety, Health, and Wellness Program*
- **NFPA 1901**, *Standard for Automotive Fire Apparatus*

Emergency Call

You are the driver/operator for Engine Company 5. While your company is operating at the scene of a large commercial structure fire, your apparatus is reassigned to the rear of the building. The incident commander has informed you that there is a hydrant somewhere at the rear of the building, and you are to connect to it and supply an aerial device that is already positioning for a defensive attack. As you get to the rear of the large building, you see numerous parked cars, dumpsters, and obstacles blocking a clear path. You maneuver through the area and locate the hydrant at the end of a long alley. Your officer asks you to back the apparatus down the alley so you can lay the supply hoseline from the hydrant to a position closer to the aerial apparatus.

1. Have you been trained to operate the fire apparatus in narrow alleyways?
2. Do you know how to complete a confined-space turnaround?
3. What are the proper hand signals for backing the apparatus?

Introduction

The most fundamental task of a driver/operator is actually "driving" the fire apparatus to and from emergency incidents. The driver/operator must safely get the members of the crew, the fire apparatus, and the equipment that it carries to the scene of the incident. This response should not be taken lightly. Fire apparatus are not designed like many other vehicles on the road. They are usually bigger and heavier, which changes the characteristics of the vehicle—and, therefore, changes how it should be driven. Do not assume that the fire apparatus can be driven like your own personal vehicle. Fire apparatus can be very dangerous machines when individuals who have not been properly trained in safe and efficient operational techniques drive them. It takes training and time to become a skilled fire apparatus driver. New driver/operators should not attempt the same maneuvers that more experienced drivers may perform until they are capable of doing so with confidence.

This chapter discusses how to properly prepare to drive the apparatus, start the apparatus, perform several basic maneuvers, and shut down the fire apparatus. It also covers the use of seat belts—essential safety equipment on the fire apparatus that protects both the driver/operator and the other members of the company.

Preparing to Drive

360-Degree Inspection

Before entering the cab and starting the apparatus, you must complete a preliminary inspection of the fire apparatus, also known as a 360-degree inspection. A 360-degree inspection is a quick check of the fire apparatus and its surroundings to ensure that the apparatus is prepared for a response, either to an emergency or to a nonemergency. Failure to complete this inspection may result in damage to life and/or property. For example, an open compartment door may be sheared off by the fire station walls as the fire apparatus leaves the bay. Unsecured equipment stored on the outside of the fire apparatus may fly off and strike a civilian. The preliminary inspection must be performed every time that you move the fire apparatus, regardless of the emergency. Remember—complacency kills.

If the fire apparatus is responding from inside the fire station, the first step in a preliminary inspection is to open the fire apparatus bay door. While the door is opening, continue with the inspection—do not waste valuable time waiting for the door to open later. Walk around the fire apparatus, and physically check that the cab doors are completely shut. All compartments should be checked to confirm that they are secure for travel. Ground ladders and equipment mounted to the exterior must be properly secured. Many fire apparatus have an interior warning light or buzzer to notify you that a compartment is open or not completely latched. Inspect the hose for any signs that it may come loose during a response. Remove any cups, equipment, or debris that may have been improperly placed on the running boards, front bumper, or tailboard. Visually verify that the area underneath the fire apparatus is free of debris. Your review should take only a matter of seconds. By making this inspection a habit, you will ensure that the fire apparatus is safe to respond.

To perform a 360-degree inspection, follow the steps in SKILL DRILL 6-1.

Starting the Apparatus

After the 360-degree inspection is complete, you will enter the cab and initiate the sequence to start the fire apparatus. Modern fire apparatus are usually powered by a diesel engine. This engine requires a significant amount of current during the starting process. Before starting the fire apparatus, always ensure that unnecessary electrical loads are shut off (i.e., headlights, heater, and air conditioning). Verify that the **parking brake** is set. This brake is required by National Fire Protection Association (NFPA) 1901, *Standard for Automotive Fire Apparatus*, to hold the fire

SKILL DRILL 6-1

Performing a 360-Degree Inspection

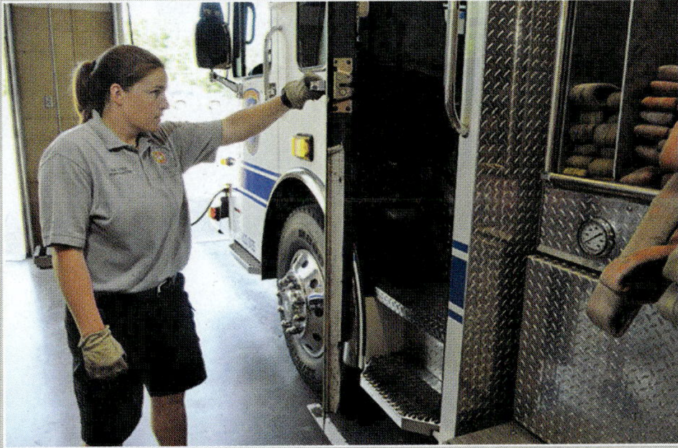

1 Open the fire apparatus bay door completely.

Walk completely around the fire apparatus.

Check that all doors are secured.

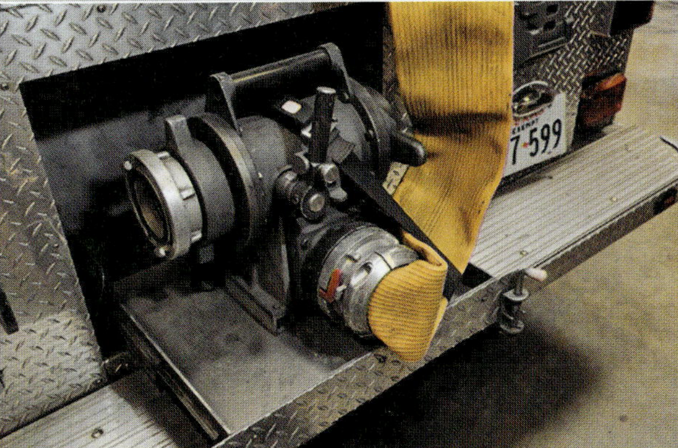

2 Check that all compartment doors are secured.

Check that all exterior-mounted equipment is properly secured.

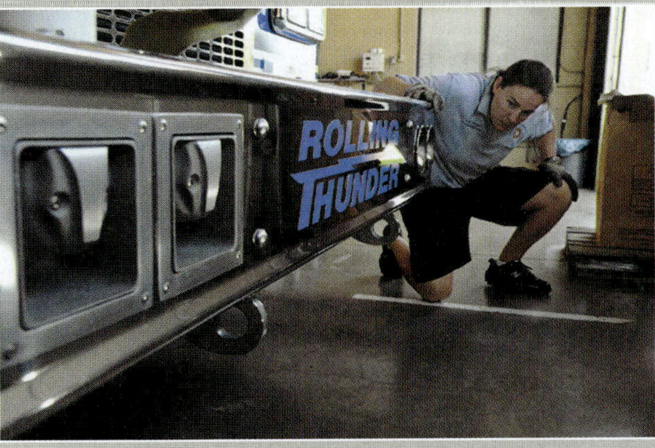

3 Remove any debris from the running boards, front bumper, and tailboard.

Check that the area underneath the fire apparatus is clear of debris.

Check that the area in front of the fire apparatus is clear and free of debris.

apparatus on at least a 20 percent grade. If the fire apparatus has an automatic transmission (most modern fire apparatus do), make sure it is in the neutral position.

For most fire apparatus, the battery selector switch is turned on next. The **battery selector switch** is used to disconnect all electrical power to the fire apparatus to prevent discharge while it is not in use. Once the power has been transferred to the electrical system, in some fire apparatus that electrical system will initiate the system check sequence. A **system check sequence** is a series of checks that an electrical system performs to ensure that all systems are functioning properly before the fire apparatus is started. This check usually takes just a few seconds to complete. If the fire apparatus is started without allowing the system check sequence to finish, it may cause intermittent alarms to occur. For any nonemergency response, always allow the prove-out sequence to continue until the cycle is complete. During an emergency situation, this time delay may not be practical, however.

Once the system check sequence is complete, the fire apparatus is ready to start. Some newer models are equipped with an ignition switch and one or two starter switches. The **ignition switch** delivers operational power to the chassis; engage this switch. The **starter switch** engages the starter motor for cranking. If two starter switches are available, they are provided for redundancy. Engage either or both of these switches to operate the starter motor. When the engine starts, release the starter switch. If the engine does not start within 30 seconds (or in accordance with the manufacturer's recommendations), release the starter switch, and allow the starter motor to cool off for 2 minutes before attempting to start it again.

During the daily fire apparatus inspection, you should have adjusted all of the seats and mirrors in preparation for your operation of the apparatus. If they are not adjusted correctly, readjust them now while the fire apparatus is not in motion. It is very dangerous to attempt to make any changes to the seating or mirror configurations while operating a moving vehicle. Many driver/operators prefer to adjust the mirrors so that the side of the fire apparatus is barely in view of the mirror; this way they can see the side of the apparatus if necessary and can observe any objects to the side of the vehicle FIGURE 6-1.

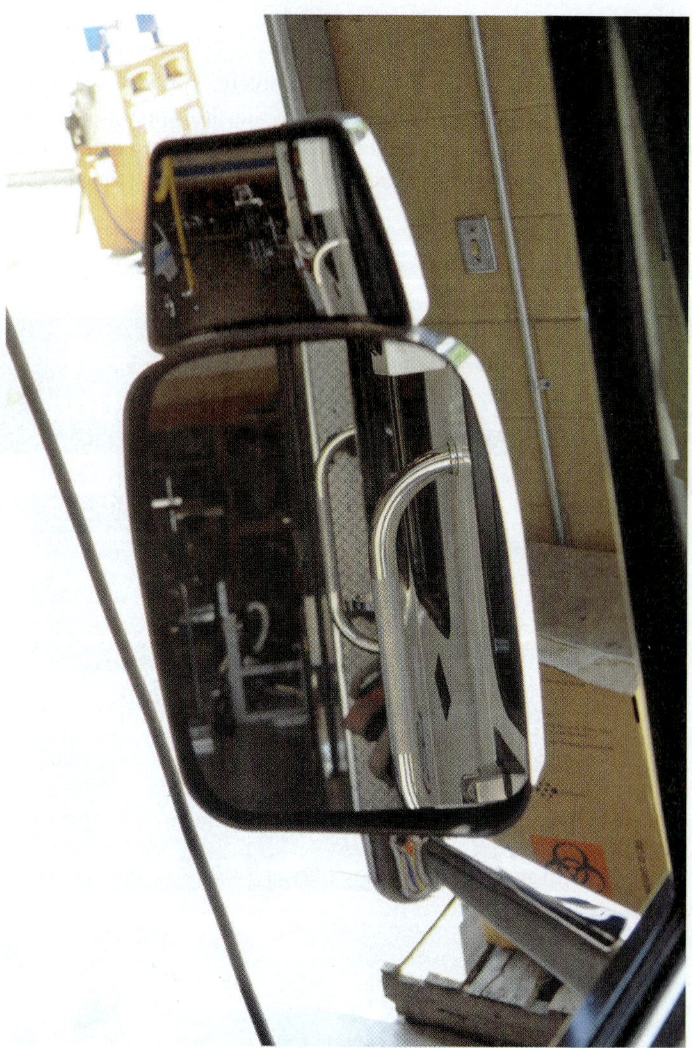

Figure 6-1 Adjust the fire apparatus mirrors for safety.

Before you leave for the incident, you must look over the instrument panel. The following items on the instrument panel should always be checked:

- Fuel. The **fuel gauge** indicates the amount of fuel in the apparatus tank. All fire apparatus should be maintained in a constant state of readiness. No fire apparatus fuel tank should ever drop below the halfway level. Always monitor the fuel gauge during operations.
- **Air pressure gauges**. These gauges identify the air pressure stored in the tanks or reservoirs of apparatus equipped with an air braking system. This air pressure is used to slow down and stop the apparatus while it is responding on the roadway. NFPA 1901 requires that the fire apparatus have a quick build-up capability so that if the apparatus has a completely discharged air system, it is able to move within 60 seconds of start-up. On a chassis that cannot be equipped with a quick recharge air brake system, an onboard automatic electric compressor or a fire station compressed-air shoreline hookup is permitted so as to maintain full operating air pressure while the vehicle is not running. The fire apparatus is also required to have a warning alarm to indicate a low level of air pressure in the system. This alarm is activated when the pressure falls below 60 psi (414 kPa) and remains active until adequate pressure has built up to release the parking brake. For most fire apparatus equipped with air braking systems, the normal operating pressure for those systems is between 100 and 120 psi (690 and 827 kPa). Always consult the manufacturer's recommendations to determine the appropriate pressure.
- **Voltmeter**. The voltmeter measures the voltage across the battery terminals of the apparatus and gives an indication of the electrical condition of the battery

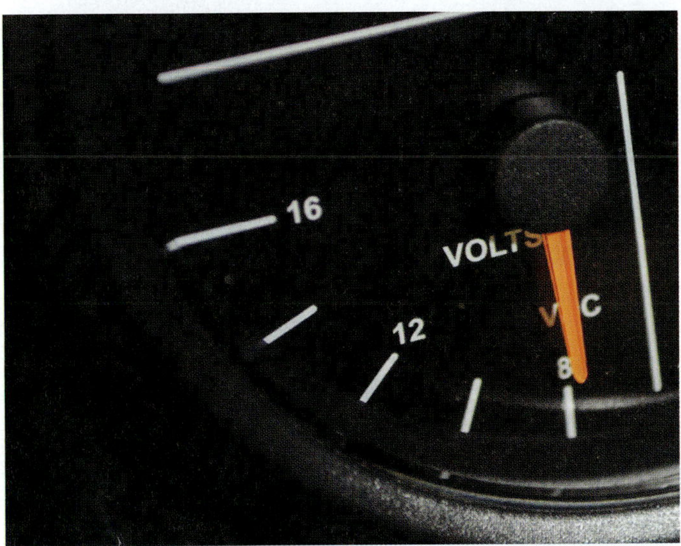

Figure 6-2 A voltmeter.

FIGURE 6-2. Operating voltage while the alternator is charging may vary among vehicles depending on the regulator setting. The voltmeter allows for direct observation of the system voltage. If this kind of monitoring is provided, an alarm will sound if the system voltage drops below 11.8 V for 12-V nominal systems or below 23.6 V for 24-V nominal systems for more than 120 seconds. Newer apparatus are extremely sensitive to drops in voltage; it is imperative that the correct voltage be maintained at all times. Many apparatus are equipped with onboard chargers for various pieces of auxiliary equipment, such as flashlights, thermal imaging cameras, and mobile data computers. It is imperative that such apparatus be plugged into shore-line electrical power when parked in the bays of the firehouse to keep this equipment fully charged.

- **Oil pressure gauge**. This gauge identifies the pressure of the lubricating oil in the engine. When the fire apparatus is started, it should provide a reading within a few seconds. If it does not, stop the engine and have a trained technician check the oil pressure.

Seat Belt Safety

Before the fire apparatus moves, you must visually check that all members are wearing a seat belt. You should never move an emergency vehicle with members unsecured. NFPA 1901 requires that all seats of fire apparatus be enclosed and provided with an approved seat belt.

NFPA 1500, *Standard on Fire Department Occupational Safety, Health, and Wellness Program*, requires the driver/operator not to move the fire apparatus until all persons on the vehicle are seated and secured with seat belts in approved riding positions. While the vehicle is in motion, fire fighters shall not release or loosen their seat belts for any purpose, including the donning of personal protective equipment (PPE) or self-contained breathing apparatus (SCBA).

SAFETY TIP

Newer fire apparatus have alarms to notify you if a fire fighter is not wearing a seat belt. Some fire apparatus will not move unless a weight sensor indicates that all fire fighters are properly wearing their seat belts.

SAFETY TIP

NFPA standards are not exclusive to emergency vehicle responses; they apply at all times. During funeral processions, parades, or public relations/education events, standing or riding on the tailboard, side-steps, running board, or any other exposed position should be specifically prohibited. This action is unprofessional and needlessly jeopardizes the safety of fire fighters and the members of the public whom they serve. Whenever the fire apparatus moves, everyone should be seated and belted—no exceptions!

Getting Under Way

Once all members are secure in the cab of the fire apparatus, verify once again that all exterior compartment doors, ladder racks, telescoping scene lights, and any other fire apparatus–mounted equipment are secure FIGURE 6-3. Some fire apparatus are equipped with compartment-door indicator lights. These lights are activated only if the fire apparatus compartment doors are open and the parking brake is in the off position. Other fire apparatus may have a digital display that shows any open compartment doors or other equipment that may be damaged if the vehicle moves FIGURE 6-4. A 360-degree inspection is always required to ensure safe operation; use these apparatus-mounted systems only as a secondary resource. Double-check the sides of the fire apparatus by using the mirrors.

Interior compartment doors also need to be secured in the closed position while the apparatus is responding to an incident. Otherwise, the items that are stored in these

Voice of Experience

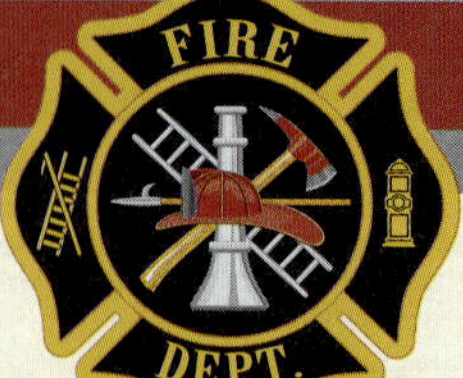

When I began my career in the fire service, I was trained as a driver/operator in an urban area with wide streets and plenty of lanes. Later in my career, my wife and I decided to relocate to the southern part of our state, which happens to be more rural. When I joined my current department, I felt confident in my abilities as a driver/operator and informed the chief that I was ready to drive as soon as he was ready to let me. Back then, our certification process was nonexistent.

During training one day, the chief decided that he was ready to let me drive and prove my abilities. I confidently assumed the driver's seat and began the work of proving to the chief that I was everything that I claimed to be behind the driver's wheel. Just as I had predicted, everything went fine, and there were no problems in my driving proficiency. However, during this evaluation time, we spent all of our time on wider "in-town" roads and kept off the narrower country roads.

Finally, it was time for me to drive beyond the confines of training. My sergeant told me where we were going. I was familiar with the road and knew that it was one of the narrowest in our district, but I felt confident that I could handle it. We turned onto the narrow road, and at first there were no issues; however, there was no oncoming traffic yet, either.

Then it happened: I met my first oncoming vehicle. Unfortunately, the driver of that vehicle did not feel like yielding to our much larger fire engine. I moved over to the side of the road a little bit more than I should have and accidentally dropped the rear tire into a shallow ditch. I thought that my heart was going to jump out of my chest and that my sergeant was going to pass out.

Luckily, we were able to get the rear tire back up onto the road without any incident or damage, but I learned that day that there is a huge difference between driving a large fire engine in the city and driving one in the country. I also learned to never yield too much road. If a motorist decides not to give me enough room, I stop and allow the car to pass before I proceed. It's better to get there a few seconds later than not at all.

Jesse Vacra
New Mexico Firefighters Training Academy
Socorro, New Mexico

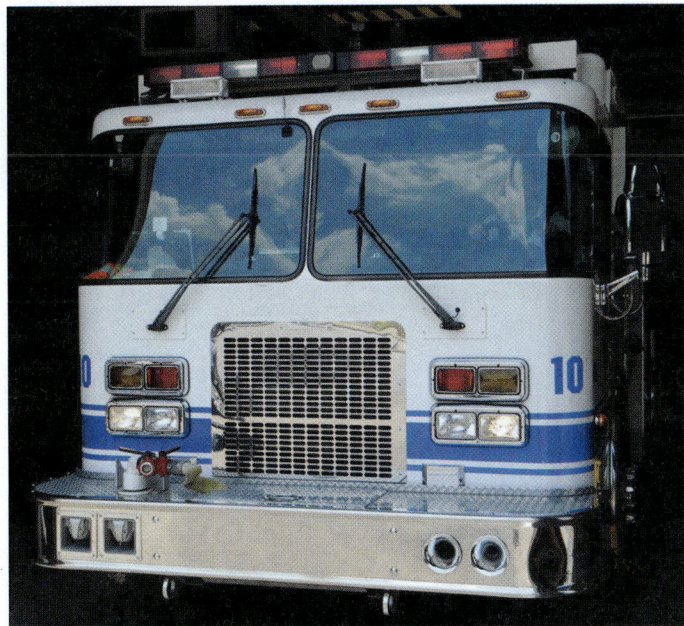

Figure 6-3 Before leaving the bay, the driver/operator must verify that all exterior compartment doors, ladder racks, telescoping scene lights, and any other fire apparatus–mounted equipment are secure.

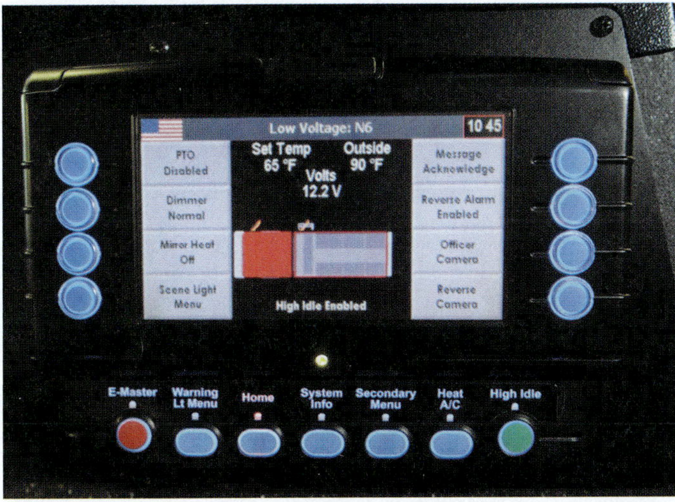

Figure 6-4 The fire apparatus may have a digital display that shows open compartment doors or other equipment that may be damaged if the vehicle moves.

compartments may fly out if the fire apparatus becomes involved in an accident. No fire fighter should ever be injured because someone failed to secure equipment that is stored inside the cab. In particular, equipment such as axes and Halligan tools should never be stored in the cab unless they are secured in an approved bracket. If a compartment or mounting system is provided for equipment, use it!

Whenever possible, allow the engine to warm up for 3 to 5 minutes. This will help extend the life of the fire apparatus and may prevent future breakdowns, as operating a cold engine and transmission under very hard conditions (emergency response) may have a damaging effect to the engine. Of course, this kind of warm-up may not always be feasible depending on the nature of the emergency.

Turn on the headlights whenever the fire apparatus is moving, not just during the night. Research has shown that a vehicle is easier for other drivers and pedestrians to identify during any conditions if it has its headlights on.

Once the overhead garage door is fully open, you may drive the fire apparatus out of the station. Be aware that other fire apparatus at the station may be leaving at the same time or that the exhaust extractor system and electrical cords may not eject properly. For these reasons, you should not exceed 5 mi/h (8 km/h) while pulling out of the fire station.

Look to the sides of the fire apparatus, and ensure that the cords and extractor are clear. Always remember to close the doors after clearing the building. If responding in an emergency mode, activate the emergency lights and audible warning devices at this time.

To start a fire apparatus and ensure that it is ready for a response, follow the steps in SKILL DRILL 6-2.

SAFETY TIP

According to a Texas State Fire Marshal's Office Fire Fighter Fatality Investigation Report, a fire fighter fell from a moving fire apparatus while responding to a structure fire. On April 23, 2005, fire fighter Brian Hunton of the Amarillo Fire Department was riding in the left-rear seat of a Ladder 1 apparatus when the door opened and he fell out. Hunton struck his head on the street and sustained severe head injuries; he died two days later. During the response, he had been donning his SCBA and not wearing his seat belt.

All fire fighters are responsible for their own safety. During an emergency response, all members should wear their seat belts. This type of accident is preventable with the proper use of seat belts. Each fire department should have a standard operating procedure (SOP) in place that requires the use of seat belts, and this policy must be enforced by all members. Requiring fire fighters to wear seat belts is a simple rule that could prevent 10 to 15 fatalities every year.

DRIVER/OPERATOR TIP

Driving a fire apparatus while wearing cumbersome turnout pants and boots can be very difficult for some fire fighters. For this reason, some fire departments do not require their driver/operators to dress in turnout gear while driving to an incident. Evaluate your ability to safely operate the fire apparatus while wearing turnout pants and boots. If you do not feel safe operating under these conditions, notify your supervisor, and determine the best course of action. Remember—safety always comes first.

SKILL DRILL 6-2

Starting a Fire Apparatus NFPA 1002, 4.3.1, 4.3.1(B)

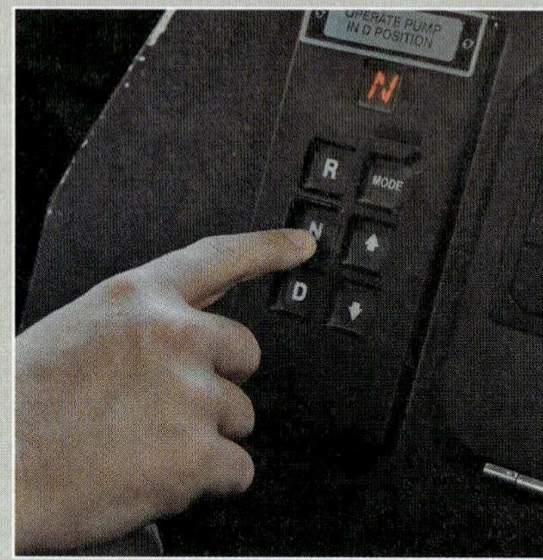

1 Enter the fire apparatus cab.

Verify that the parking brake is set in the "on" position.

Check that the transmission is in the neutral position.

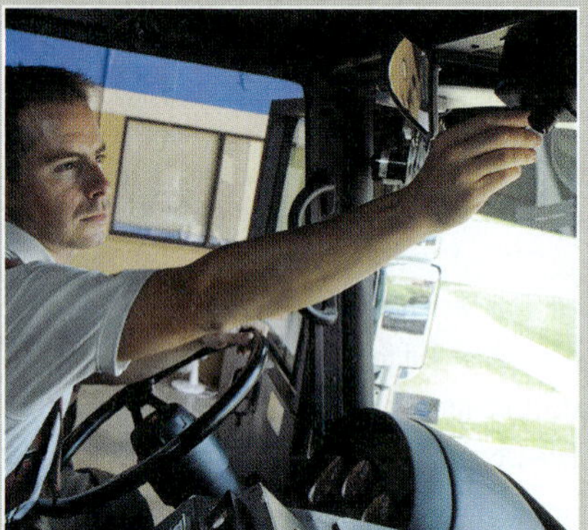

2 Verify that any unnecessary electrical loads (including the air conditioner/heater and headlights) are turned off before activating the battery.

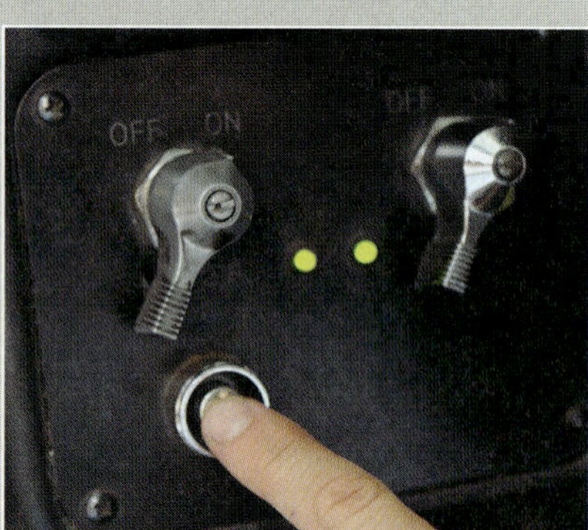

3 Turn on the battery selector switch.

Allow the apparatus to complete the system check sequence.

Engage the ignition switch.

Engage the starter switch.

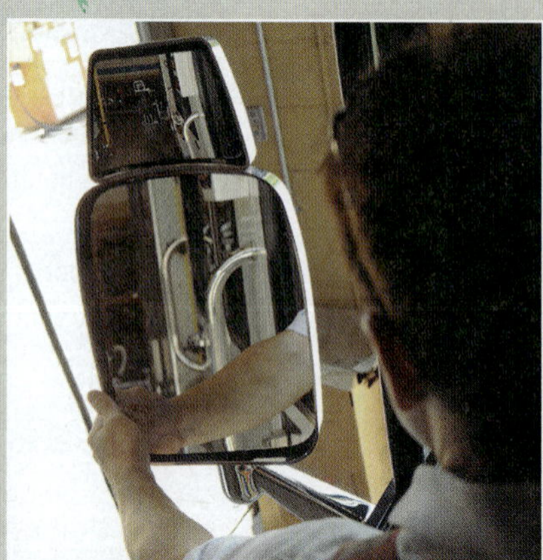

4 Adjust the seat and mirrors, if necessary.

Check the gauges: fuel, air pressure, voltmeter, and oil pressure.

SKILL DRILL 6-2 Continued

Starting a Fire Apparatus NFPA 1002, 4.3.1, 4.3.1(B)

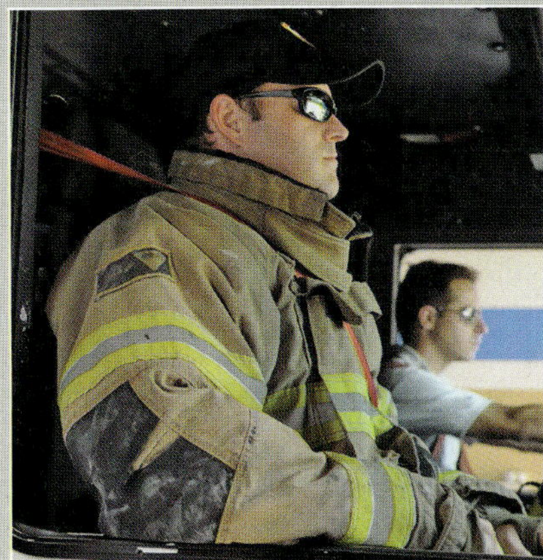

5 Ensure that each crew member is wearing a seat belt before moving the fire apparatus.

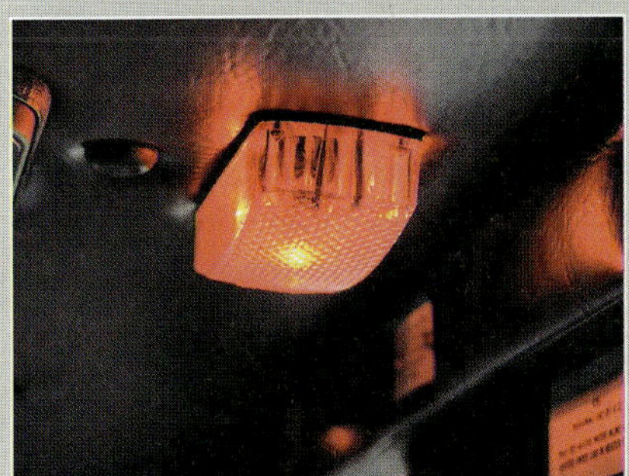

6 Check the compartment-door indicator light, if applicable, to ensure that no compartments are open.

Turn on the headlights.

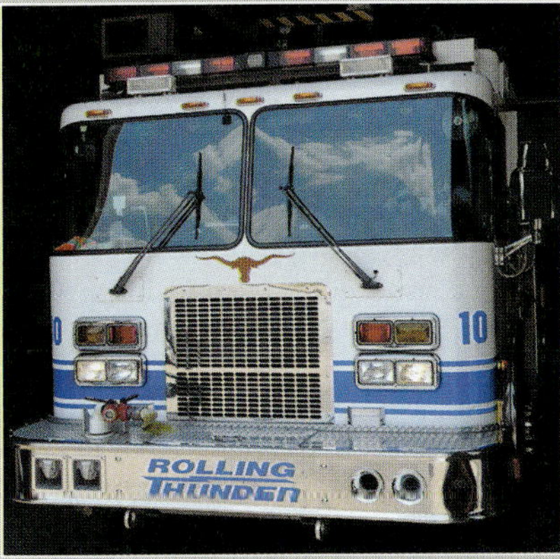

7 Allow the engine to warm up before moving, if applicable. Place the transmission in "drive."

Release the parking brake.

Activate the emergency lights and audible warning devices.

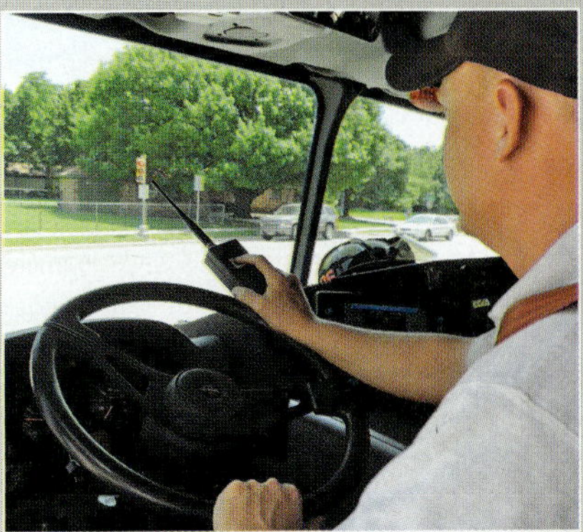

8 Drive the fire apparatus out of the fire station at a speed less than 5 mi/h (8 km/h). Check the sidewalk to make certain that all pedestrian traffic has stopped.

Activate any signal control system to stop traffic in front of the fire station.

Close the fire station doors with the remote control to ensure security.

Driving Exercises

Riding in a fire apparatus as it is responding to an emergency scene can be very exciting. Driving the fire apparatus to a scene is even more exciting. You may develop a rush of adrenaline while operating the fire apparatus on the roadway. This excitement, however, should not make you lose sight of the task at hand—transporting the fire apparatus and your crew members to the emergency scene in a safe and efficient manner. Do not drive the fire apparatus faster than existing conditions permit or at a speed greater than can be maintained with safety. At all times, you must be able to maintain control of the fire apparatus. Do not allow the situation or other members of the crew to push you into driving the fire apparatus at a speed or in a manner beyond your abilities. Instead, always use common sense and good judgment. A speedy response is achieved through a safe and efficient means of operation—not by taking unnecessary risks. Never endanger life or property, under any circumstances.

During the emergency response, you may have to maneuver the fire apparatus around objects at the scene or parked vehicles that are blocking access to a preferred location. This type of maneuver is done at a reduced speed with an emphasis on the safety of pedestrians, other objects, and the fire apparatus. NFPA 1002, *Standard for Fire Apparatus Driver/Operator Professional Qualifications*, requires that all driver/operators complete a serpentine exercise that simulates these conditions. The exercise measures the driver/operator's ability to maneuver in close quarters without stopping the fire apparatus.

Performing a Serpentine Maneuver

As part of the serpentine maneuver exercise, a minimum of three marker cones are spaced 30 to 38 ft (9 to 12 m) apart in a line. The spacing of the marker cones should be equal to the fire apparatus' wheelbase. The space on the sides of the marker cones must provide adequate space for the fire apparatus to travel freely. To perform the serpentine maneuver, drive the fire apparatus along the left side of the marker cones in a straight line, and stop with the fire apparatus just past the final marker cone. You are now in position to begin the exercise. Back the fire apparatus to the left of marker cone 1, to the right of marker cone 2, and to the left of marker cone 3. Once the front of the fire apparatus is past marker cone 3, drive the fire apparatus forward between the marker cones by passing to the right of marker cone 3, to the left of marker cone 2, and to the right of marker cone 1.

During the entire exercise, the marker cones should not be struck, and the fire apparatus should move in a continuous motion, except when required to change direction of travel. A spotter is necessary for this exercise. To perform the serpentine exercise, follow the steps in **SKILL DRILL 6-3**.

Performing a Confined-Space Turnaround

When responding to an incident, you may inadvertently pass a street on which you should have turned. When this situation occurs, the best course is to drive the fire apparatus around the block rather than try to turn the fire apparatus around in the confines of a roadway. Other motorists may be confused by your actions as you attempt to move a large fire apparatus around 180 degrees, only to proceed back in the direction from which you just came. However, even seasoned driver/operators can go down a wrong road or find themselves in a position where they need to turn around and go the other way.

NFPA 1002 requires that all driver/operators complete an exercise that simulates these circumstances, during which they turn a fire apparatus 180 degrees within a predetermined area where the apparatus cannot complete a U-turn. This exercise, which is called a confined-space turnaround, measures your ability to turn the fire apparatus around in a confined space without going outside a set boundary. It is completed in a 50 ft × 100 ft (15 m × 31 m) area, where marker cones may be used to identify the set boundary. The fire apparatus enters the area through an opening, no more than 12 ft (4 m) wide, in the center of one of the 50-ft (15-m) sides. The fire apparatus proceeds forward, turns around 180 degrees, and returns through the same opening. You may maneuver the fire apparatus forward and reverse as many times as needed to accomplish the task, but the fire apparatus must remain inside the set boundary lines. During the entire exercise, the fire apparatus must remain within the marked boundary and move in a continuous motion, except when required to change direction of travel. A spotter is necessary for this exercise.

To perform the confined-space turnaround exercise, follow the steps in **SKILL DRILL 6-4**.

Performing a Diminishing Clearance Exercise

Once at the scene, you may have to operate the fire apparatus in tight quarters. Sometimes other fire apparatus, trees, storefront signs, or buildings can obstruct your path. However, the most common obstruction on an emergency scene is parked cars.

LISTEN UP!

When operating the fire apparatus, you must always drive with "**due regard** for the safety of others." This statement or something similar is found in most state laws that pertain to emergency vehicle operations. An emergency vehicle operator may have the right to disregard certain traffic laws but does not have the right to jeopardize the safety of other motorists or pedestrians. For example, some fire departments and local laws allow emergency vehicles to exceed the speed limit on roads and highways. Usually, certain conditions must be met to operate in this way—namely, light traffic and good weather conditions. If the emergency vehicle operator exceeds the speed limit under adverse conditions, he or she is not "driving with due regard for the safety of others." During the entire response, you must be constantly aware of other motorists and pedestrians as well as your own safety.

SKILL DRILL 6-3

Performing the Serpentine Exercise NFPA 1002, 4.3.3, 4.3.3(B)

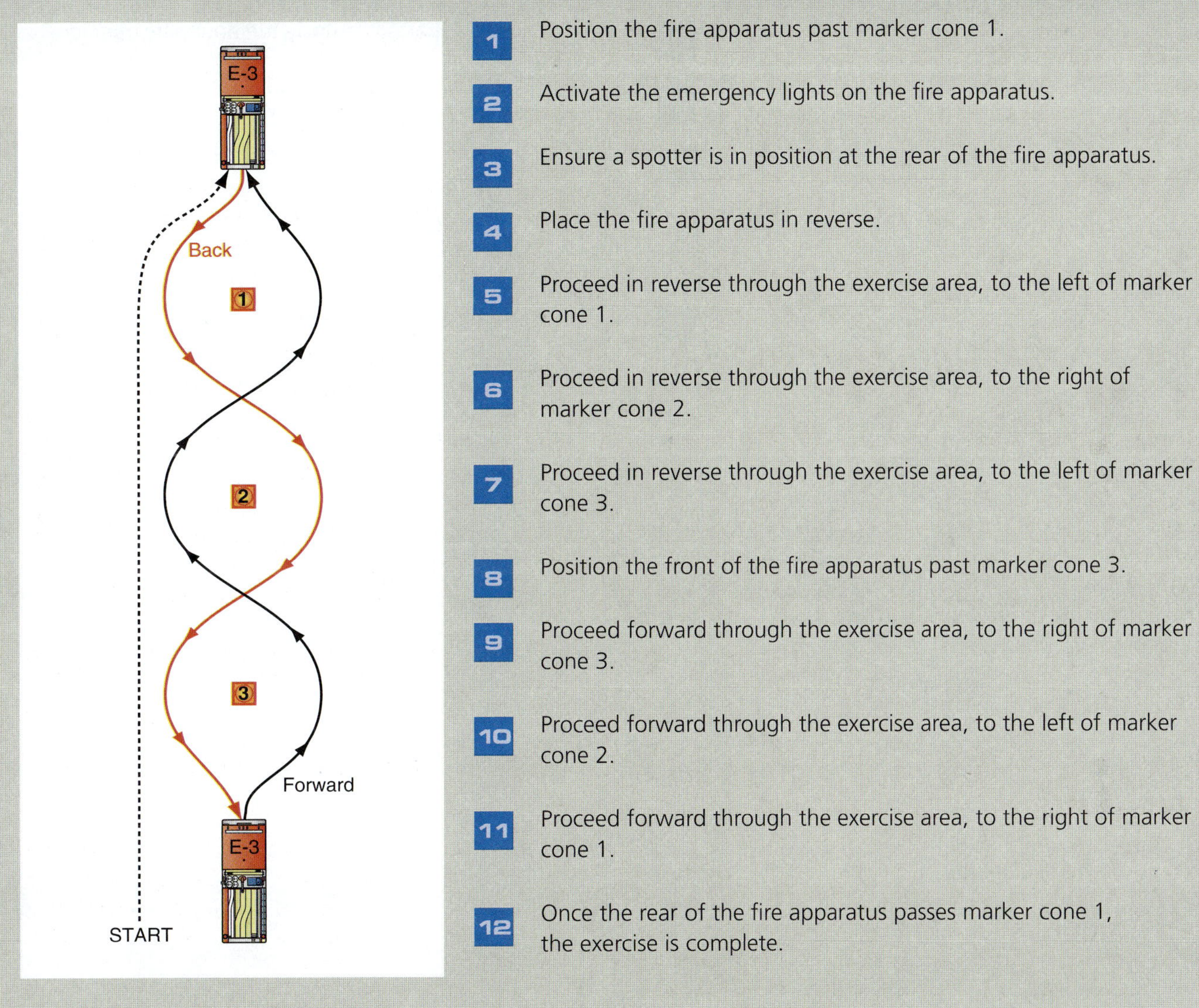

1. Position the fire apparatus past marker cone 1.
2. Activate the emergency lights on the fire apparatus.
3. Ensure a spotter is in position at the rear of the fire apparatus.
4. Place the fire apparatus in reverse.
5. Proceed in reverse through the exercise area, to the left of marker cone 1.
6. Proceed in reverse through the exercise area, to the right of marker cone 2.
7. Proceed in reverse through the exercise area, to the left of marker cone 3.
8. Position the front of the fire apparatus past marker cone 3.
9. Proceed forward through the exercise area, to the right of marker cone 3.
10. Proceed forward through the exercise area, to the left of marker cone 2.
11. Proceed forward through the exercise area, to the right of marker cone 1.
12. Once the rear of the fire apparatus passes marker cone 1, the exercise is complete.

Any one of these obstructions may restrict the horizontal or vertical clearance of the fire apparatus and create challenges for you as the driver/operator. During these situations, you must judge the distance you have available to maneuver the apparatus through openings and not cause any damage.

NFPA 1002 requires that all driver/operators complete an exercise that simulates a restricted horizontal and vertical clearance for a fire apparatus. This "diminishing clearance" exercise measures your ability to maneuver the fire apparatus in a straight line and judge the distance between the fire apparatus

DRIVER/OPERATOR TIP

The National Fallen Firefighters Foundation (NFFF) summarizes the issues pertaining to vehicle safety:

- It's not a race.
- Safe is more important than fast.
- Stop at red lights and stop signs! There are no excuses.
- If they do not get out of your way, do not run them over! Think and react carefully.

SKILL DRILL 6-4

Performing a Confined-Space Turnaround NFPA 1002, 4.3.4, 4.3.4(B)

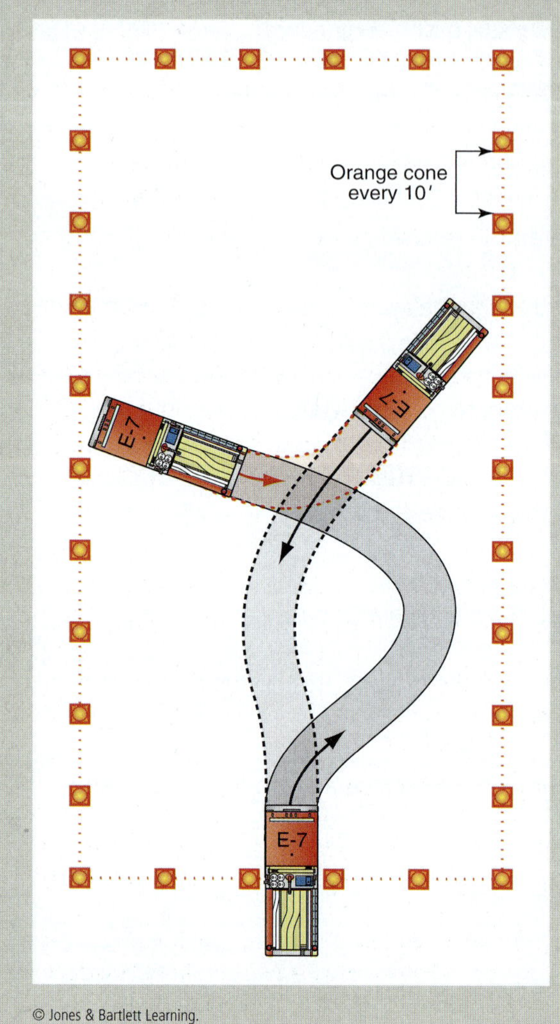

1. Position the fire apparatus outside the boundary opening.
2. Proceed forward through the opening.
3. Maneuver the fire apparatus so that it is turned 180 degrees. This will require driving forward, swinging the tail of the apparatus almost 90 degrees, and then maneuvering forward. "Forward, swing, forward."
4. Proceed forward through the opening and out of the set boundary.

and an object in front of it. The fire apparatus should proceed at a speed that requires your quick judgment. It moves forward down two rows of marker cones to form a lane 75 ft (23 m) long. The lane's width diminishes from a starting point of 9 ft 6 inches (2.9 m) to a width of 8 ft 2 inches (2.5 m). Marker cones identify the lane's boundaries. To perform the exercise successfully, you must proceed forward down the lane without striking the marker cones. Bring the apparatus to a complete stop 50 ft (15 m) past the last marker cone at a predetermined finish line. No portion of the fire apparatus can protrude past this set line. The fire apparatus then proceeds in reverse past the point where it entered the diminishing clearance exercise.

> **SAFETY TIP**
>
> The use of sirens during gridlock merely confuses other drivers when they have nowhere to move their cars. Use the public address system and give the drivers directions.

During the course of the fire apparatus moving forward and reversing in the diminishing clearance exercise, a vertical crossbar prop is positioned to determine your ability to judge the height of the fire apparatus. This crossbar may be positioned

SAFETY TIP

A prompt, safe response can be achieved by adhering to the following guidelines:

- Leave the station in a standard manner:
  - Perform a 360-degree walk around the fire apparatus. Check for open compartments.
  - Quickly mount the fire apparatus.
  - Make sure that all personnel are on board and are seated with seat belts on.
  - Make sure the station doors are fully open.
  - Close the fire station doors with a remote control upon leaving.
  - Drive defensively and professionally at reasonable speeds.
  - Know where you are going.
  - Use warning devices to move around traffic and to request the right-of-way in a safe and predictable manner.

  Do not:
- Leave your quarters before the crew has mounted the apparatus safely and before the fire station doors are fully open.
- Drive too fast for the current conditions.
- Drive recklessly or without regard for safety.
- Take unnecessary chances with negative right-of-way intersections.
- Intimidate or scare other drivers.

DRIVER/OPERATOR TIP

According to a National Incident for Occupational Safety and Health (NIOSH) report:

> On August 14, 2004, a 25-year-old female career fire fighter (the victim) died when she apparently fell from the tailboard and was backed over by an engine. The victim and her crew had been released from the scene of a residential fire. The road was blocked by other apparatus, so the victim's crew began backing to an intersection approximately 300 ft (90 m) away so as to then proceed forward. The victim took her position on the tailboard as the "tailboard safety member" and signaled the driver to begin backing. A captain acting as the "traffic control officer" guided the backing operation from the road on the driver's side, behind the apparatus, by using hand signals. When the captain turned and walked into the intersection to stop cross-traffic, the victim apparently fell from the tailboard and was run over by the engine. Members on the scene provided advanced life support, and the victim was transported to a local hospital, where she was pronounced dead.

You should always be aware of the hazards involved with moving fire apparatus. Even when the situation is not deemed urgent, remain alert to your surroundings. An injury can occur at any time—not just during emergency situations.

at several heights, including one that is lower than the fire apparatus. You must be capable of judging the vertical and horizontal clearances of the fire apparatus.

During the entire exercise, the fire apparatus must remain within the marker cones and move in a continuous motion, except when required to change direction of travel. A spotter is necessary for this exercise.

To perform the diminishing clearance exercise, follow the steps in SKILL DRILL 6-5.

Returning to the Station

When returning to the fire station, you cannot become complacent. Operating an emergency vehicle on the roadway can be dangerous even when driving back from a call. You may be fatigued and unable to react appropriately. Civilian drivers may think that the fire apparatus is responding to an emergency and unexpectedly stop in front of it. Some civilian drivers, while trying to be courteous, may wave or invite the fire apparatus into traffic ahead of them. While their intentions are good, you must always obey the rules of the road and be cautious of other drivers. Do not allow anyone to force you into traffic.

When the fire apparatus returns to the firehouse, it should be allowed to cool whenever possible. This should take place on the ramp of the firehouse rather than inside the facility, as the high exhaust temperatures can cause serious damage to exhaust removal hoses and equipment. This practice helps extend the life of the engine and transmission. If the fire apparatus is driven hard everywhere it goes and does not have adequate time to cool down before being shut off, damage to the power train may occur over time.

Reversing the Fire Apparatus

For most fire departments, the largest number of fire apparatus accidents are related to backing up fire apparatus. Very few fire departments respond with only one member on the fire apparatus. If two or more

SKILL DRILL 6-5
Performing a Diminishing Clearance Exercise NFPA 1002, 4.3.5, 4.3.5(B)

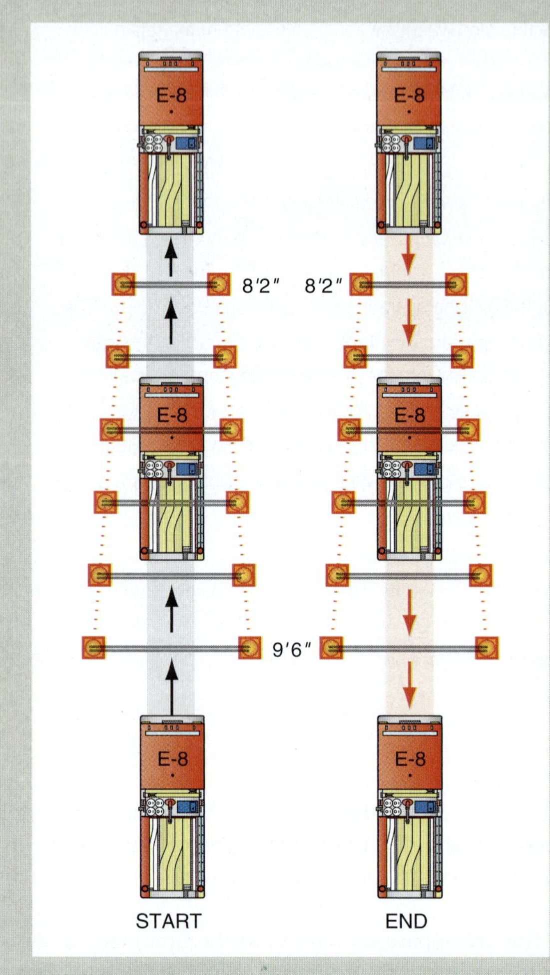

1. Position the fire apparatus at the opening of the diminishing clearance. Proceed forward through the lane. Stop the fire apparatus at the finish line.
2. Proceed in reverse through the lane. Identify any vertical heights on the crossbar that may strike the fire apparatus.

members are on the fire apparatus, this type of accident is entirely preventable. Every fire department should have an SOP that covers fire apparatus backing procedures. In turn, each member of the fire department needs to be trained and held accountable for these procedures.

Most modern fire stations are now built with drive-through bays so that fire apparatus do not have to back into the station. While this arrangement may reduce the number of backing-up accidents at the station, it may also contribute to backing-up skills becoming rusty.

Whenever an emergency vehicle is backing up, its emergency lights should be turned on, and the driver/operator should use a spotter to assist with the procedure. A **spotter** is a person who guides the driver/operator into the appropriate position while the apparatus is operating in a confined space or in reverse mode. The spotter should always be in the driver/operator's full view FIGURE 6-5. No vehicle should be backed into an intersection, around a corner, into the fire station, or in traffic unless emergency lighting is used and a spotter precedes it to safely direct such movement. During poor-visibility conditions, rear apparatus spotlights may be used as necessary. Never hesitate to use more than one spotter to assist with backing-up maneuvers if the situation warrants. If the driver/operator cannot see the spotter at any time, the vehicle should be stopped.

It is your responsibility to ensure that all spotters know in advance what is expected, where you intend to back up the fire apparatus, and which signals will be used. Before backing up the fire apparatus, roll down the windows and turn off any audio equipment to ensure any orders to stop the fire apparatus given

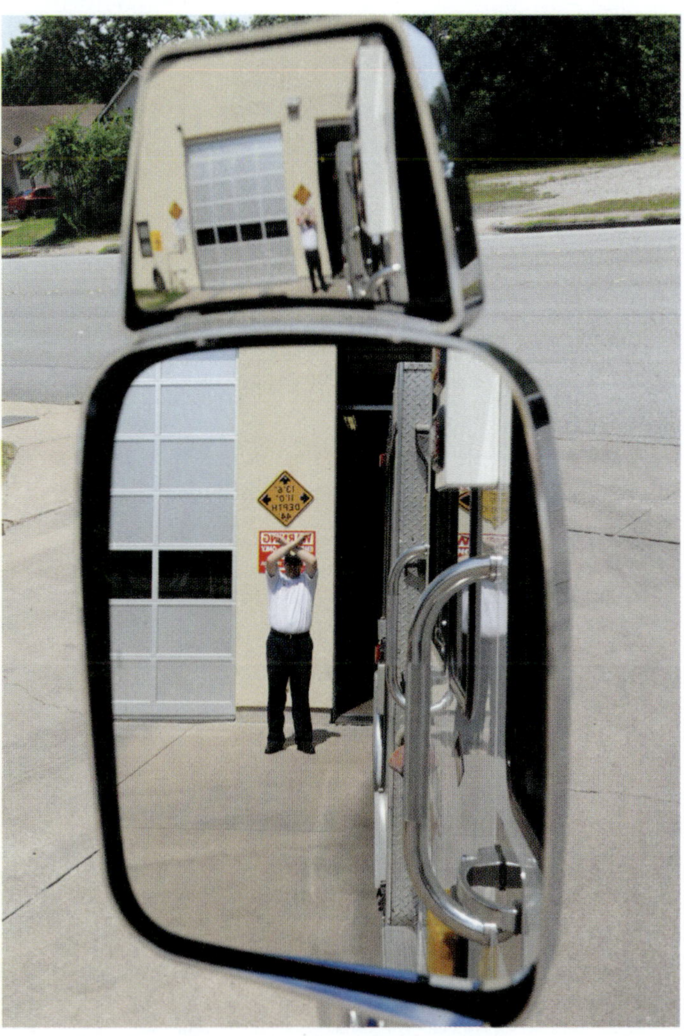

Figure 6-5 The spotter should always be in your full view.

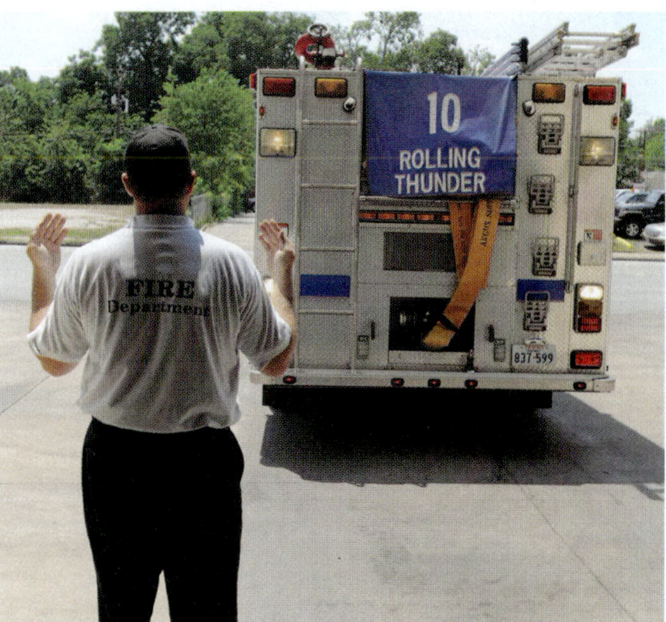

Figure 6-6 Arm placement when the spotter is directing the fire apparatus in a straight line.

by the spotter are clearly heard and understood. The spotter should use a portable radio to communicate with you. Any verbal communication between the driver/operator and the spotter should take place via radio.

The following are some suggested procedures for spotters:

- The rear spotter must stay behind and to the left of the fire apparatus. This spotter should position his or her body as a landmark for you to line up on. The spotter should always be able to see you in the side mirror. If the spotter cannot see you, then you cannot see the spotter. Stop immediately!
- Any spotter can give a loud "Stop!" order directly to you when it is deemed necessary.
- During high noise conditions, one spotter must be equipped with a radio to inform you to stop. Select an appropriate radio channel for this communication.
- All verbal signals must be loud enough and clear enough to be heard by you.
- All hand signals must be in "large" movements and as simple as possible. Signals given in front of the body can be difficult to see.
- While the fire apparatus is backing up at night or in limited-visibility conditions, the spotters should use flashlights to illuminate the surrounding area and hand signals.
- When the spotter is directing the fire apparatus backward or forward in a straight line, the spotter should have both arms extended forward and slightly wider than the body, parallel to the ground. The palms should face the direction of desired travel. The spotter bends both arms repeatedly toward the head and chest to direct the fire apparatus FIGURE 6-6.
- When the spotter is directing the fire apparatus either to the right or to the left while it is moving, the spotter should have the directional arm extended from the side of the body, parallel to the ground, indicating the direction in which to travel. The motioning arm should be extended in the opposite direction (palm upward) and repeatedly bent toward the head, indicating the desired direction of travel FIGURE 6-7.
- To provide the driver/operator with a visual reference for the distance to the stopping point, the spotter should have both arms extended sideways with elbows bent upward at 90 degrees. The spotter's palms should face forward, hands above the head, and the spotter should bring the elbows forward as the distance narrows.

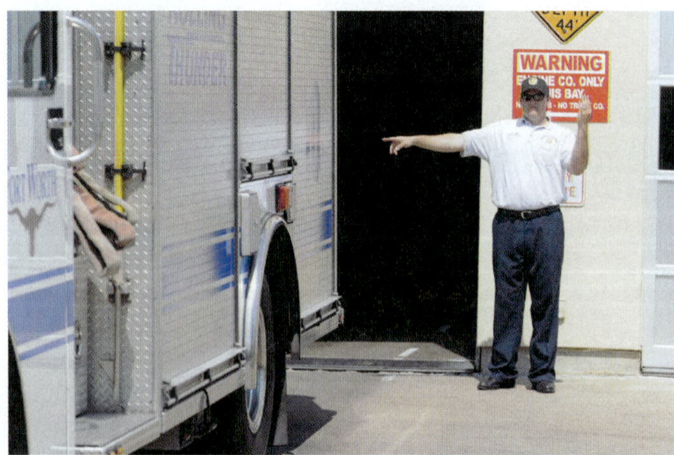

Figure 6-7 Arm placement when the spotter is directing the fire apparatus right or left.

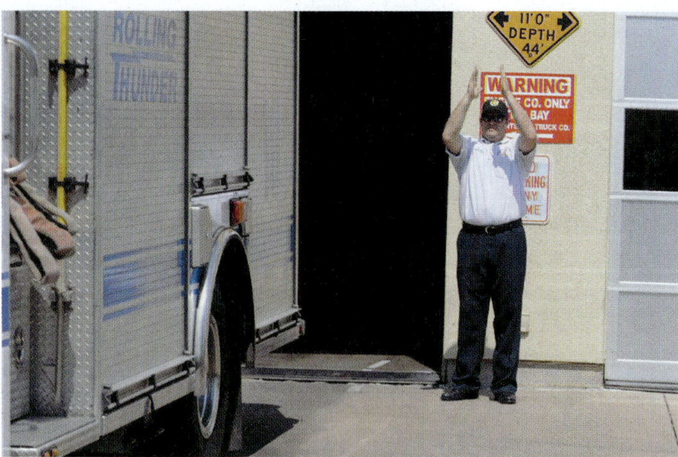

Figure 6-8 This spotter is indicating how much room the driver/operator has to maneuver before he or she needs to stop.

As the elbows reach the straightforward position, the spotter's hands continue coming together above the head to indicate that the stopping point is being reached. Upon reaching the stopping point, the spotter should give a loud "Stop!" signal FIGURE 6-8.

- The spotter may signal to stop the fire apparatus when it has reached the desired objective or if the safety of the operation is compromised. To do so, the spotter crosses the arms at the wrist (forearms) above the head and then maintains this position until the fire apparatus comes to a complete stop. While motioning with the arms, the spotter should also shout as loudly as possible, "Stop!" These actions should catch your attention and cause you to bring the fire apparatus to a halt FIGURE 6-9.

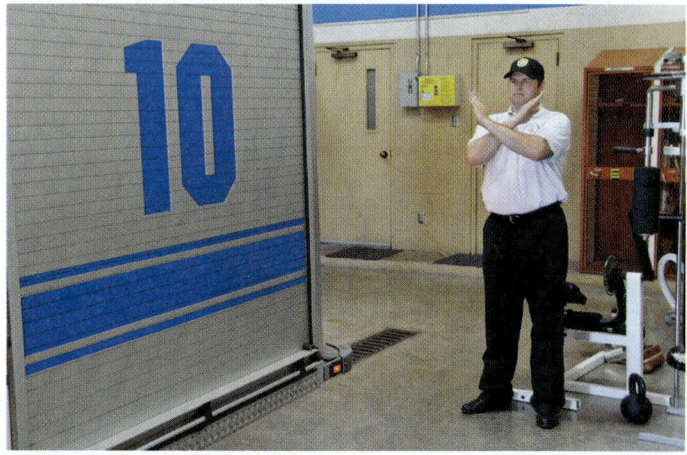

Figure 6-9 The signal to halt.

In most circumstances, the driver/operator is able to operate the fire apparatus in reverse without receiving instructions from a spotter. In these cases, it is the spotter's responsibility to ensure that the driver/operator does not hit anything or anyone. Regardless of the number of spotters utilized, you should receive directions only from one spotter in the rear of the vehicle and, if utilized, from one spotter to the front of the fire apparatus. If the fire apparatus is equipped with a rear-mounted camera, you should use it as well FIGURE 6-10. This technology should not take the place of an actual spotter but simply serves to augment your ability to see what is behind you.

NFPA 1002 requires that all driver/operators complete an exercise that simulates backing up a fire apparatus into a fire station, known as the station parking procedure drill. A fire apparatus bay is simulated by allowing for a 20-ft (6-m) minimum setback from a street that is 30 ft (9 m) wide; barricades are placed at the end of the setback, spaced 12 ft (3.7 m) apart to simulate the garage door. The setback distance should accurately reflect those distances found during normal duties. A marker placed on the ground indicates the proper position of the left-front tire of the fire apparatus once stopped and parked. A reference line may be used to facilitate using the fire apparatus mirrors. The minimum depth of the fire apparatus bay is determined by the length of the fire apparatus. During the entire exercise, the fire apparatus must remain within the marked boundary and should move in a continuous motion, except when required to change direction of travel. A spotter is necessary for this exercise.

To perform the procedure for backing a fire apparatus into a fire station bay, follow the steps in SKILL DRILL 6-6.

Although it is not recommended, during an emergency situation a fire apparatus may have to be backed up without a spotter. In this situation, you should do a preliminary inspection; check for obstructions, vertical and horizontal clearances, and power lines, and ensure that all compartments, doors, latches, and gates are closed. Proceed with extreme caution, and back the unit just far enough to where it can be turned around and then driven forward.

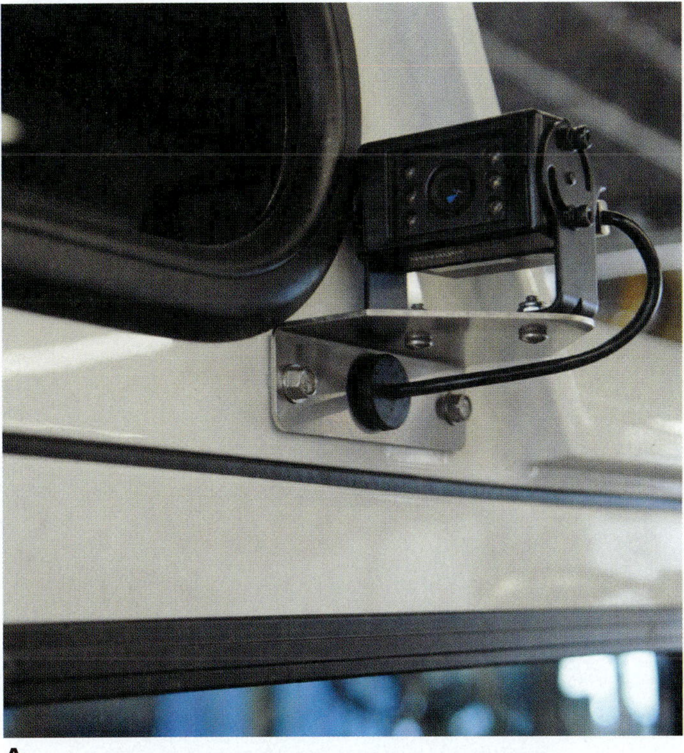

A

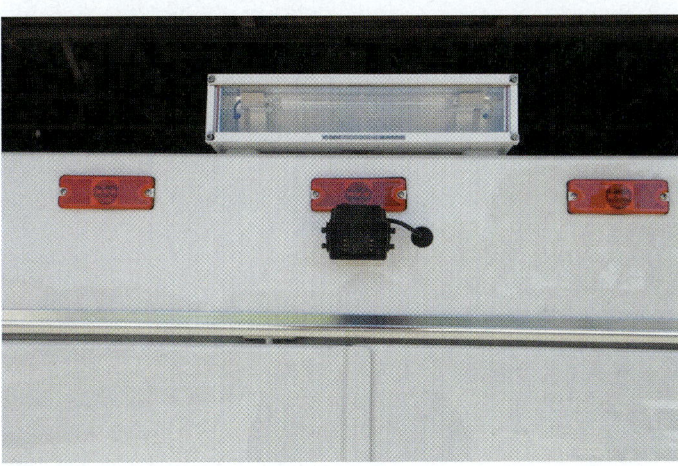

B

Figure 6-10 A camera is an important piece of safety equipment. **A.** Side-mounted camera. **B.** Rear-mounted camera.

LISTEN UP!

Some fire apparatus may be equipped with a 15- to 20-ft (4.5- to 6.1-m) coiled wire and push button for the spotter to use while the fire apparatus is being operated in reverse. This device plugs into the rear of the fire apparatus and allows the spotter to directly communicate with the driver/operator. Wireless intercom headsets are found more commonly with modern apparatus.

SAFETY TIP

At night, spotters should use flashlights. You should stop immediately if the spotter disappears from the rear-view mirror.

Shutting Down the Fire Apparatus

Once the fire apparatus is inside the fire station, it should be properly shut down. All of the electrical loads should be turned off first, including the headlights, air conditioner/heater, emergency lights, and any other electrical load that has an on/off switch. If these switches are left in the "on" position, the components will put an unnecessary load on the system the next time the fire apparatus is started.

Next, shift the transmission into neutral, and engage the parking brake. If needed, allow the fire apparatus to cool down before shutting it off. This is best done with the fire apparatus sitting at an idle rate for 3 to 5 minutes. Allowing the apparatus to cool down is best accomplished on the ramp, rather than in the firehouse. Repeatedly operating the apparatus in the firehouse can cause damage to the exhaust removal hoses due to excessive temperature (particularly with newer diesel engines). The engine's lubricating oil and coolant fluid are able to carry heat away from the combustion chamber, bearings, shafts, and other engine components when the engine is run at idle speed. This cool-down step is particularly important with turbocharged engines, because the delicate bearings and seals inside the turbocharger are subject to the high heat of combustion exhaust gases. This heat is carried away by normal oil circulation while the engine is operating. If the engine is abruptly stopped, however, the turbocharger temperature may increase considerably and perhaps result in seized bearings or loose oil seals. Failure to adequately cool the engine for the proper length of time before shutdown can lead to reduced engine life and engine component failure.

Finally, turn the ignition and battery switches to the off position. Reconnect any electrical shore lines, exhaust, and extractor systems.

As the driver/operator, you are responsible for the readiness of the fire apparatus at all times. Before anything else is done at the station, the fire apparatus must be returned to a ready state. Any equipment that was used during the emergency must be replaced, cleaned, or repaired. If the call was for emergency medical services (EMS) and only a few bandages were used, then replace them. If the fire apparatus returned from a small rubbish fire and the onboard water tank is now low, then fill the water tank **FIGURE 6-11**. If the SCBA and other equipment need to be cleaned after crew members responded to a structure fire, then clean these items and return the equipment to service.

To perform the procedure for shutting down and securing a fire apparatus, follow the steps in **SKILL DRILL 6-7**.

SKILL DRILL 6-6

Backing a Fire Apparatus Into a Fire Station Bay NFPA 1002, 4.3.2, 4.3.2(B)

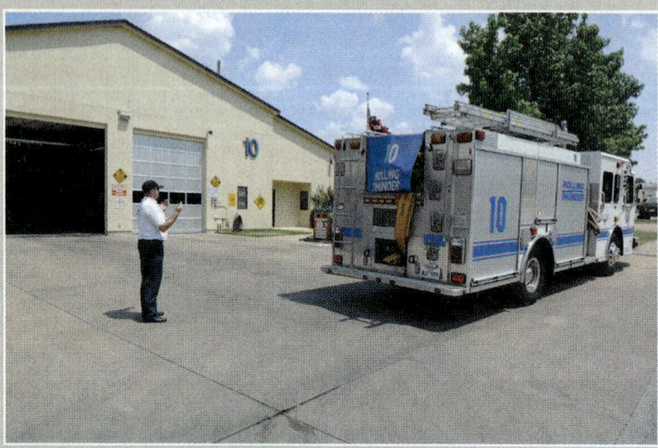

1 Position the rear of the fire apparatus past the fire station bay's opening at a 90-degree angle to the station. Ensure a spotter is correctly positioned behind the fire apparatus.

Activate the emergency lights.

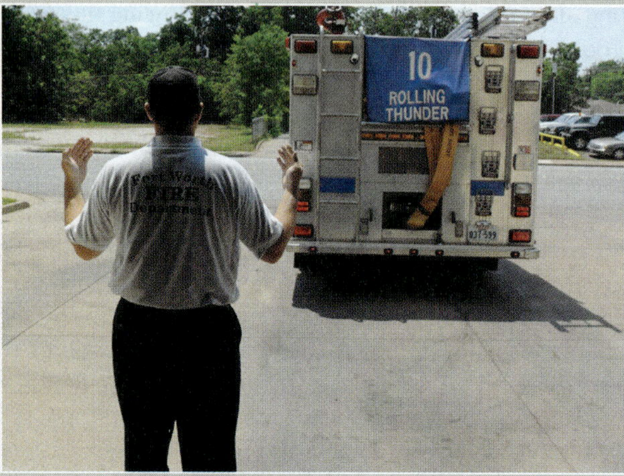

2 Turn off any fire apparatus–mounted stereo equipment.

Disengage the parking brake, if set.

Shift the transmission to reverse.

Proceed in a reverse mode, and turn the fire apparatus to align it with the objective.

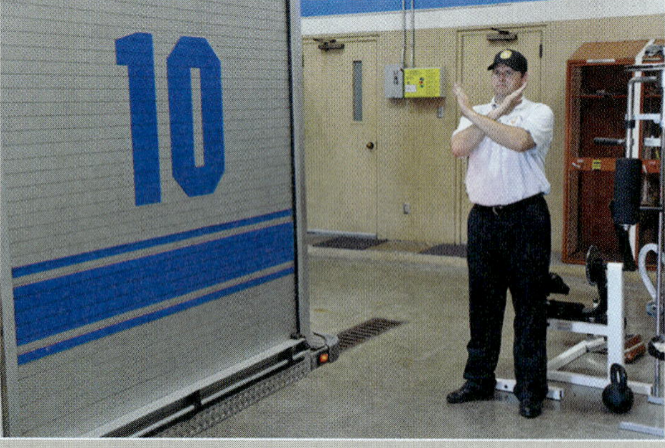

3 Continue backing the fire apparatus until it has reached the desired objective or the spotter signals "Stop."

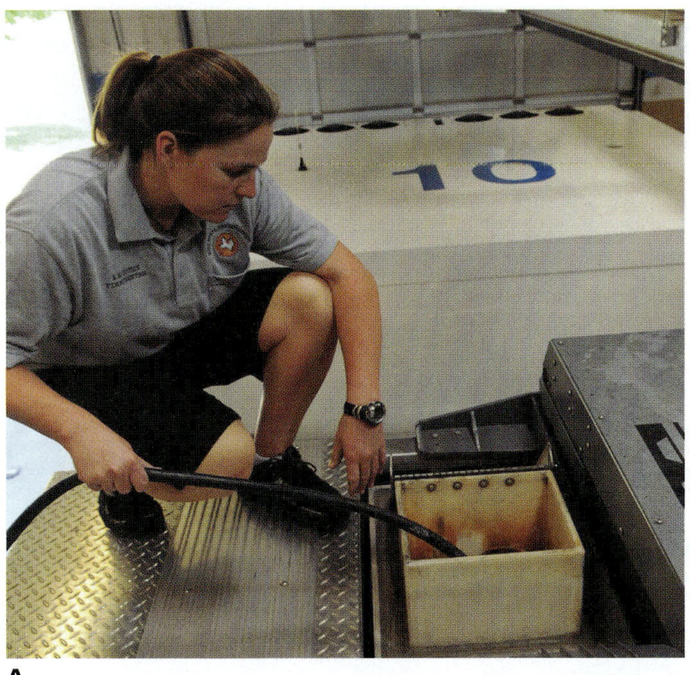

A

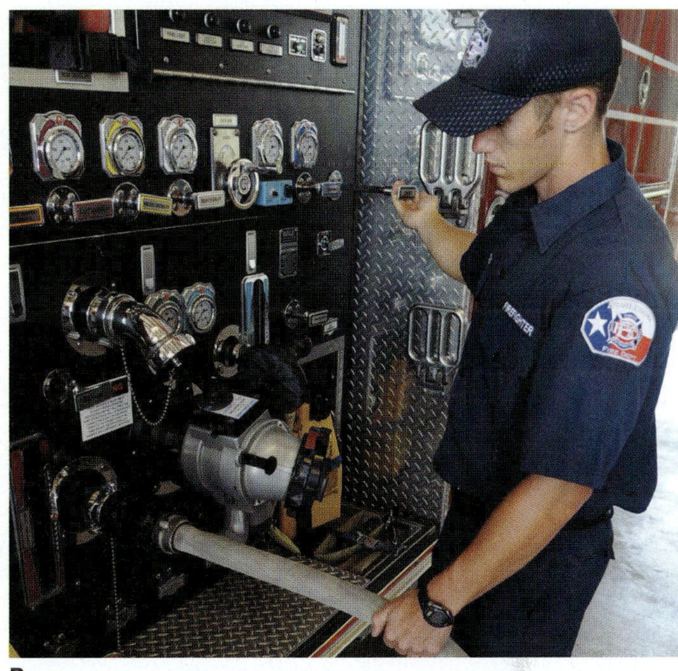

B

Figure 6-11 Fill the onboard tank if it is low. This can be done two ways: **A.** with a garden hose or **B.** with a fire department hoseline.

SKILL DRILL 6-7

Shutting Down and Securing a Fire Apparatus NFPA 1002, 4.3.1, 4.3.1(B)

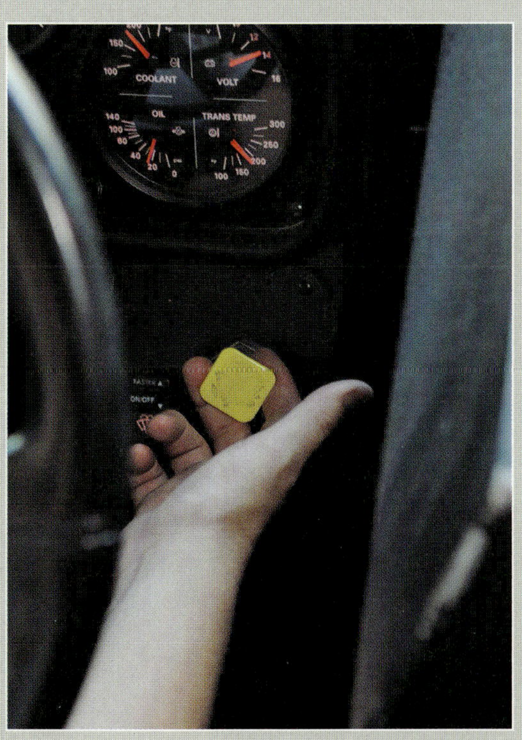

1. Turn off the emergency lights, headlights, and any other electrical loads.

   Shift the transmission into neutral.

   Engage the parking brake.

(continued)

SKILL DRILL 6-7 Continued

Shutting Down and Securing a Fire Apparatus NFPA 1002, 4.3.1, 4.3.1(B)

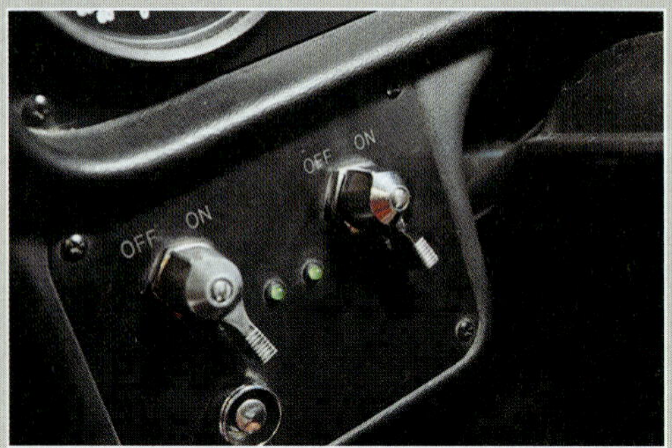

2 Ensure that the apparatus has adequately cooled down before shutting it off.

Turn the ignition switch to the "off" position.

Turn the battery to the "off" position.

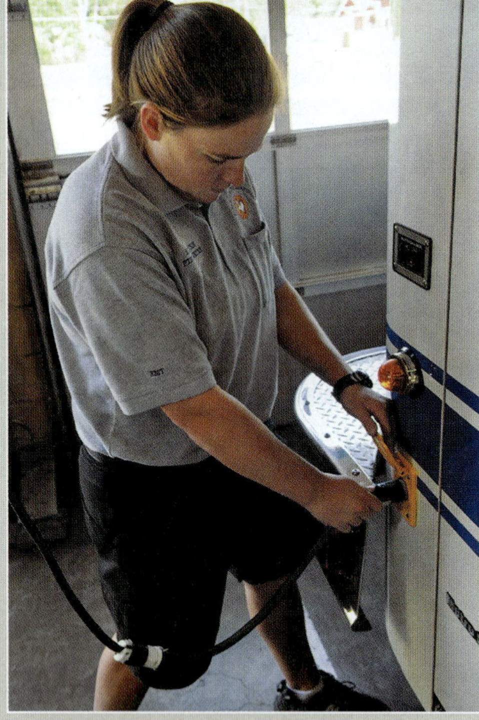

3 Reconnect any applicable electrical cords and extractor systems.

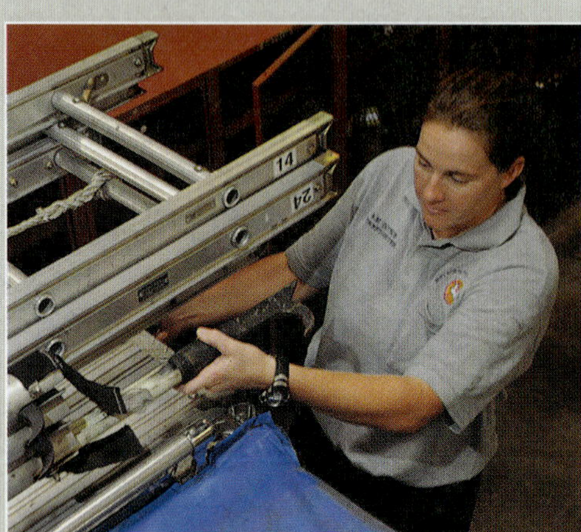

4 Replace, clean, and repair any used equipment.

After-Action REVIEW

IN SUMMARY

- The driver/operator must complete a preliminary inspection before the fire apparatus is considered ready to depart for the response.
- The driver/operator should follow the recommended starting sequence for the fire apparatus.
- Before the fire apparatus can get under way, you must ensure that all company members are seated and wearing seat belts, so as to satisfy NFPA 1500.
- While responding to the scene, the driver/operator may need to complete several maneuvers so that the fire apparatus can access the incident. NFPA 1002 requires the driver/operator to complete several exercises to prove his or her skill in managing these situations.
- As a driver/operator, you should not become complacent when returning to the station.
- Follow safe procedures when backing up the fire apparatus. Always use spotters to assist with backup operations.
- When operating a fire apparatus in reverse, stop immediately if you lose sight of the spotter.
- Follow the standard sequence for shutting down the fire apparatus.

KEY TERMS

air pressure gauges Gauges that identify the air pressure stored in the tanks or reservoirs of an apparatus equipped with a pneumatic braking system.

battery selector switch A switch used to disconnect all electrical power to the vehicle, thereby preventing discharge of the battery while the vehicle is not in use.

due regard The care exercised by a reasonably prudent person under the same circumstances.

fuel gauge A gauge that indicates the amount of fuel in the fire apparatus' fuel tank.

ignition switch A switch that engages operational power to the chassis of a motor vehicle.

oil pressure gauge A gauge that identifies the pressure of the lubricating oil in the fire apparatus engine.

parking brake The main brake that prevents the fire apparatus from moving even when it is turned off and there is no one operating it.

spotter A person who guides the driver/operator into the appropriate position while operating in a confined space or in reverse mode.

starter switch The switch that engages the starter motor for cranking.

system check sequence A series of checks that an electrical system completes to ensure that all of the systems are functioning properly before the fire apparatus is started.

voltmeter A device that measures the voltage across a battery's terminals and gives an indication of the electrical condition of the battery.

REFERENCES

National Fire Protection Association (NFPA) 1002, *Standard for Fire Apparatus Driver/Operator Professional Qualifications*. 2017. http://www.nfpa.org/codes-and-standards/all-codes-and-standards/list-of-codes-and-standards/detail?code=1002. Accessed December 27, 2017.

National Fire Protection Association (NFPA) 1500, *Standard on Fire Department Occupational Safety, Health, and Wellness Program*. 2018. http://www.nfpa.org/codes-and-standards/all-codes-and-standards/list-of-codes-and-standards/detail?code=1500. Accessed December 27, 2017.

National Fire Protection Association (NFPA) 1901, *Standard for Automotive Fire Apparatus*. 2016. http://www.nfpa.org/codes-and-standards/all-codes-and-standards/list-of-codes-and-standards/detail?code=1901. Accessed December 27, 2017.

On Scene

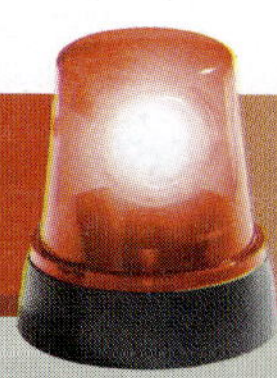

While your company is returning to the firehouse from the last fire, your company officer commends you and the other members of the crew for performing so well. He is pleased with how you maneuvered the apparatus around the rear of the fire building and set the apparatus in a position to adequately perform its task. He asks that you explain some of the training that you received from the department's training division on how to drive a fire apparatus.

1. Which switch delivers operational power to the chassis?
   - A. Starter switch
   - B. Ignition switch
   - C. On switch
   - D. Chassis switch
2. NFPA 1901 requires that a fire apparatus be capable of moving within _____ seconds of starting up.
   - A. 30
   - B. 40
   - C. 50
   - D. 60
3. Who on the apparatus is responsible to ensure all personnel are seated with their seat belts fastened while the apparatus is in motion?
   - A. The company officer
   - B. The driver/operator
   - C. The fire fighter
   - D. Everyone on the apparatus
4. Who is responsible for ensuring that the spotters know in advance what is expected when the apparatus is being backed up?
   - A. The fire chief
   - B. The company officer
   - C. The training officer
   - D. The driver/operator
5. Whenever possible, you should allow the engine to warm up for _____ minutes.
   - A. 1 to 2
   - B. 3 to 5
   - C. 5 to 7
   - D. 7 to 10

CHAPTER 7

Emergency Vehicle Driving

KNOWLEDGE OBJECTIVES

After studying this chapter, you will be able to:

- Describe pre-emergency response dispatch information.
- Discuss the various mapping systems used in the fire service.
- Discuss emergency vehicle operations laws.
- Describe the effects of vehicle control during a liquid surge on the roadway. (**NFPA 1002, 4.3.1, 4.3.1(A), 4.3.6, 4.3.6(A)**)
- Describe the effect of a wet roadway on the braking reaction time. (**NFPA 1002, 4.3.1, 4.3.1(A), 4.3.6, 4.3.6(A)**)
- Describe the effect of the fire apparatus' load on the control of the vehicle on a wet roadway. (**NFPA 1002, 4.3.1, 4.3.1(A), 4.3.6, 4.3.6(A)**)
- Describe the risk of a fire apparatus roll-over due to the effects of the apparatus' high center of gravity. (**NFPA 1002, 4.3.1, 4.3.1(A), 4.3.6, 4.3.6(A)**)
- Describe general steering reactions of a fire apparatus. (**NFPA 1002, 4.3.1, 4.3.1(A), 4.3.6, 4.3.6(A)**)
- Describe the effect of speed in controlling a fire apparatus on the roadway. (**NFPA 1002, 4.3.1, 4.3.1(A), 4.3.6, 4.3.6(A)**)
- Describe the effect of centrifugal force in controlling a fire apparatus on the roadway. (**NFPA 1002, 4.3.1, 4.3.1(A), 4.3.6, 4.3.6(A)**)
- Describe the applicable laws and regulations in operating a fire apparatus. (**NFPA 1002, 4.3.1, 4.3.1(A), 4.3.6, 4.3.6(A)**)
- Describe the principles of skid avoidance when operating a fire apparatus. (**NFPA 1002, 4.3.1, 4.3.1(A), 4.3.6, 4.3.6(A)**)
- Describe the principles of safe night driving of a fire apparatus. (**NFPA 1002, 4.3.1, 4.3.1(A), 4.3.6, 4.3.6(A)**)
- Discuss proper shifting and gear patterns of a fire apparatus. (**NFPA 1002, 4.3.1, 4.3.1(A), 4.3.6, 4.3.6(A)**)
- Describe how to safely cross intersections, railroad crossings, and bridges. (**NFPA 1002, 4.3.1, 4.3.1(A), 4.3.6, 4.3.6(A)**)
- Describe the weight and height limitations of a fire apparatus for both roads and bridges. (**NFPA 1002, 4.3.1, 4.3.1(A), 4.3.6, 4.3.6(A)**)
- Describe how to control the fire apparatus using defensive driving techniques under emergency conditions. (**NFPA 1002, 4.3.6, 4.3.6(A), 4.3.6(B)**)
- Explain how fire stations receive and process dispatch information. (**NFPA 1002, 4.4.1**)
- Identify the information in a typical dispatch message. (**NFPA 1002, 4.4.1**)
- Describe your responsibilities as you approach an emergency scene.
- Describe Level I and II staging procedures.

92

- Identify potential hazards while approaching emergency incidents.
- Describe the driver/operator's role when positioning the fire apparatus to operate at various emergency incidents.
- Describe how to operate a fire apparatus safely through an intersection. (**NFPA 1002, 4.3.1, 4.3.1(A), 4.3.6, 4.3.6(A)**)
- Describe how to operate a fire apparatus across a railroad crossing. (**NFPA 1002, 4.3.1, 4.3.1(A), 4.3.6, 4.3.6(A)**)
- Describe how to operate a fire apparatus on a curve, either left or right. (**NFPA 1002, 4.3.1, 4.3.1(A), 4.3.6, 4.3.6(A)**)
- Describe how to operate a fire apparatus on a section of limited-access highway with an entrance and exit ramp. (**NFPA 1002, 4.3.1, 4.3.1(A), 4.3.6, 4.3.6(A)**)
- Describe how to operate a fire apparatus while passing other vehicles. (**NFPA 1002, 4.3.1, 4.3.1(A), 4.3.6, 4.3.6(A)**)
- Describe how to operate a fire apparatus on a downgrade requiring a down-shift and braking. (**NFPA 1002, 4.3.1, 4.3.1(A), 4.3.6, 4.3.6(A)**)
- Describe how to operate a fire apparatus on an upgrade requiring a gear change to maintain speed. (**NFPA 1002, 4.3.1, 4.3.1(A), 4.3.6, 4.3.6(A)**)
- Describe how to operate a fire apparatus and travel safely under either an underpass or a low-clearance bridge. (**NFPA 1002, 4.3.1, 4.3.1(A), 4.3.6, 4.3.6(A)**)
- Describe how to maintain safe following distances when operating a fire apparatus. (**NFPA 1002, 4.3.1, 4.3.1(A), 4.3.6, 4.3.6(A)**)
- Describe how to accelerate in a fire apparatus. (**NFPA 1002, 4.3.1, 4.3.1(A), 4.3.6, 4.3.6(A)**)
- Describe how to decelerate in a fire apparatus. (**NFPA 1002, 4.3.1, 4.3.1(A), 4.3.6, 4.3.6(A)**)
- Describe how to turn in a fire apparatus. (**NFPA 1002, 4.3.1, 4.3.1(A), 4.3.6, 4.3.6(A)**)
- Describe how to operate the fire apparatus safely under adverse driving conditions. (**NFPA 1002, 4.3.1, 4.3.1(A), 4.3.6, 4.3.6(A)**)
- Describe the operational limits of the fire apparatus.

SKILLS OBJECTIVES

After studying this chapter, you will be able to:

- Identify dispatch information.
- Perform the alley dock exercise with the fire apparatus. (**NFPA 1002, 4.3.4, 4.3.4(B)**)

Additional NFPA Standards

- **NFPA 1001**, *Standard for Fire Fighter Professional Qualifications*
- **NFPA 1500**, *Standard on Fire Department Occupational Safety, Health, and Wellness Program*
- **NFPA 1561**, *Standard on Emergency Services Incident Management System and Command Safety*
- **NFPA 1620**, *Standard for Pre-incident Planning*
- **NFPA 1901**, *Standard for Automotive Fire Apparatus*

Emergency Call

You have been assigned to the position of driver/operator and are working your first shift in a new fire station. It has been a few hours since your shift began. So far, you have checked and washed the apparatus and completed training. You have just sat down to eat lunch when you hear the tones go off. As the dispatch comes in at the station, your heart begins to race. You quickly write down the incident address and look up the exact location on the station's map before going to the apparatus bay.

1. How should you respond to this call?
2. Which other units may be responding?
3. How should you position the apparatus upon arrival?

Introduction

Driving a fire apparatus to an emergency is one of the most exciting tasks driver/operators will perform. It can also be one of the deadliest tasks that they will perform. Each year fire fighters are killed and injured while responding to and from emergency incidents. Data trends indicate that fewer fire fighters are dying on the fireground, both in actual numbers and in relative terms; however, more are being killed while responding to emergency incidents or performing duties other than fighting fires. Each time a company rolls out of the station to respond to a call, the fire fighters put their lives at risk. This chapter discusses the laws and regulations that pertain to driving the fire apparatus to an emergency scene. It also discusses safe driving practices for driver/operators to follow so that they can do their job successfully—that is, get fire fighters to the emergency scene to help others.

Pump/Water Supply Operator

In the fire service, **response** comprises a series of actions that begin when a crew is dispatched to an alarm and end with the crew's arrival at the emergency incident. Response actions include receiving the alarm, donning protective clothing and equipment, mounting the apparatus, and transporting equipment and personnel to the emergency incident quickly and safely. Because fire crews must be ready to react immediately to an alarm, preparations for response begin long before the alarm sounds. These preparations include checking personal equipment, ensuring that the fire apparatus is ready, and making sure that all equipment carried on the apparatus is ready for use. Driver/operators also should be familiar with their response district, know the buildings under their protection, and understand their department's standard operating procedures (SOPs). Other response actions for the apparatus driver include considering road and traffic conditions, determining the best route to the incident, identifying nearby hydrant locations or water sources, and selecting the best position for the apparatus at the incident scene.

Pre-Emergency Vehicle Response

Most emergency responses start with the dispatch for an emergency. The driver/operator and the rest of the crew will receive a message about the emergency that indicates the type of emergency, the location of the emergency incident, and the assigned tactical radio frequency. The driver/operator then locates the emergency scene on a map using the information given during the dispatch and determines the most efficient response route using the department's mapping system. In addition, the driver/operator determines the fire apparatus response mode for the emergency based on the information in the dispatch.

Dispatch

Pump/Water Supply Operator

The emergency response process begins when an alarm is received at the fire station. Fire personnel should be familiar with the dispatch method or methods used by their departments. In many fire departments, a local or regional communications center dispatches individual units. In smaller departments, the dispatcher may be located at the fire station or another location.

Although radio, telephone, and public address systems are often used to transmit information to fire stations, the use of computer terminals and printers to transmit dispatch messages is increasing. Some fire departments still use a system of bells to transmit alarms. Although volunteer or rural departments may use outdoor sirens or horns to summon personnel to an emergency, most volunteer fire personnel receive dispatch messages over pagers or cell phones.

The **communications center** gives the information for the emergency to responders in the form of a dispatch. **Dispatch** is the process of sending out emergency response resources promptly to an address or incident location for a specific purpose. This step is usually performed by a telecommunicator at the communications center. The communications center must have at least two separate ways of notifying each fire station—a primary method and a backup method. The primary method may consist of a hard-wired circuit, a telephone line, a data link, a microwave link, or a radio system.

The majority of fire departments use verbal messages to alert those units that are responding to the incident. This dispatch may be announced from speakers located in the station or via an apparatus-mounted radio. In some fire departments, response vehicles may be equipped with **mobile data terminals (MDTs)**—that is, computers located on the fire apparatus FIGURE 7-1. With this approach, the dispatch information

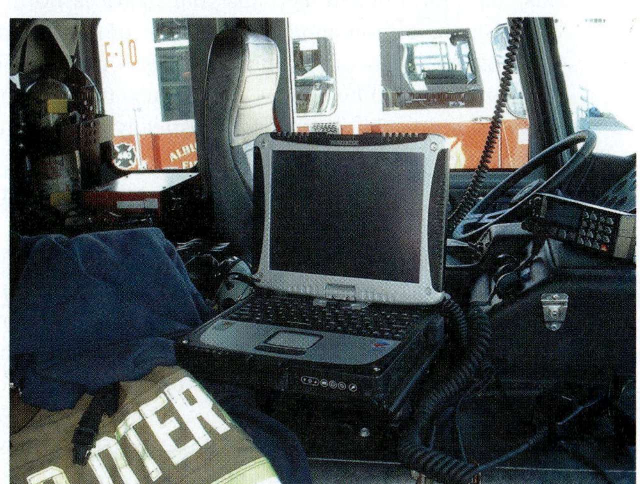

Figure 7-1 A mobile data terminal.
Courtesy of Paul W. Dow.

can be transmitted to the fire apparatus through both the radio speakers and the MDT. Sensitive information may be transmitted only to the MDT, without announcing it over a radio frequency, as radio communications may be monitored by the media.

When dispatched for an emergency, whether the message is delivered at the fire station or in the fire apparatus, you should always pay attention to the following information:

- **Type of emergency.** This may be a structure fire, emergency medical services (EMS) call, or nonemergency call for service. The information given will determine how you will respond—that is, emergency mode or nonemergency mode. Each fire department should have a predetermined response mode for all types of incidents to which its personnel will respond. For example, when dispatched to a structure fire, the unit may respond to the scene with lights and sirens. In contrast, if the fire apparatus is dispatched to a non-life-threatening call, it may respond without lights and sirens. Always follow your local SOPs in determining the mode of response.
- **Location of the emergency.** Each dispatch includes the physical address of the emergency. Usually, the dispatch also contains information such as cross streets, the geographical location of the response district, and possibly grid numbers to locate the incident on a map. These data are used to pinpoint the location of the incident.
- **Description of the incident.** The dispatcher should clearly describe what is happening at the incident. This information may include the victim's condition during an EMS incident or the location of a fire in a multistory occupancy.
- **Other responding units.** You should be familiar with your fire department's normal response to emergencies. If your fire apparatus is dispatched to a structure fire in your response district and the units that normally respond with your company are not dispatched as well, this can be a problem. Perhaps your district's normal backup units are on another call or out of service for training. Although other units may respond in their place, there could be a delay in response time. At the scene of a fire, this factor can drastically change the tactics of the initial units.
- **The assigned tactical radio frequency.** Each fire department should be capable of assigning units to a separate radio channel for on-scene tactical communications. During the initial dispatch to a structure fire or as part of other multicompany responses, most fire departments assign a tactical channel to the responding units. You need to ensure that you are on the correct channel while responding.
- **Additional information from the dispatcher.** Most dispatchers provide some additional information to a responding fire apparatus while the unit is en route to the call. This information can be used to determine the appropriate action to take while responding to the incident. For example, if the dispatcher advises that the scene is a violent one, you might adjust your response. In some fire departments, responding units are required to stage several blocks from the scene until it is deemed safe by the local police department. During this type of response, the driver/operator would turn off the emergency lights and siren so that the unit is not identified until the scene is safe to enter.

As a driver/operator, you should carry a writing utensil and a notepad at all times. When a call goes out, you can then write down the information from the initial dispatch, especially the location of the emergency. Some calls and their locations may become well known to fire fighters—but that is no excuse to become complacent. Even veteran driver/operators can be stumped with an unusual address or location in their response area. Being prepared can help avoid confusion and ensures that valuable time is not wasted by asking for the communications center to retransmit the information. Write it down the first time!

Pump/Water Supply Operator

When an alarm is received, the crew's response should be prompt and efficient. Responding fire fighters should walk briskly to the apparatus. There is no need to run; the objective is to respond quickly, without injuring anyone or causing any damage. Follow established procedures to ensure that stoves, faucets, and other appliances at the station are shut off. Wait until the apparatus bay doors are fully open before leaving the station.

Maps

Because it can take years to learn a response area, you must be familiar with your maps. Some fire departments may not have maps for their response area but instead rely solely on the fire fighters' knowledge of the response area. While this approach may be effective for some fire departments, most have a map that driver/operators can use to locate incidents.

Fire department maps may be accessed several different ways. The most common type of map is found at the fire station. Usually it takes the form of a large paper map, which may be placed in various areas around the station. Most such maps show details of the fire station's primary response area, and some are color-coded to identify the response districts of other fire stations FIGURE 7-2. Paper maps may utilize a grid system that divides the entire response area into more specific areas, with these areas being sectioned off according to the fire station's response area. For example, in the Albuquerque (New Mexico) Fire Department, the entire city and surrounding county are divided into fire boxes. These areas may be several square blocks or several square miles, depending on the density of the

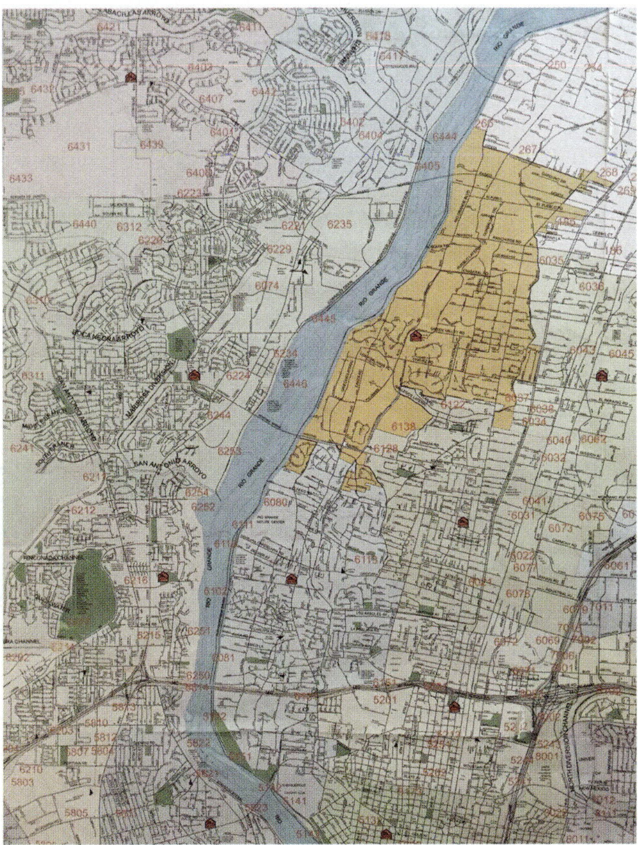

Figure 7-2 Some firefighting-specific maps are color-coded.
Courtesy of Paul W. Dow.

area. Each fire station has any number of fire boxes within its response area. When a call is dispatched, the incident's location is identified with an address and a fire box. This practice allows Albuquerque fire fighters to look on the map and locate first the station's response area, then the fire box, and finally the actual street address of the call.

Before you leave the station, you should reference the station-mounted map. Knowing where you are going saves valuable time during the response.

Smaller versions of the station-mounted maps may also be found on the fire apparatus. These maps are sometimes grouped with all of the neighboring districts' response areas. When responding to out-of-station calls, these maps can prove very useful. While such maps may not be as detailed as those found at the fire station, they are still effective.

You should never try to read a map while responding to an emergency. Firefighting is a team activity: Another member of the crew should reference the map and guide you.

Another map that some fire departments are now using is found on the MDT. When used in tandem with a **global positioning system (GPS)**, the MDT may be capable of pinpointing the exact location of the emergency in relation to your location. A GPS device uses satellite technology to locate the fire apparatus anywhere in a specified area. Some fire departments use this technology to dispatch the closest unit to an incident. When a call is dispatched, the information is transmitted to the MDT, so the location of the emergency appears on the screen and aids the driver/operator in locating the scene. Of all of the maps, this one is usually the easiest to update and may be the most current.

All of these maps used by fire fighters may have similar features. Sometimes they identify the sites of hydrants, enabling crews to locate a water supply while en route to the fire scene. The maps may also identify parks, schools, and other important features of the response area.

Whichever type of map your fire department uses, it is important to select a safe and efficient route when responding to each call. The goal is for the fire apparatus to arrive at the correct location in a safe and timely fashion. This responsibility will always fall upon you as the driver/operator.

To identify the critical information received from the dispatch, locate the emergency scene, and determine the proper route on the map and the response mode, follow the steps in SKILL DRILL 7-1.

SKILL DRILL 7-1
Determining the Fire Response Mode

1. Start with the dispatch information for an emergency. Using a notepad, document the type of emergency, the location of the emergency incident, and the assigned tactical radio frequency (if applicable).
2. Locate the emergency scene on a map using the information given during the dispatch.
3. From the fire station, determine the most efficient response route using the map.
4. Determine the fire apparatus response mode for this emergency, using the information from the dispatch.

DRIVER/OPERATOR TIP

Never hesitate to reference your station's map!

Pump/Water Supply Operator

Riding the Apparatus

Don your PPE before mounting the apparatus; do not attempt to dress while the apparatus is on the road. Your seat belt should be fastened whenever the apparatus is moving. Wait until you dismount at the incident scene to don any protective clothing that was not donned prior to mounting the apparatus.

All equipment should be properly mounted, stowed, or secured on the fire apparatus. Unsecured equipment in the crew compartment can prove dangerous if the apparatus must stop or turn quickly, because a flying tool, map book, or PPE can seriously injure a fire fighter.

Be careful when mounting and dismounting apparatus—the steps on fire apparatus are often high and can be slippery. Follow the steps in SKILL DRILL 7-2 to mount an apparatus properly.

Pump/Water Supply Operator

SKILL DRILL 7-2

Mounting Apparatus NFPA 1002, 5.2.1(B)

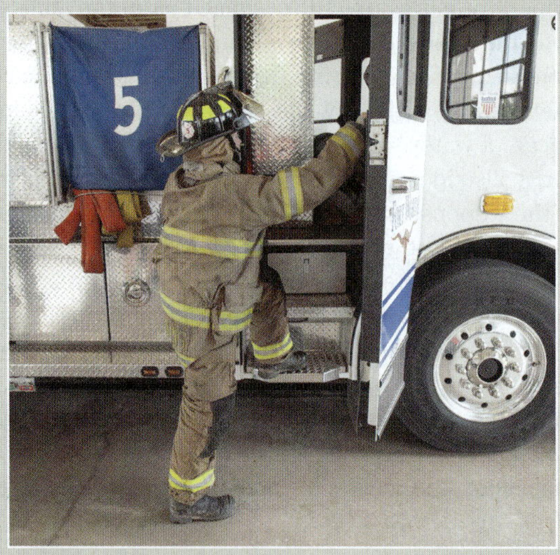

1. When mounting (climbing aboard) fire apparatus, always have at least one hand firmly grasping a handhold and at least one foot firmly placed on a foot surface. Maintain the one hand and one foot placement until you are seated.

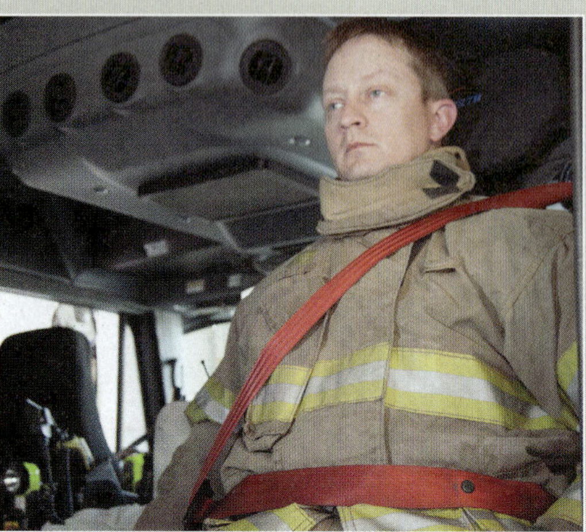

2. Fasten your seat belt, and leave it fastened until the apparatus is stopped at its destination. Don any other required safety equipment for the response, such as hearing protection and intercom.

All personnel must be seated in their assigned riding positions with seat belts and/or harnesses fastened before the apparatus begins to move. National Fire Protection Association (NFPA) 1500, *Standard on Fire Department Occupational Safety, Health, and Wellness Program*, and NFPA 1001, *Standard for Fire Fighter Professional Qualifications*, require all fire fighters to be in their seats, with seat belts secured, whenever the vehicle is in motion. Do not unbuckle your seat belt to don any clothing or equipment while the apparatus is en route to an incident.

The noise produced by sirens and air horns can have long-term, damaging effects on fire personnel's hearing. For this reason, your department should provide hearing protection for personnel riding on fire apparatus—and all crew members should use it. Some of these devices include radio and intercom capabilities so that crew members can talk to one another and hear information from the dispatcher or the incident commander (IC).

During transport, limit conversation to the exchange of pertinent information. Listen for instructions from the IC, for instructions from your company officer, and for additional information about the incident over the radio. As the driver/operator, your attention should be focused on driving the apparatus safely to the scene of the incident.

The ride to the incident is a good time for the crew to consider any relevant factors that could affect the situation. These factors could include the time of day or night, the temperature, the presence of precipitation or wind, the type of occupancy, the type of construction, and the location and type of incident.

Emergency Vehicle Laws

No member of any fire department should be allowed to drive an emergency vehicle or fire apparatus until that person has completed a training course approved by the fire department. Simply allowing any member to drive these vehicles without the proper training is irresponsible. Several Emergency Vehicle Operations courses are available, and each fire department should ensure that its members are trained to operate the fire apparatus that they will be driving. The days of allowing anyone with a driver's license to jump into the front seat and pilot the fire apparatus to the emergency scene are behind us. The fire service can and should provide personnel with qualified training to ensure that all driver/operators drive safely and act responsibly while operating emergency vehicles.

Each fire department is governed by federal regulations as well as by different state laws and local regulations. Some of these laws and regulations are very detailed and descriptive; others are vague and leave much of their interpretation to the members of the fire department. All members of the fire department should be familiar with applicable federal, state, provincial, and local regulations governing the operation of emergency vehicles, including their department's own procedures. A lack of knowledge regarding the applicable emergency vehicle driving laws is not an excuse for disobeying them. As the driver/operator of a fire apparatus, you must understand that you will be held responsible for your actions while driving an emergency vehicle. Driver/operators who are found to be at fault for an accident involving a fire apparatus may be prosecuted in both criminal and civil court—which can create many problems for those members both at work and at home. As a driver/operator, you must understand the local laws and regulations with which you must comply.

The use of sirens and warning lights does not automatically give the right-of-way to the fire apparatus. These devices simply request the right-of-way from other drivers, based on their awareness of the emergency vehicle's presence. You must take every step possible to make your presence and intended actions known to other drivers, and you must drive defensively so that you are prepared for unexpected and inappropriate actions from other vehicles. The driver/operator of a fire apparatus is not the only person allowed to use the roadway even under emergency conditions: You must follow many of the same laws as any other driver on the road.

Many states provide certain privileges to emergency vehicle driver/operators while they are responding to an emergency. They also specify the conditions under which these privileges are granted. For example, in New Mexico, the motor vehicle code states that the following four privileges may be granted as long as the emergency vehicle sounds an audible signal and the vehicle is operating with its emergency lights activated; all other laws apply during the emergency vehicle's response:

1. **Park or stand irrespective of the provisions of the motor vehicle code.** This privilege allows for the driver/operator to position the fire apparatus in the roadway to block the scene and provide for the safety of the fire fighters and those involved in the emergency.
2. **Proceed past a red or stop signal or stop sign but only after slowing down as necessary for safe operation.** The fire apparatus should come to a complete stop before proceeding through the intersection.
3. **Exceed the maximum speed limits as long as the driver/operator does not endanger life or property.** Many fire departments allow fire apparatus to exceed the posted speed limit by only 10 mi/h (16 km/h) during an emergency response and only in light traffic and good weather conditions.
4. **Disregard regulations governing direction of movement or turning in specified directions.** This provision allows the driver/operator to drive or position the vehicle against the flow of traffic. This maneuver should be done only in a safe and controlled manner. Some fire departments refer to this practice as "bucking" traffic and strictly prohibit it. Other fire departments allow moves against the normal flow of traffic to be made within one block of an incident and only for the purpose of positioning the fire apparatus.

These laws do not relieve you of the duty to drive with due regard for the safety of all persons, nor do they protect you from the consequences of reckless disregard for the safety of others. Each driver/operator is accountable for his or her own actions.

Other state or local laws that may apply to emergency vehicle operators include the following provisions:

- Comply with any lawful order or direction of any police officer invested by law with the authority to direct, control, or regulate traffic.
- Bring the apparatus to a complete stop, and do not proceed until it is confirmed that it is safe to do so, such as at any stop signal (i.e., sign, light, or traffic officer), blind intersections, intersections where the operator cannot see all lanes of traffic, stopped school buses with red warning lights flashing, and unguarded railroad crossings.
- Do not leave the scene of an accident in which you are involved.

DRIVER/OPERATOR TIP

State laws and many other rules and regulations may be defined in greater detail by local fire departments. Each driver/operator is responsible for knowing the state and local laws governing the operation of fire apparatus.

LISTEN UP!

"Due regard" is a legal term. As the driver/operator of a fire apparatus, you should ask yourself, "Would a reasonably careful person performing similar duties under the same circumstances react in the same manner?" If you are performing in an unsafe manner and putting others at risk, you are not driving with due regard for the safety of others. Be aware that you will be held responsible for your actions. Drive safely or do not drive at all.

Emergency Vehicle Driving

Pump/Water Supply Operator

The fire apparatus driver/operator must always exercise caution when driving to an incident. Fire apparatus can be very large, heavy, and difficult to maneuver. Operating an emergency vehicle without the proper regard for safety can endanger the lives of both the fire fighters on the vehicle and any civilian drivers and pedestrians encountered along the way. Although the impulse to respond as speedily as possible is understandable, safety should never be compromised to achieve a faster response time.

An emergency vehicle must always be operated with due regard for the safety of everyone on the road. Although most states and provinces permit drivers of emergency vehicles to disobey specific traffic regulations when responding to emergency incidents, driver/operators must always consider the potential actions of other drivers before making such a decision. For example, traffic laws require other drivers to yield the right-of-way to an emergency vehicle. There is no assurance, however, that other drivers will do so when an emergency vehicle approaches. The driver/operator must also anticipate which routes other units responding to the same incident will take.

When starting the emergency response, you should accelerate slowly and in a controlled manner. Allow the engine to gradually build up speed instead of flooring the accelerator from a stopped position. Both of your hands should remain on the steering wheel at all times unless you are operating air horns, sirens, or other essential equipment. For this reason, you should check and memorize the position of instruments and controls before moving the fire apparatus. It should never be necessary to search for instruments or controls while the fire apparatus is in motion, as this behavior will draw your attention away from the road. Taking your eyes off of the roadway for too long to search for controls may result in a collision.

Pump/Water Supply Operator

Prohibited Practices

For safety's sake, SOPs often prohibit specific actions by other crew members during response. As noted previously, fire fighters must remain seated with their seat belts securely fastened while the emergency vehicle is in motion. Never unfasten your seat belt to retrieve or don equipment. Do not dismount the apparatus until the vehicle comes to a complete stop.

In addition, no one should ever stand up while riding on apparatus. Likewise, no member should hold on to the side of a moving vehicle or stand on the rear step. When a vehicle is in motion, everyone aboard must be seated and belted in an approved riding position.

Level of Response

Local jurisdictions determine which level of response is appropriate for nonemergency and emergency incidents. During an emergency response, the fire apparatus should be driven with both the emergency lights and the sirens activated—a practice commonly referred to as a **Code 3 response**. When the fire apparatus is operating with only the emergency lights and no audible siren, it is engaging in a **Code 2 response**. During normal operations or nonemergency responses, the fire apparatus does not have any emergency lights or sirens operating; this situation is considered a **Code 1 response**. A Code 2 response is usually prohibited in many fire departments because it does not properly alert other drivers to the presence of the fire apparatus. Although some fire fighters might argue that the sirens are unnecessary at 3:00 AM when the streets may be empty of traffic, sirens should still be used to alert others of the fire apparatus' approach and to avoid any potential liability should an accident occur.

During a nonemergency response, the apparatus should be operated in a nonemergency mode (without lights and sirens) and obey all traffic laws. This includes units that are en route to move up or to fill an empty station.

Passing Vehicles

The fire apparatus should be driven with the intention of passing other vehicles on the left side. On streets with multiple lanes, the fire apparatus should be driven in the far left lane to provide ample room for the other drivers to pull to the right and stop. Weaving in and out of the other vehicles should be avoided. This action confuses other drivers and may cause a collision with other vehicles as they try to avoid the fire apparatus. Always attempt to pass other vehicles on the left side. Any deviation from this should be done with extreme caution.

When operating the fire apparatus on straight sections of roadway, you must remain in your own lane **FIGURE 7-3**. Some driver/operators have a tendency to occupy parts of two lanes. This practice should be avoided, because it confuses other drivers by not making your intentions clear while traveling down the road. When making lane changes, use your turn signal, and try to remain in the far left lane until you need to turn. While performing a two-lane change, make sure that you clear each lane individually before proceeding. Be aware that other vehicles may attempt to race or even pass the fire apparatus while you are responding to the scene.

Fire apparatus that are following each other to an emergency should maintain an adequate distance to avoid a rear-end collision. Overtaking and passing other vehicles during an emergency response should be attempted with extreme caution and should be done only on the left side.

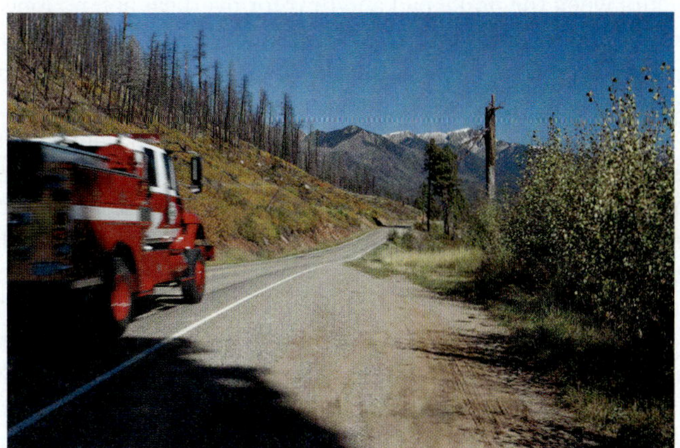

Figure 7-3 When operating the fire apparatus on straight sections of roadway, you must remain in your own lane.
© AlanHaynes.com/Alamy Images.

Defensive Driving Practices

While responding to the incident, you should yourself ask the following questions:

- Can I stop this fire apparatus?
- What will I do if someone pulls in front of me?
- Is another vehicle in my blind spot?
- Am I too close to the vehicle in front of me?

All of these questions relate to the need to operate the fire apparatus in a safe manner and to drive defensively. If you drive cautiously and anticipate that the unexpected may happen, then you will be more prepared when it does. Defensive drivers are safer than aggressive drivers. To drive defensively, you must always be aware of your surroundings. Scan the area in front of the fire apparatus to determine which hazards may lie ahead. Is another vehicle about to pull in front of the fire apparatus? If you are checking the road ahead, then you will see any potential problems and be better prepared to avoid a collision.

While traveling behind other vehicles, consider how close you can safely be to the vehicles ahead. While driving in good weather conditions (during daylight with good, dry roads and low traffic volume), you should ensure a safe distance from the vehicle ahead of you by following the "3-second rule." This distance will change depending on the speed at which the fire apparatus is traveling and the road conditions. To determine the appropriate following distance, first select a fixed object on the road ahead such as a sign, tree, or overpass. When the vehicle that you are following passes the object, slowly count, "One one-thousand, two one-thousand, three one-thousand." If you reach the object before completing the count, then you are following too closely. Making sure that there are at least 3 seconds between the fire apparatus and the car ahead of it gives you enough time and distance to respond to any problems that occur ahead of you. While responding in poor driving conditions (e.g., in inclement weather, in heavy traffic, or at night), you should double the 3-second rule to 6 seconds, for added safety. As the driving conditions worsen, you will, in turn, have to increase the distance that you travel behind other vehicles.

During the response, consider how fast you are going in relation to the street on which you are traveling. Although many fire departments allow fire apparatus to travel faster than the speed limit, it may not always be safe to do so. For example, in a residential neighborhood, the speed limit is usually 25 mi/h (40 km/h) or less. In such an area, small children and other pedestrians might be present, so you must adjust your speed accordingly.

Being able to control the fire apparatus and stop when required should be your goal. The distance that it takes for you to recognize the hazard, process the need to stop the fire apparatus, apply the brakes, and then come to a complete stop is referred to as the **total stopping distance**. The distance that the fire apparatus travels after you recognize the hazard, remove your foot from the accelerator, and apply the brakes is referred to as the **reaction distance**. The distance that the fire apparatus travels from the time that the brakes are activated until the fire apparatus makes a complete stop is known as the **braking distance**. These distances are very important for you to consider while responding in the fire apparatus, and they will differ for each fire apparatus depending on several factors:

- **The size and weight of the fire apparatus.** The more weight the fire apparatus is carrying, the more energy it will take to bring it to a complete stop. Larger vehicles generally have a greater total stopping distance than smaller vehicles that are traveling at the same speed.
- **The fire apparatus' overall condition, including brakes, tires, and suspension.** Fire apparatus that are maintained in optimal condition are capable of coming to a complete stop more quickly than fire apparatus that are poorly maintained. Tires should always have adequate tread life and be inflated to the proper pressure. The brakes should be capable of stopping the fire apparatus as required. The suspension system of the fire apparatus should not allow excessive bounce; this will prevent the tires from making the proper contact with the road and delay the braking process.
- **The speed at which the fire apparatus is traveling.** Faster speeds will require the fire apparatus to travel a greater distance before it comes to a stop.
- **The surface condition of the road.** Dry, paved roads provide the best surface for both driving and stopping conditions. By comparison, when roads are wet or covered with ice and snow, they have less friction with the tires of the apparatus. The lower the friction value, the longer it will take for the fire apparatus to come to a complete stop.

Driver/operators must also be aware of the term **liquid surge** and know how it relates to driving, especially for fire apparatus that carry water. Liquid surge is the movement of liquid inside a container as the container is moved. As the fire apparatus accelerates or decelerates, the water carried inside the tank on the fire apparatus will slosh around. This movement can be very hazardous owing to the large amount of water that is carried on many fire apparatus. If the fire apparatus has to brake quickly, then the liquid surge will try to force the fire apparatus forward—putting additional strain on the fire apparatus' braking system and increasing the total stopping distance. To reduce the effects of liquid surge, the water tanks on fire apparatus are designed with baffles inside them. These plates inside the tank slow down the movement of the water and displace some of the energy transferred during the movement of the fire apparatus.

As a driver/operator, you should know how to prevent the fire apparatus from skidding. Skids can happen whenever the tires lose grip on the road. This problem can be caused by slippery surfaces, a too-sudden change in speed or direction, or lack of tire maintenance. A road that is safe under good conditions may, in contrast, be very dangerous when it is wet or covered with snow or ice. Traveling at high speeds even under normal conditions will increase the possibility of a skid if the fire apparatus must complete a turn or stop suddenly. If the fire apparatus is responding in rain or snow conditions, this problem is even more profound. Auxiliary engine brakes can sometimes cause loss of control of vehicles in rainy and icy conditions. The activation of the engine brake can cause the vehicle to pull to one side, and the driver/operator could potentially lose control. Most original equipment manufacturers (OEMs) recommend turning secondary braking off in wet and icy conditions. Although adverse weather conditions such as rain and ice contribute to skidding, poor driving skills are the main cause of skidding. If the fire apparatus begins to skid, take the following actions:

- **Stay off the brake.** Until the vehicle slows, your brakes will not work and could cause you to skid more.
- **Steer.** Turn the steering wheel in the direction you want the vehicle to go. As soon as the vehicle begins to straighten out, turn the steering wheel back the other way. If you do not do so, your vehicle may swing around in the other direction and you could start a new skid.
- **Continue to steer.** Continue to correct your steering, left and right, until the vehicle is again moving down the road under your control.

Maintaining Control on Hills, Turns, and Curves

While driving down hills, you should rely on the engine and the auxiliary braking device to slow down the fire apparatus. If only the fire apparatus brakes are used to control the speed of the fire apparatus, they may heat up to the point where they become ineffective in stopping the fire apparatus. This situation, commonly referred to as **brake fade**, occurs when the brake drums become hot and expand away from the brake shoes so that the stroke of the slack adjusters becomes less effective. Brake fade also occurs when the brake pad and/or rotor overheat and no longer produce sufficient friction to slow the apparatus. To avoid this problem, you should use the brakes only in short, 5- to 10-second bursts rather than as a continuous application.

Also, while traveling down a steep slope, you may need to use the auxiliary braking system and down-shift the transmission to a lower gear. To complete this action properly, shift into one gear lower than the gear that would be used when going up the hill. Down-shifting will make it easier to control the fire apparatus and will save wear on the brakes.

When traveling up hills, you should avoid over-throttling the fire apparatus. This action will result in a loss of power while the engine works to catch up to the amount of work that is being demanded. Instead, you should slowly build up speed and use the lower gears of the transmission until adequate horsepower is achieved. To do so, you may have to manually shift the transmission into these lower gears while climbing a hill.

When making left or right turns, make sure that you have enough clearance to completely make the turn without striking curbs, trees, and other objects that may be in the blind spot of the fire apparatus. Fire apparatus may be top heavy from aerial ladders, water, and other equipment. To avoid the potential for roll-over owing to the apparatus' load, you must slow down before making the turn—90 percent of braking should be done in a straight line before entering a corner. How fast you take a turn will depend on the road conditions and the type and design of the apparatus. If you are turning right from the far left lane, you may not be able to see whether vehicles on your right have completely stopped. In this case, you should have the fire officer or other crew member in the front seat look out the window into the blind spot and determine whether it is clear to proceed with the turn. When you are alone, you will have to slow down, make your intentions very clear to other motorists, and proceed with extreme caution while making such a turn.

When turning to the left, you should turn wide enough to make the turn but not so wide that you travel into an outside lane and strike another vehicle. During the response, you may have to make a U-turn to position the fire apparatus or maneuver down a one-way street. In such a case, you should make sure that the area is wide enough to complete the turn and that adequate clearance for both the front and the rear of the fire apparatus is available. Remember, the back of the fire apparatus will swing out away from the turn. Therefore, if the vehicle is too close to the outside curb, the back end may swing out and strike objects such as poles, trees, and parking meters along the curb. With some fire apparatus, you may not realize you are turning too fast until it is too late. When in doubt, slow down.

Curved roadways are found all over this country—in the mountains, along the coastlines, and in urban areas of major cities. Curved sections can be found on small dirt roads and on highway entrance and exit ramps. No matter where they are, curved roadways can pose a very serious problem for emergency vehicles. Many of these ramps are designed with extreme curves and can be difficult to judge when traveling at normal speeds. As a driver/operator, you must realize that traveling on these curves with a fire apparatus is very different from traveling on the same route with a passenger car.

Driver/operators of fire apparatus should be familiar with the term **centrifugal force**, including how it relates to driving on curved roads. Centrifugal force is the tendency for objects to be pulled outward when rotating around a center. The fire apparatus is subject to this force when making a turn; the centrifugal force will try to keep the fire apparatus going in a straight line while you are making the turn. If it is to avoid losing control, the fire apparatus must have proper traction with the roadway. To keep the fire apparatus in the turn without allowing centrifugal force to pull the vehicle off the road, you should slow down before the curve and brake gently while making the turn.

Driving along curves will also severely affect the weight transfer of the fire apparatus. As with any vehicle, the weight carried on a fire apparatus is usually distributed among all of the tires of the apparatus while it travels down the road. The weight on the front axle, however, is not the same as the weight on the rear axle; typically, one-third of the weight is on the front axle, and two-thirds of the weight is on the rear axle. There is also a 7 percent allowance from side to side—meaning the left-side weight may differ from the right-side weight. This keeps the vehicle's center of gravity in the middle of the vehicle, depending on its height and weight. When the apparatus travels on a curve, however, the center of gravity will shift, causing the weight of the fire apparatus to shift to one side or the other. If this shift of weight is too great, the fire apparatus will roll over. Remember to slow the fire apparatus down well before entering a turn; otherwise, you risk losing control of the vehicle.

Every curve in a road has a **critical speed**. If the fire apparatus is traveling faster than the critical speed, it will not be capable of completing the turn and will go off the road or roll over. Either way, you will lose control of the fire apparatus and wreck. To determine the critical speed, you should know how sharp the curve is and how slippery the road conditions are. As the curve gets sharper and the road more slippery, the critical speed goes down; as a consequence, the fire apparatus must travel around the curve at a slower speed. This does not have to be a complicated process. For example, if it is raining and the roads are slippery, you will not be able to drive around the curve at the same speed as if it were dry. Once the fire apparatus is beyond the critical speed, it is too late to try to correct the problem. Prevention is the key—so slow down **FIGURE 7-4**.

Night Driving

Responding to an emergency during the night is usually more difficult than during the day. The streets and landscape are difficult to see, and the reduced visibility makes the response area look dramatically different. Landmarks and street signs that are easily seen during the day may be missed as you respond in darkness. The lights of other vehicles, street lights, and traffic signals can make it difficult to maneuver the fire apparatus along the roadway.

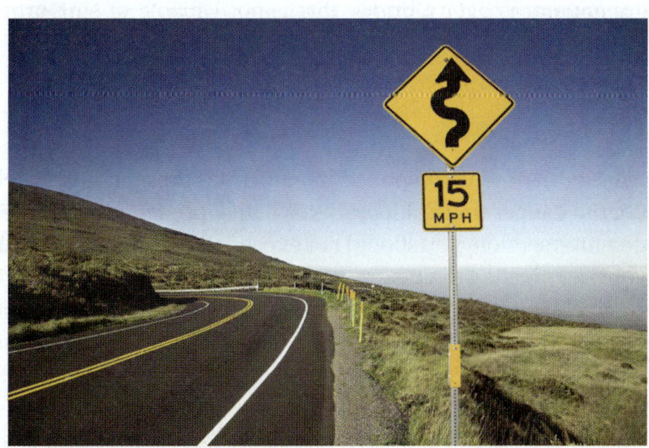

Figure 7-4 When approaching a curve, slow down!

To reduce the risks of responding during the night, follow these guidelines:

- Keep your eyes constantly scanning the roadway. Scan carefully for pedestrians, cyclists, and animals on the road.
- To avoid glare from oncoming lights, glance to the right edge of the road.
- Keep the fire apparatus' front windshield and headlights clean.
- Keep the interior cab lights off, and adjust the instrument panel lights to a low setting.
- Many fire apparatus cabs are equipped with red lights inside the cab. These lights should be used during the night because they do not interfere with your vision during the response.
- Stay alert at night. You must be well rested and prepared to operate the fire apparatus.
- Slow down, and increase your following distance.

Bridges and Overpasses

Bridges and overpasses are obstacles that you must be aware of before the emergency response begins. Know beforehand which overhead obstructions your fire apparatus can safely pass beneath. Fire apparatus are required by NFPA 1901, *Standard for Automotive Fire Apparatus*, to have labels in the cab that identify the height of the vehicle. You should ensure that the fire apparatus is capable of fitting underneath any obstacle before attempting to navigate it. When in doubt, find another access point or use a spotter to prevent damaging both the obstacle and the fire apparatus.

Another potential problem concerning bridges is their weight limitation. Some bridges are not designed to carry the heavy loads associated with certain fire apparatus. You should identify these potential problems and, if they present obstacles to the fire apparatus, access the scene of the emergency from another route or use smaller fire apparatus to respond to the scene. Under no circumstances should you attempt to operate a fire apparatus over a bridge that is not capable of supporting its weight.

Intersections

During an emergency response, intersections present the greatest potential danger to fire apparatus. When approaching and crossing an intersection, you should not exceed the posted speed limit. If you are traveling too fast, you will not be able to stop in time to avoid a collision. Also, do not assume you have the right-of-way simply because you are using the emergency warning lights and sirens: Other drivers may not see or hear the fire apparatus as you approach the intersection. Scan the intersection for possible hazards such as right turns on red, pedestrians, and vehicles traveling fast or weaving through traffic. Observe the traffic in all four directions: left, right, front, and rear. Proceed through the intersection only when you can account for all lanes of traffic at the intersection. In multilane intersections, you should clear each lane individually before proceeding. In some cases, other vehicles may block your view or the view of other drivers. As a consequence, you might think the lane is cleared and completely

SAFETY TIP

Because of their design, diesel engines have very little compression of backpressure to assist in stopping the fire apparatus. Auxiliary braking systems, however, provide braking torque through the driveline to the rear wheels. Use of an auxiliary brake reduces brake wear, reduces brake heat build-up, and can help minimize the occurrence of brake fade during heavy or frequent braking. Be aware that an auxiliary braking system should not be used during slippery road conditions or inclement weather; doing so may cause the rear wheels to lock up, resulting in a loss of control of the fire apparatus.

Several types of auxiliary braking devices are available for diesel-powered engines. The most popular include the following options:

- **Compression brake.** The compression brake is a mechanical system added to the engine valve train that is electronically actuated. This system alters the operation of the engine's exhaust valves so that the engine works as a power-absorbing air compressor.
- **Transmission retarder.** An efficient means of slowing a vehicle down, the transmission retarder utilizes the transmission fluid to create backpressure that assists in slowing the fire apparatus. The application of this type of device will help avoid engine damage. If the transmission fluid is overheated, however, major transmission damage can result.
- **Exhaust brake.** A shutter valve activated in the exhaust system just behind the turbocharger will engage this type of device. The closed valve causes a build-up of pressure in the exhaust system, which then passes back through the turbocharger and the valves and into the combustion chamber of the cylinder. The pressure build-up creates braking horsepower, which is then used to slow the vehicle down. With a transmission that offers the same type of direct interface, this system is quite efficient because the same horsepower used to keep the vehicle in motion can help slow it down. The maximum efficiency is reached at the maximum engine speed (rpm) for which the exhaust brake is rated.
- **Electromagnetic retarder.** This device is the most efficient, but most expensive, means of slowing a fire apparatus. When engaged, the electromagnet around the driveshaft creates an opposing magnetic field around the driveshaft that causes the driveshaft to resist turning, thereby slowing the fire apparatus. The system may be applied in stages either manually or by combinations of brake and accelerator pedal settings. Any heat that is generated by this system is dissipated by cooling fins on the retarder.

miss another vehicle that is proceeding through the intersection. In some cases, you may have to slow down to less than 5 mi/h (8 km/h) while in the intersection and visually clear each lane of traffic before proceeding.

At all intersections with green lights or where the fire apparatus has the right-of-way, you should slow down as necessary to ensure safe operation by disengaging the throttle and pressing the brake pedal. This strategy ensures that you are ready for any potential hazard—that you are driving defensively. When approaching an intersection where all lanes of traffic are blocked with other vehicles, you should turn off all sirens and horns at least 200 ft (60 m) before the stopped traffic is reached. Leave the emergency lights on and bring the fire apparatus to a stop at least 100 ft (30 m) from the nearest vehicle in traffic. This stance will let the civilian drivers know that you are still there and responding to an emergency but will not "push" them into the intersection. Never encourage or force traffic to proceed against red lights or to advance into dangerous traffic conditions. Instead, stay in the far left lane so that when the light turns green or the left green arrow is activated, you can proceed with lights and sirens through the intersection. The fire apparatus should come to a complete stop at all uncontrolled intersections, stop signs, and yellow and red lights. Proceed through the intersection only after it has been determined that the other vehicles have stopped and that it is safe to do so.

Many jurisdictions use **traffic signal preemption systems** at intersections to assist fire apparatus during the emergency response. These systems can change the signal from red to green for an emergency vehicle as it approaches the intersection. A flashing light on the fire apparatus, also known as an **emitter**, will trigger a **receiver** on the traffic signal and change the light to allow the fire apparatus to secure the right-of-way through these intersections in as safe and efficient a manner as possible. In jurisdictions using this type of traffic control system, each emergency vehicle is equipped with an emitter, which is usually mounted next to the emergency lights, and which emits visible flashes of light or invisible infrared pulses at a specified frequency. A receiver device is mounted on or near intersection traffic control devices to recognize the signal and preempt the normal cycle of traffic lights. Once the emergency vehicle passes through the intersection and the receiving device no longer senses the remote triggering device, normal operation of the intersection's traffic signals resumes. Such a system provides the fire apparatus with the benefit of a quicker response. Be aware that these intersections will require a heightened level of awareness and understanding. Other fire apparatus that are responding to the same emergency scene may also trigger this system from another direction and proceed through the intersection at the same time.

An encounter by the public with an emergency response vehicle en route to an emergency is not a normal, everyday occurrence. This fact is clearly evident from the confusion that is often witnessed when fire apparatus approach civilian traffic at intersections controlled by traffic signal preemption systems. For example, while the traffic signal preemption system cycles the light through the normal sequence of yellow and then red, an approaching fire apparatus is typically unable to determine how long the light was green for cross traffic. An unusually short green light for cross traffic may appear to that traffic as a malfunctioning light, encouraging the civilian drivers to run a yellow light. Proceed only after ensuring that it is safe to do so: A green light given as a result of traffic signal preemption system activation should not be assumed to be safe until verified visually, in all directions.

When a green light is given to the responding fire apparatus due to a traffic signal preemption system's activation well in advance, the driver/operator must still slow down as necessary to ensure safe operation. If the system is not granted a green light on approach, you should come to a complete stop just before the intersection to ensure safe operation. This delay will provide time for the system to activate the traffic signal, allow the intersection to clear completely, and give those civilian drivers who are either inattentive or prone to running yellow lights a chance to clear through.

As is the case with all intersections, when approaching a traffic signal preemption system–controlled intersection where all lanes are blocked, turn off all sirens and horns but leave the emergency lights on. Depending on your department, the system may be operational only when the vehicle's emergency lights are activated and the **parking brake** is in the off position. When activation has been granted and the green light delay occurs, activate sirens and horns for a few seconds to give the civilian vehicles time to clear the intersection completely.

Railroad Crossings

The driver/operator must obey all railroad crossing signals when responding to emergencies. Whenever you approach an unguarded railroad crossing, you should bring the fire apparatus to a complete stop before entering the grade crossing. Do not assume that the track is devoid of any trains in an attempt to continue the response. While stopped at the crossing, turn off all sirens, roll down the windows, operate the fire apparatus at an idle, and listen for the sound of an oncoming train. Railroad crossings must be treated with the same caution as any other intersection. Remember that with the siren activated, it may be difficult to hear a train horn or crossing bells. At intersections with railroad crossbars, you should never proceed between the crossbars in an attempt to continue the response. In this situation, you may have to alert the dispatch center or other responding units of a delayed response due to an inability to cross the railroad tracks safely.

Approaching the Scene of an Emergency

All emergency scenes have one thing in common: They are dynamic in nature. A scene can go from bad to worse in a matter of seconds. For this reason, everyone should always be cautious. As a driver/operator approaching the scene, you should slow down, identify the correct address/location, and recognize any potential hazards. If you take all three of these actions, you can make the scene safer for the members of your crew and anyone else in the immediate area.

Slow Down

When fire apparatus are responding to an emergency, the commotion usually attracts a lot of attention from the public. People are naturally curious about what is going on and may want to help. This is especially true in residential neighborhoods. Children may dart out into traffic, individuals may try to flag down fire apparatus, or people may stop their cars in the middle of the street. Some individuals even become so preoccupied with watching the emergency that they do not pay attention to their surroundings. This is why it is so essential for you to slow down and proceed with the utmost caution, especially in the last few blocks before reaching the emergency FIGURE 7-5.

Identify the Address/Location

Responding to the wrong location can not only be embarrassing but may also lead to loss of property and even lives. This type of mistake may be avoided by writing down the address when the call is dispatched. If you forget the address, you can reference the information that you wrote down earlier. Although some fire departments have onboard computers that can be used to locate the incident, it is always better to have a hard copy as a backup.

Once the apparatus is in the vicinity of the emergency, all crew members aboard the fire apparatus should help in locating the address. In some response areas, identifying the location of the incident may be difficult to do even during daylight hours. At night, the task is usually even more challenging. That is why everyone on the fire apparatus should be looking for the correct location. Firefighting is a team concept. Although the driver/operator is responsible for delivering the members of the company to the scene, you may need some assistance along the way.

In large apartment complexes, especially garden-style apartments, finding the location can be even more difficult. Unfortunately, not every apartment complex is numbered the same way. While some may have a letter to identify the building and a number for the actual apartment, others use the exact opposite addressing system FIGURE 7-6. Knowing the response district and having access to current maps can make all the difference. This information is best obtained before the emergency.

In rural areas, many fire departments rely on the knowledge of the fire department members. They may use local landmarks and old terminology to locate an emergency site. While this approach is not the preferred method to find emergency locations, in some jurisdictions it is the only way. In these situations, it is critical to have someone guide responders from other outside agencies to the scene as they seek the correct location. This may involve staging a unit on a main street to direct others down a dirt road that lacks a sign.

Locating the correct location may involve more than just looking for a physical address. Some calls may be dispatched to an area and not a specific address. When trying to locate an emergency scene, the entire crew should look for some of the following signs:

- Civilians attempting to wave them down
- Smoke in the area FIGURE 7-7
- Police cars with their emergency lights on
- Large crowds of people
- Congested streets that normally are devoid of traffic
- Residential lights that are flickering on and off during the night
- Headlights from a car that is off the roadway

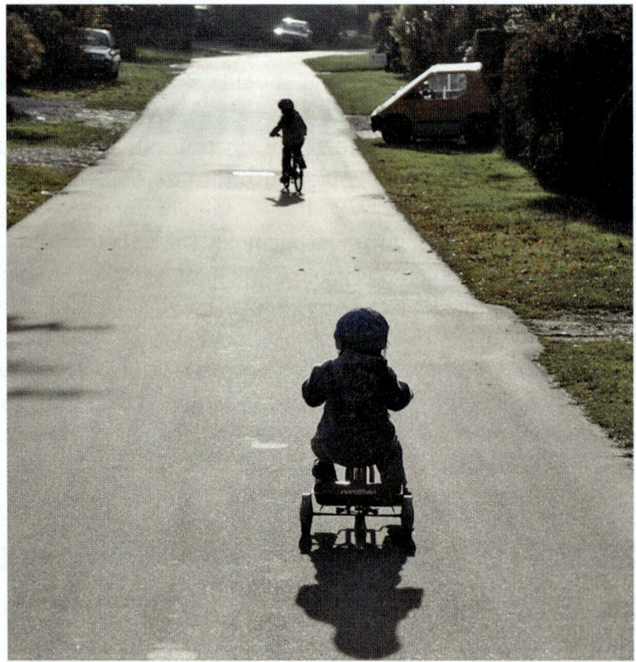

Figure 7-5 Slow down as you approach the scene—you never know who else is on the road.

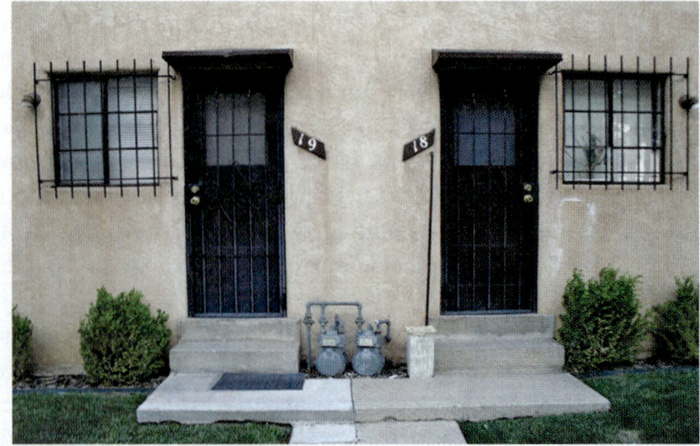

Figure 7-6 Not every apartment complex is numbered the same way.

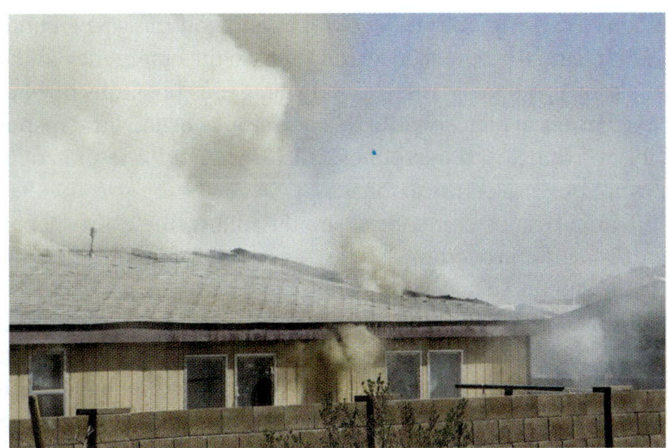

Figure 7-7 Smoke can help you in locating the incident.

Recognize Potential Hazards

Recognizing potential hazards while approaching the incident can be difficult sometimes. You may respond to the same types of calls over and over. This routine may become monotonous, and it is easy for some members to become complacent. By constantly being on the lookout for hazards, you can ensure the safety of your crew. Some of the hazards that you may encounter include fallen power lines in the area, scenes involving violence, large amounts of pedestrian traffic, and debris in the roadway from a motor vehicle accident (MVA). While these hazards may be easily mitigated, failure to recognize them could put the crew's safety at risk. Do not become complacent; always be aware of your surroundings.

Fire Scene Positioning

Pump/Water Supply Operator

From the moment that fire crews arrive at an emergency incident scene, their department's SOPs and the structured Incident Command System (ICS) must guide all of their actions. Fire personnel should always work in assigned teams (companies or crews) and be guided by a strategic plan for the incident. Teamwork and disciplined action are essential to provide for the safety of all personnel and the effective, efficient conduct of operations.

The command structure plans, coordinates, and directs operations. Personnel responding to an incident on an apparatus constitute the crew assigned to that vehicle and take direction from their company officer, who ensures that their actions are coordinated with the overall plan. Fire personnel who take action on their own, without regard to SOPs, the command structure, or the strategic plan, are **freelancing**. This type of activity—whether it is done by individual fire fighters, groups of fire fighters, or full companies—is unacceptable. Freelancing cannot be tolerated at any emergency incident. The safety of every person on the scene can be compromised by personnel who do not work within the system.

Fire companies and personnel must not respond to an emergency incident scene unless they have been dispatched or have an assigned duty to respond. Unassigned units and individual personnel arriving on the scene unexpectedly can overload the IC's ability to manage the incident effectively. Individuals who simply show up and find something to do are likely to compromise their own safety and create more problems for the command staff. All personnel must operate within the established system, reporting to a designated supervisor under the direction of the IC.

While approaching a fire scene, you should attempt to view at least three sides of the structure. To do so, you may have to drive slightly past the structure. This positioning gives the crew on the fire apparatus a better **size-up** of the building—including the company officer, who may have to share initial size-up information with other responding units.

Every fire department should train its members on proper staging procedures. Always follow your fire department's staging procedures. Some fire departments require that the first engine, ladder, and battalion chief go directly to the fire scene. With only a few necessary units at the scene, the IC can begin to orchestrate strategies and tactics without being overwhelmed. Eventually, specific tasks will be assigned to each unit by the IC. If tasks have not been delegated within a reasonable amount of time, the responding fire apparatus should attempt to contact the IC for an assignment.

Proper Positioning

As the first-arriving units are approaching the incident, the emphasis should be on the proper positioning of the fire apparatus. This initial placement should allow members to effect an investigation and allow for future operations. In most cases, it requires parking near the main entrance to the building. Stay outside with your fire apparatus, monitor all radio traffic, and await orders from the IC. While the other members of the crew are completing an investigation of the building's interior, you should further size up the incident from the exterior and prepare for any needed operations. This effort may include the following steps:

- Determining the best position to spot other incoming fire apparatus
- Locating the nearest hydrant
- Locating the sprinkler system or standpipe connection **FIGURE 7-8**
- Preparing equipment that may be requested by the officer or IC, such as carbon monoxide detectors, thermal imaging cameras, and positive-pressure ventilation fans
- Observing any potential hazards on the scene

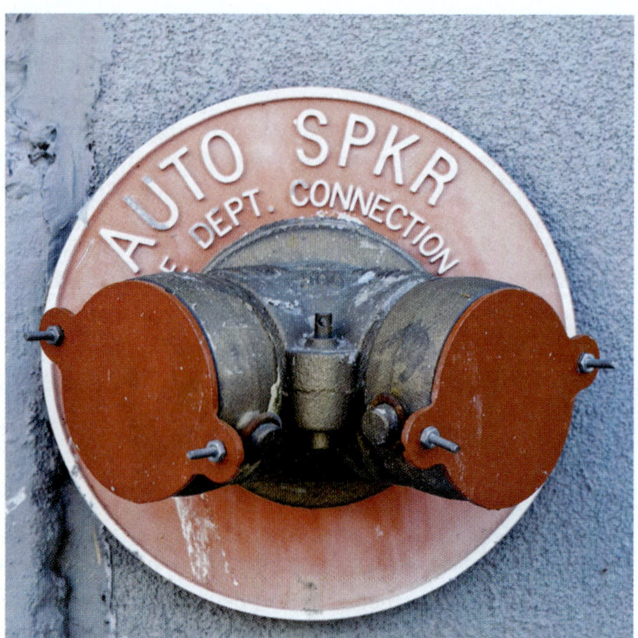

Figure 7-8 A fire department connection.

Always follow your department's SOPs and chain of command. Do not make decisions or issue orders when you do not have the authority to do so. Obtain information about the incident and relay it through the chain of command.

Working Fire

When the fire apparatus arrives at a working fire, the driver/operator must position it for maximum potential benefit. Unfortunately, there is usually a natural inclination to drive the fire apparatus as close to the fire as possible, which often results in positioning of fire apparatus that is both dysfunctional and dangerous. The placement of all fire apparatus on the fireground should take into account the following considerations:

- Your fire department's SOPs
- A direct order from the IC
- A conscious decision on the part of the company officer based on existing or predictable conditions

Efficient fire apparatus placement must begin with the arrival of the first-responding fire apparatus. This vehicle will set the tone for the entire incident. If the initial fire apparatus is placed in the optimal position, then other fire apparatus will follow suit. In contrast, improper placement of the first-arriving units will create a problem that will have to be tolerated for the remainder of the incident. First-arriving fire apparatus should park at maximum advantage and go to work; later-arriving fire apparatus should be placed in a manner that builds on the initial plan and allows for expansion of the operation. Remember that firefighting is a team concept. Driver/operators who are already on the scene should communicate to those who are en route to the emergency and let them know in advance the most advantageous positions in which to place their vehicles. While this decision is usually the responsibility of the IC, all personnel will be affected if later-arriving units are positioned erroneously.

Later-arriving companies should follow their fire departments' staging procedures. Everyone must maintain an awareness of which site access provides the best tactical options and ensure that the immediate fire area does not become congested with fire apparatus. When possible, an access lane should be maintained down the center of the street. Park unneeded units out of the way. Fire apparatus that are not working should be left in the staging area or parked where they will not compromise access. Take advantage of the equipment on fire apparatus already in the fire area instead of bringing in more fire apparatus—many times only additional personnel are needed to address the incident.

When fire apparatus are on a fire scene, they are classified into one of two categories:

- **Working.** These fire apparatus are actually in use on the fire scene. The fire apparatus or the equipment that they carry is actively being used.
- **Parked.** These fire apparatus are not being used on the fire scene. Their only reason for being on scene, for the time being, is to transport personnel to the scene of the fire. No significant amounts of tools or equipment from such fire apparatus are actively being used. Given these facts, the fire apparatus should remain in the appropriate staging area or be positioned so that they do not compromise the access route of other incoming units.

Staging

NFPA 1561, *Standard on Emergency Services Incident Management System*, identifies the need to provide a standard system to manage reserves of responders and other resources at or near the incident. If too many units arrive at the incident without direction, their presence may lead to possible freelancing and confusion. At such a chaotic scene, the IC will have great difficulty controlling the personnel and maintaining discipline. Accountability of all personnel on scene may also be complicated if it is not known when units arrived or who was given an assignment.

To avoid this dilemma, later-arriving fire apparatus should stay in an uncommitted position and await orders from the IC, a practice commonly referred to as **staging**. Staging is the standard procedure used to manage uncommitted resources at the scene of an incident. Its objective is to provide a standard system of initial placement for responding fire apparatus, personnel, and equipment prior to their assignment at tactical incidents **FIGURE 7-9**. Staging also provides a way to control and record the arrival of subsequent resources

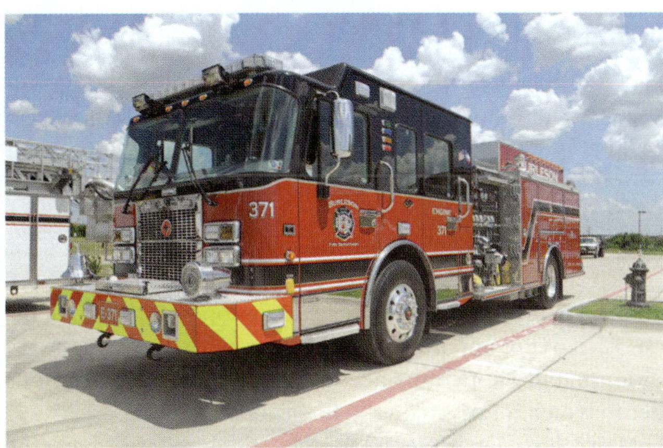

Figure 7-9 The objective of staging procedures is to provide a standard system of initial placement for responding fire apparatus, personnel, and equipment prior to their assignment at tactical incidents.

LISTEN UP!

Once at the scene of the incident, do not place the front of the fire apparatus too close to the rear of another fire apparatus. This will block in fire apparatus and may prohibit some equipment from being accessed, such as ground ladders carried on an aerial apparatus. Most modern aerial apparatus carry their ground ladders in the rear compartment. To remove the ladders, there must be a clear area behind them greater than the nested length of the ground ladder; for a 35-ft (11-m) extension ladder, this can be as much as 20 ft (6 m). Likewise, poor positioning of fire apparatus can cause problems in accessing the hose that is carried on the apparatus. If too many units are confined into a tight space together, the fire fighters will have a difficult time deploying the attack lines around other apparatus. Do not block other operations with your fire apparatus. Remember—hoselines can be extended; ladders cannot.

and eventually their assignment to specific locations or functions within the Incident Management System (IMS).

When used successfully, proper staging of fire apparatus can accomplish the following goals:

- **Reduce unnecessary radio traffic.** During the first few critical moments of a structure fire, vital information is disseminated to all members who are responding. The IC will give a size-up of the incident. First-arriving units may request a water supply or additional resources to be sent to a specific location. Now is not the time to clutter the radio channel with needless radio traffic.
- **Reduce excessive apparatus congestion at the scene.** When too many fire apparatus are cluttering the scene, matters can become both dangerous and confusing. By placing fire apparatus in an uncommitted location close to the immediate scene, the IC can evaluate conditions prior to assigning companies. This will allow time for command personnel to formulate and implement a plan without undue confusion and pressure.
- **Provide the IC with a resource pool.** The IC may then assign units and resources at his or her leisure. These units should be ready to deploy as required by the IC.

Level I Staging

Many fire departments use two levels of staging. Generally, **Level I staging** is in effect for all first alarm assignments, or incidents involving three or more units. For example, during a working structure fire response, all units continue responding to the scene until the first-in unit reports its arrival on the scene. Following its arrival and assumption of command, the first-in unit begins the assignment of the remainder of the dispatch. During Level I staging, the only units that proceed directly to the scene of a working structure fire are the first-due engine, ladder, and chief FIGURE 7-10. These units initiate appropriate operations as directed by their department's SOPs or by the IC. All other units stage in their direction of travel, uncommitted, approximately one block from the scene. A position that supports the maximum number of tactical options with regard to access, direction of travel, water supply, and other considerations is preferred. Staged units announce their arrival, report their company designation, and identify their staged location/direction (e.g., "Engine Five, South"). These units remain in position until they receive an assignment from the IC.

Level II Staging

Level II staging is utilized on second or greater alarms or when mutual aid units report to an incident. This type of staging places all reserve resources in a central location and automatically

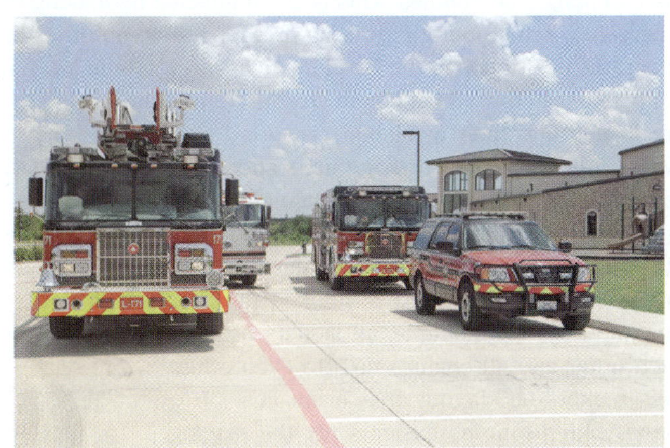

Figure 7-10 Level I staging.

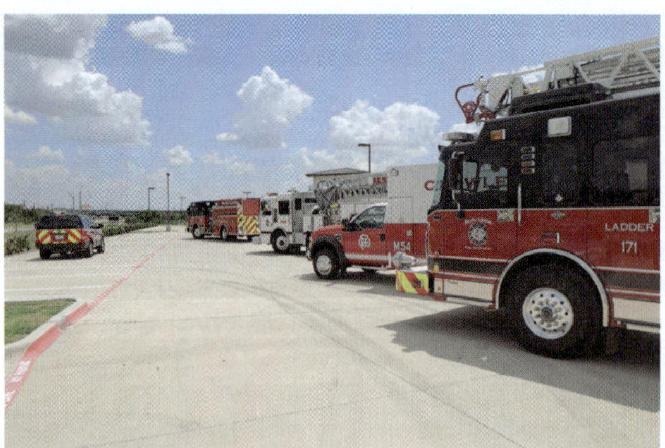

Figure 7-11 Level II staging.

requires the implementation of a staging area manager. The **staging area manager** is the person responsible for maintaining the operations of the staging area. The **staging area** is an area away from the incident where units will park until requested to enter the emergency scene **FIGURE 7-11**. This area should allow staged apparatus to access any geographic point of the incident without delay or vehicle congestion.

First alarm units that are already in Level I staging or en route to Level I staging will stay in Level I unless otherwise directed by the IC. All other responding units will proceed to the Level II staging area.

When activating Level II staging, the IC should give an approximate location for the staging area. This area should be some distance away from the emergency scene to reduce site congestion yet close enough to permit a prompt response to the incident site. Large parking lots or empty fields are excellent choices for a staging area.

The IC may designate a member of the department to serve as the staging area manager. When this position is not otherwise designated, the first fire officer whose unit enters the Level II staging area will assume this role. The staging area manager takes a position that is both visible and accessible to incoming and staged companies. This is accomplished by leaving the emergency lights operating on the fire apparatus; no other fire apparatus positioned in the Level II staging area should leave its emergency lights on. All incoming resources into the staging area are logged and their availability reported to the IC. All subsequent arriving units should report in person to the staging area manager and await assignment, a strategy that reduces unnecessary radio traffic. Within the staging area, like units should be positioned next to one another—for example, all ladders next to each other and all engines next to each other. This makes the staging area manager's job of identifying resources easier. Only the staging area manager may release resources from the staging area.

Engines and Ladders

Engine and ladder companies are the quintessential bread-and-butter apparatus of the fire service. The proper placement of ladders and engines should complement one another so as to rescue civilians and effect total fire extinguishment. Never assume that these two types of units can be positioned in the same way; instead, each unit has a specific function that should be taken into account when positioning the apparatus at a fire scene. Some fire departments have driver/operators who operate both types of fire apparatus on a regular basis. If this is the case, position the fire apparatus according to its function—not in the order in which it arrives on the fireground.

Many fire departments in the United States have both engines and ladders in their fleets. This section focuses primarily on these two indispensable pieces of equipment. Although other fire apparatus are also discussed, their presence on a fire scene is usually not as critical to its outcome.

The placement of the first-arriving engine or ladder should be based on the initial size-up and the fire department's SOPs. If the engine driver/operator arrives on scene first, he or she must choose a setup position that provides for efficient operation of the engine company as well as the first-arriving ladder apparatus. Just because your vehicle is the first fire apparatus to arrive at the scene, that fact does not mean that you are entitled to the best position on the fire scene. Instead, you must look at the big picture and imagine how the scene might unfold. An engine company occupying a spot that would be better suited for a ladder apparatus is an example of poor fire apparatus positioning and inexperience.

Usually, only the engine company responds to the fire scene with hose, water, and a fire pump on board the fire apparatus. As a consequence, the engine's placement depends on the conditions encountered upon arrival. While other responding fire apparatus may assist the engine company, it is ultimately the engine crew's responsibility to provide the water flow for fire extinguishment. This water may be supplied through handlines or master streams. It is imperative that the engine company establish a water supply that will last for the duration of the incident.

The ladder company should be positioned to support the engine company's operations and vice versa. Preplanning is the key to ensuring the optimal positioning. When positioning a ladder apparatus on the scene of a fire, the driver/operator must take into account all of the hazards that may plague the engine company as well as some additional hazards that are specific to an **aerial device** (a generic term used to describe the hydraulically powered aerial ladder or platform that is operated from the top of an aerial apparatus). Aerial ladders and aerial platforms may be used as launching points for rescue, entry, search, and ventilation operations. They may also be used to stretch hoselines to upper floors or the roof, bridge a gap, perform ladder pipe operations, and serve as observation posts from which to assess conditions. When their need is evident upon arrival, aerial devices should be raised immediately. When need for them is anticipated to arise later, these devices should be positioned for rapid setup and future use. In these situations, the driver/operator of the ladder apparatus should remain in the vicinity of the turntable until the fire is under control.

The IC may give specific instructions regarding the placement of fire apparatus and the operations to be performed. As a driver/operator, you must base your decision about placement of the fire apparatus on two conditions: rescue potential and exposures.

DRIVER/OPERATOR TIP

Each fire department should develop a procedure for the placement of initial fire apparatus that driver/operators should follow upon their arrival at an incident. Always follow your fire department's procedures, and learn the procedures for other jurisdictions covered by mutual aid agreements.

Rescue Potential

Rescue is the first priority for every responding fire apparatus. If civilians are potentially trapped inside the structure upon arrival, you should ensure that the front of the structure is available for access by the ladder apparatus. Position the fire apparatus to assist in or perform this operation. In this scenario, engine apparatus should be out of the way but preparing to go to work. For efficient and safe control, all apparatus driver/operators must work together to ensure that the aerial apparatus is positioned for maximum use and minimum stress to the aerial device. Usually, the front of the building is left available for the first-arriving ladder apparatus regardless of the conditions. It may be necessary or advantageous for ladder apparatus to circle the block and come in from the opposite end of the street, if such action will improve the fire apparatus placement.

Exposures

When exposure protection is necessary upon arrival, do not position the fire apparatus between the fire and the exposure. Doing so may cause the fire apparatus to become an exposure problem itself. Instead, position the vehicle far enough away from the exposure to remain safe but close enough to deliver fire streams for exposure protection. Regardless of the initial placement, if conditions change (i.e., rapid fire spread exposes the fire apparatus) and lead to collapse potential, then repositioning may be required and must be accomplished quickly and safely. Proper training and planning are essential in such cases.

As a driver/operator, you must always think ahead and position the fire apparatus with the idea that it might have to be repositioned at some point during the incident. Do not get blocked in or out of the fire area. Consider the collapse potential based on severe fire conditions and building construction. Many fire fighters have been killed and fire apparatus damaged because of failure to recognize a building's collapse potential. To ward off this threat, most fire departments specify a **collapse zone**—that is, a distance of 1½ times the height of the building in which fire fighters and fire apparatus must not be located in case of a building collapse. In buildings with bowstring trusses, identification of an even larger area as the collapse zone may be required. If such a building's walls and bowstring roof assembly fail, they may propel outward greater than 1½ times the height of the building. When tall buildings are involved with fire and a danger of collapse is present, a collapse zone of 1½ times the building's height may not be practical, as it would require positioning fire apparatus so far away that they may not be effective.

In some circumstances, the fire apparatus should be positioned in one of the **corner safe areas** of the fireground. In his book *Safety and Survival on the Fireground*, retired Fire Chief Vincent Dunn describes studying this area by looking at the structure from a bird's-eye view: There are four areas of the fireground that may not be covered by collapsing walls—namely, areas outside the building where two walls intersect. As the fire progresses, fire fighters must continually reevaluate the potential for building collapse. Positioning the ladder apparatus at the corner safe areas of a building affords coverage on two fronts. This strategy enables coverage of a much wider area, permitting greater access and providing observation points from which to check the stability of the building and other issues.

When positioning the fire apparatus, note the locations of street lights, traffic signals, trees, utility poles, and wires at street corners or other parts of the site. Placement of the aerial device should be oriented toward providing as much effective operating area for the basket/tip as possible on both fronts of the building.

Fire Conditions

The initial engine company needs to be positioned for the efficient deployment of the first attack line—the most important attack line on the fireground. You should not position the fire apparatus with the preconnected attack line directly in front of the building's entrance. While this positioning may simplify the attack line deployment, it will place the engine in a position that compromises the operation of other incoming fire apparatus, especially the ladder apparatus. Instead, the engine should be placed past the structure, with the front of the building being left open for the ladder company. Most engines have an excess of fire hose, whereas aerial devices have a fixed length. Do not render the aerial device useless by blocking it out just to make stretching the attack lines easier.

Water Supply

Dependent upon department procedures, the first-due engine companies approaching the scene with any evidence of a working fire in a structure may secure a water supply. The next-in engine company may be too far away or encounter a delay while responding to perform this task. In some cases, however, securing the water supply may not be the first-arriving engine company's primary task—for example, when there is an obvious critical rescue requiring the entire crew or when the exact location of the fire in a multiple-unit occupancy is unknown. Whenever possible, the supply line should consist of large-diameter hose (LDH), as this type of hose reduces the friction loss and provides an adequate water supply. Always notify other responding apparatus when laying LDH across streets and intersections, as this supply line may block other fire apparatus from reaching the scene of the fire. When laying the hose from the hose bed, always attempt to position it to the same side of the street as the hydrant.

Slope

Positioning the fire apparatus uphill from the incident may prevent future problems, such as those caused by water runoff from the fire scene. The slope of the area will usually not affect normal engine operations. NFPA 1901 requires that fire apparatus have two wheel chocks mounted in readily accessible locations, each designed to hold the fire apparatus when loaded to its maximum in-service weight on a 20 percent grade with the transmission in neutral and the parking brake released. When the pump is engaged, make sure that these wheel chocks are placed in the proper positions. If there is any doubt about the unit's ability to keep from rolling down the hill, chock it or move it!

Some sloping surfaces may not allow for adequate deployment of an aerial device. To operate with 100 percent capacity of the aerial device, some aerial apparatus stabilizers can correct for a slope and grade of only a few degrees. You may be able to park the fire apparatus in an optimal position, but if the aerial device is incapable of operating in that position, this placement is futile. You must know the limitations of the fire apparatus that you are operating and position it accordingly.

Terrain and Surface Conditions

The terrain is the landscape on which the apparatus is positioned. In many cases it may be an asphalt roadway or a concrete driveway, but sometimes it may include areas off the roadway. In these circumstances, you should position the fire apparatus with future pump operations in mind. If possible, leave the fire apparatus on the asphalt roadway or a concrete driveway that can support the weight of the fire apparatus. If this positioning is not feasible, you should prevent significant amounts of water from flowing underneath the fire apparatus if it is positioned on top of soil that is unstable or may become unstable. Otherwise, the fire apparatus may become stuck, and the ensuing mess may hamper future operations. Where the ground is of doubtful stability, as is sometimes the case with vacant lots or other unpaved areas that may have hidden voids, and if the terrain is deemed not substantial enough, ladder apparatus should be positioned elsewhere.

Wind Conditions

Upon arrival, note the wind conditions. Place the fire apparatus out of the path of oncoming smoke and heat. Too much smoke will starve the engine of fresh air and cause it to shut down **FIGURE 7-12**. Should the wind shift during the operation and compromise the engine operation, notify the IC. If possible, it may be necessary to reposition the engine at another location. While you are operating the fire apparatus, if you need self-contained breathing apparatus (SCBA) because of the smoke conditions, move the fire apparatus: If you cannot breathe the air, neither can the fire apparatus. Remaining in the original position may cause the fire apparatus to stall and render its pumping operations useless.

The wind may also affect master stream operations. When deck guns are not reliable because of heavy wind conditions, the use of portable ground monitors may be a better alternative. The wind may also limit the operations of some aerial devices on scene. Aerial devices are designed to be operated in maximum winds that vary from 35 mi/h to 50 mi/h (56 to 80 km/h), depending on manufacturer and model, without any reduction in tip load. Always refer to the operating manual to determine the recommended operational extremes.

Overhead Obstructions

Overhead wires may interfere with any aerial device's operation. Do not be intimidated by overhead wires when the situation

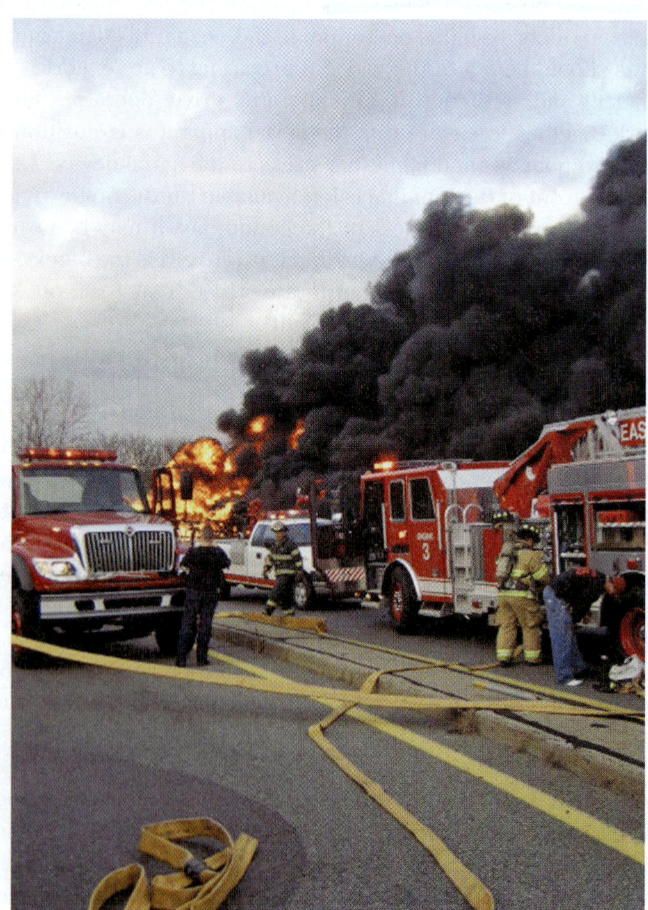

Figure 7-12 Too much smoke will starve the engine of fresh air and cause it to shut down.

clearly calls for use of the aerial device; rather, exercise caution, and be creative in your approach. The IC should have wires removed by the utility company when fire conditions warrant doing so. All aerial devices should remain a minimum of 10 ft (3 m) from all overhead wires. Do not try to guess which wires may be energized; instead, consider all wires to be live until proven otherwise.

When trees obstruct operations, it may be possible to extend or raise the aerial device through light branches. However, retraction or lowering of the boom through branches may present a problem, and some cutting may be required to overcome this obstacle. Use caution when operating around trees, as an electrical hazard should always be suspected **FIGURE 7-13**. Before an incident occurs, you should practice positioning the fire apparatus for operation with overhead obstructions in the area to become familiar with the fire apparatus' limitations and functions under these conditions. Possible alternatives may include placing the fire apparatus on sidewalks, setting it up at corners, and extending the aerial device parallel to the front of a building. The crew should also practice using this device at intersections with light posts, traffic signs or signals, intersecting overhead wires, and other obstacles to enable personnel to judge where and how fire apparatus can be positioned for maximum coverage under similar circumstances.

Auxiliary Appliances

An **auxiliary appliance** is a standpipe and/or sprinkler system. The determination of whether a building has one or both of these systems is best made during development of a preincident plan. A **preincident plan** is described by NFPA 1620, *Recommended Practice for Preincident Planning*, as a document developed by gathering general and detailed data to be used by responding personnel to determine the resources and actions necessary to mitigate anticipated emergencies at a specific facility. When creating such a preincident plan, you should locate the fire department connection, fire pump, standpipe system, and sprinkler system in the building. If this information is not readily available, you will have to rely on other members of the crew to help locate these systems, which may slow down the initial operations and result in more work for the fire fighters on scene. For example, if an engine company responds to a fire in a multistory apartment building, the crew may prefer to use the building's built-in standpipe system to establish a water supply. If you cannot identify the location of the fire department connection, the engine crew will not be able to use the standpipe to connect attack lines and, therefore, will have to stretch additional hoselines up to the fire floor. This delay in water application may cause the fire to progress past the extinguishment capabilities of a single hoseline.

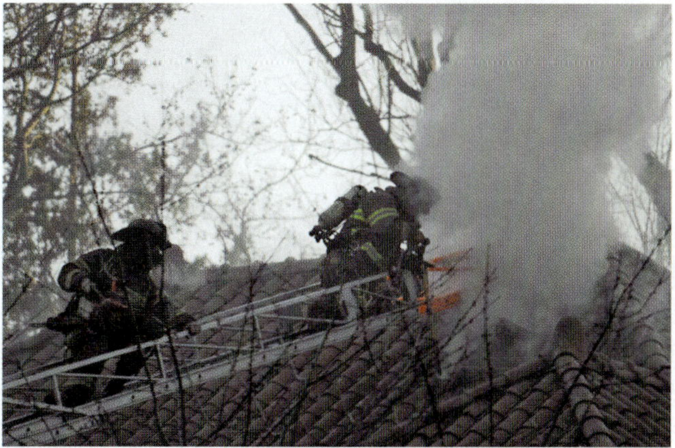

Figure 7-13 Use caution when operating around trees.

Positioning of Other Fire Scene Apparatus

Engines and ladder trucks are not the only fire apparatus required at a fire scene. Depending on the size, construction, occupancy, and involvement of the structure, a multitude of other types of fire apparatus may be needed to mount an effective response.

Specialized Fire Apparatus

Specialized fire apparatus may be equipped with an assortment of specialized equipment, such as that needed for heavy technical rescue, hazardous materials response, or mobile air supply. The personnel assigned to these fire apparatus are required to have specialized training, and their role on the fire scene is usually to provide support operations.

Specialized fire apparatus may need to be positioned close to the incident depending on the conditions. The driver/operators of these vehicles may have to be creative in their approach to the fire scene. Approaching from the same direction as all the other units may not be effective, for example. Instead, these driver/operators must listen to the radio, observe scene conditions, and identify the most efficient position for the task assigned.

Command Vehicles

The fire chief uses a **command vehicle** to respond to the fire scene. This vehicle should be positioned at a location that will allow maximum visibility of the fire building and surrounding area. It should be easily identified at the scene and placed in a logical position. The command vehicle should not restrict the movement or positioning of other apparatus at the fire scene.

Ambulances

An **ambulance** is a specially designed vehicle that is capable of transporting sick and injured patients. It is usually staffed with trained emergency technicians and/or paramedics. These vehicles should be parked in a safe position that will provide the most effective treatment and transportation of fire victims and firefighting personnel, while not blocking other apparatus or interfering with firefighting operations. Ambulance drivers are also responsible for positioning their vehicles with a clear route of egress. During large fire scenes, these emergency vehicles may be staged with other apparatus in a Level II staging area. When requested, they will respond to the scene. Once on the fire scene, the ambulance driver may stay with the vehicle while other personnel load the patient into the vehicle. This practice ensures that the patient is picked up as close to the scene as possible without compromising fire scene operations if the ambulance needs to be relocated.

Traffic Safety on the Scene

Pump/Water Supply Operator

An emergency incident scene presents several risks to fire personnel in addition to the hazards of fighting fires and performing other duties. One of these dangers is traffic, particularly when the incident scene is on a street or highway. Traffic safety should be a major concern for the first-arriving units because approaching drivers might not see emergency workers or realize how much room fire fighters need to work safely.

The first unit or units to arrive at the incident scene have a dual responsibility. Not only must personnel focus on the emergency situation facing them, but they must also consider approaching traffic, including other emergency vehicles, and other, less obvious hazards. Always check for traffic before opening doors and dismounting the apparatus, and watch out for traffic when working in the street. Follow departmental SOPs to close streets quickly and to block access to areas where operations are being conducted.

One of the most dangerous work areas for fire fighters is on the scene of a highway incident, where traffic can be approaching at high speeds. Place traffic cones, flares, emergency scene signage, the traffic safety officer, and other warning devices far enough away from the incident to slow approaching traffic and direct it away from the work area. Placement of emergency vehicles on the scene is also critical. With proper placement, such vehicles can act as a barrier between oncoming traffic and the scene. Many fire departments have specific SOPs covering required safety procedures for these incidents.

Positioning at an Intersection or on a Highway

Operating at an emergency scene that is located either on or adjacent to a highway or intersection is extremely dangerous. Personnel should understand and appreciate the high level of risk to which fire fighters are exposed when they are working in or near moving vehicles. According to the NFPA, 69 fire fighters were killed in the line of duty in 2016, and the second leading cause of death was vehicle crashes. In 2016, 19 fire fighters died in vehicle accidents, the majority of whom died while responding to or returning from incidents TABLE 7-1. This type of fire fighter fatality is not uncommon; indeed, it happens every year. Each call near a roadway should be treated with caution. Always consider moving traffic to pose a threat to scene safety.

Each day, emergency responders are exposed to motorists of varying abilities, with or without licenses, with or without legal restrictions, and driving at speeds from creeping along to going well beyond the speed limit. Some of these motorists have visual impairments, and some are impaired because of the use of alcohol and/or drugs. On top of everything else, motorists often become distracted by the incident and look at the scene and not the road. Their lack of attentiveness while passing a roadside emergency scene may affect emergency responders' safety as they work at the scene.

When the fire apparatus arrives at the scene, other crew members may have a desire to quickly dismount the apparatus and go to work. The driver/operator should not allow personnel to exit the cab until the driver/operator is satisfied with the position of the fire apparatus. To achieve this goal, it may be necessary to angle the fire apparatus off of a roadway. Only when the unit is parked and ready should the other members be allowed to exit the vehicle.

Four actions that all personnel can take to protect themselves and other crew members while operating in traffic conditions include never trusting traffic, engaging in proper protective parking, reducing motorist vision impairment, and wearing high-visibility reflective vests.

Never Trust Traffic

Everyone must have a healthy respect for all vehicles. Do not assume that because vehicles are moving around an emergency

Table 7-1 Fire Fighter Deaths by Cause of Injury

Cause	Percent
Overexertion, stress, medical	42%
Vehicle accidents	25%
Falls	10%
Struck by objects	6%
Other	6%
Fatal assault	4%
Structural collapse	4%
Struck by vehicles	3%

Source: National Fire Protection Association, Fire Fighter Fatalities in the United States, 2016.

scene that the danger is gone. Anytime that the scene is located near moving traffic, there is a potential danger to all personnel. Fire personnel should exit the apparatus on the curb side or the nontraffic side whenever possible. Always look before stepping out of the fire apparatus or into any traffic areas on scene. When walking around fire apparatus parked adjacent to moving traffic, keep an eye on traffic, and walk as close to the fire apparatus as possible. Never turn your back to oncoming traffic for extended periods of time.

Engage in Proper Protective Parking

This aspect of safety relies on your ability as the driver/operator. As you position the fire apparatus, think about the consequences of your actions. Never allow convenience to compromise safety. Always position your apparatus to protect the scene, victims, and emergency personnel and to provide a protected work area. When possible, position the fire apparatus at a 45-degree angle away from the curbside to direct motorists around the scene FIGURE 7-14. Initial fire apparatus placement should always allow for adequate parking of other fire apparatus and a safe work area for emergency personnel. Allow enough distance between the fire apparatus and the scene to prevent a moving vehicle from knocking fire apparatus into the work areas.

Reduce Motorist Vision Impairment

During an emergency, the need for emergency lights is evident. At the incident, emergency lighting may still be needed when the safety of personnel is otherwise compromised. Never hesitate to operate emergency lighting at a scene. However, understand that emergency vehicle lighting provides a warning only and does not ensure effective traffic control; the latter consideration entails protecting the emergency scene from oncoming traffic by redirecting, blocking, or stopping all moving vehicles.

While most state laws require only one lighted lamp exhibiting red light visible under normal atmospheric conditions from a distance of 500 ft (150 m), many fire apparatus exceed this requirement. Unfortunately, the use of too many lights at a scene may create a dangerous situation. An excess of emergency lights flashing can cause a carnival effect and create confusion for motorists. Limit the number of fire apparatus operating emergency lights to only those blocking oncoming traffic—and even these fire apparatus may not need all of their emergency lights to be on.

If provided, use directional arrows at the rear of the apparatus to direct any oncoming traffic FIGURE 7-15. Even when

LISTEN UP!

Each colored emergency light on the fire apparatus serves a specific purpose and results in a different reaction from other motorists. The following list identifies the lights' colors and the expected reactions:

- **Red.** For most civilians, a red light identifies the need to stop. Unfortunately, it may also attract those drivers who are under the influence of drugs and/or alcohol as well as fatigued drivers.
- **Blue.** A blue light identifies the fire apparatus as being associated with either fire or police. States may have different laws dictating who can and cannot use blue lights on their vehicles. A blue light has good visibility during both daytime and nighttime operations.
- **Amber.** An amber light signals danger or caution. This color is widely used by other services to get drivers' attention. Many experts believe it to be the best warning light for the rear of emergency vehicles. It may deter those drivers who are fatigued or who are under the influence of drugs or alcohol. During foggy conditions, an amber-colored light is more readily visible than other colored lights.
- **Clear.** Clear light is associated with caution. Although it provides good visibility, such a light should normally be shut off at an emergency scene, to prevent blinding other drivers. For the same reason, it should not be used at the rear of the fire apparatus.

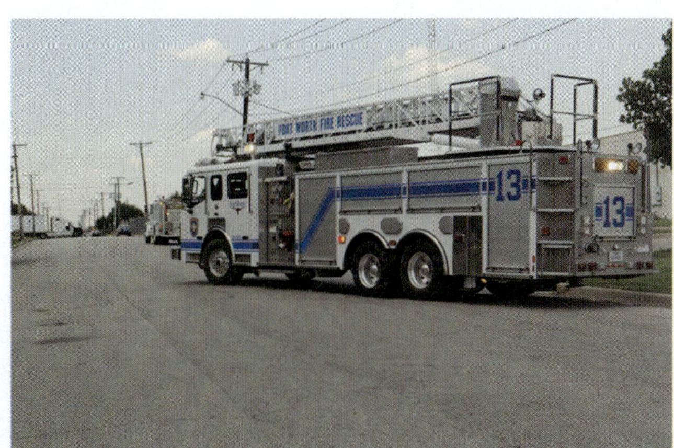

Figure 7-14 An example of proper protective parking.

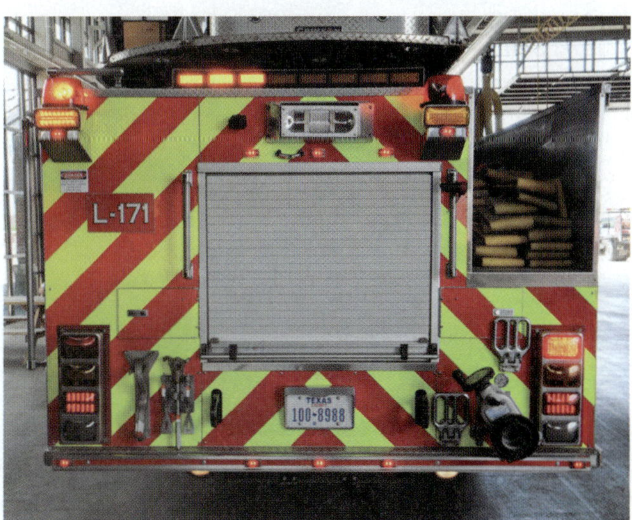

Figure 7-15 Use of directional arrows to divert the flow of traffic.

doing so, recognize that it is safer to divert traffic with advanced placement of signs and traffic cones than to rely on warning lights on fire apparatus to reroute oncoming vehicles.

Pump/Water Supply Operator

Dismounting a Stopped Apparatus

When the apparatus arrives at the incident scene, the driver/operator will park it in a location that is both safe and functional. All crew members must wait until the vehicle comes to a complete stop before dismounting. Always check for traffic before opening the door or stepping out of the apparatus. During the dismount, watch for other hazards that could be present—for example, ice and snow, downed power lines, uneven terrain, or hazardous materials. Be careful when dismounting apparatus, as the increased weight of PPE and adverse conditions can contribute to slips, strains, and sprains. Use handrails when mounting or dismounting the apparatus. Follow the steps in SKILL DRILL 7-3 to dismount an apparatus safely.

Wear High-Visibility Reflective Vests

Turnout gear does not adequately identify emergency personnel who are operating in or near traffic conditions. The reflective trim on the turnout gear may be dirty, covered with other equipment, or missing. To effectively identify themselves, emergency personnel should wear reflective vests compliant with American National Standards Institute (ANSI)/International Safety Equipment Association (ISEA) 107, American National Standard for High-Visibility Safety Apparel and Accessories. These vests should be retroreflective and fluorescent. Each fire department should require all personnel operating under these conditions to wear such vests. Some manufacturers make reflective vests out of flame-retardant material that may be worn over turnout gear.

Manual on Uniform Traffic Control Devices

The U.S. Department of Transportation's Federal Highway Administration publishes the *Manual on Uniform Traffic Control Devices for Streets and Highways (MUTCD)*. Under federal

Pump/Water Supply Operator

SKILL DRILL 7-3

Dismounting a Stopped Apparatus NFPA 1002, 5.2.1(B)

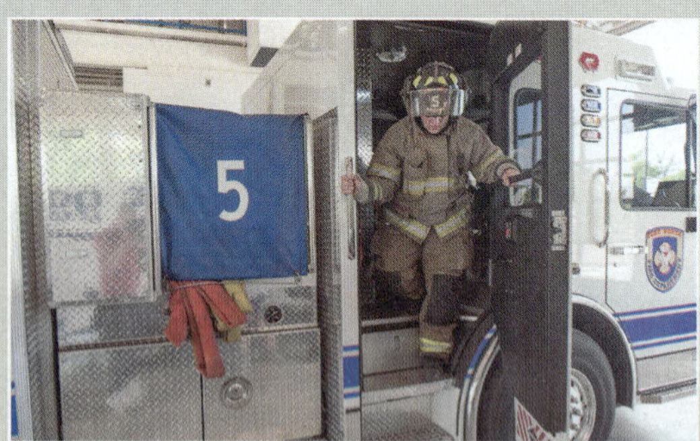

1 Become familiar with your riding position and the safest way to dismount.

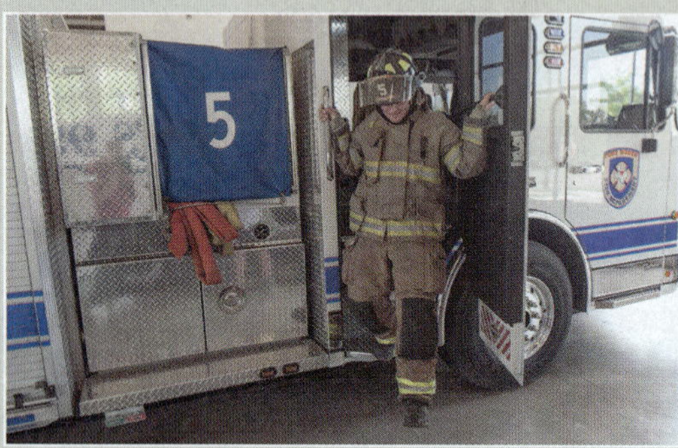

2 Maintain the one hand and one foot placement when leaving the apparatus, especially on wet or potentially icy roadway surfaces.

SAFETY TIP

The International Safety Equipment Association has identified three classes of safety vests:

- **Class 1.** This vest has the lowest level of visibility. It is generally worn in environments where speeds do not exceed 25 mi/h (40 km/h), by parking lot attendants, roadside maintenance workers, delivery vehicle drivers, and warehouse workers.
- **Class 2.** This category includes the most popular style of safety vest. It is commonly worn in environments where traffic is moving in excess of 25 mi/h (40 km/h), by construction workers, utility workers, school crossing guards, and emergency responders. A fire-retardant Class 2 safety vest is also available for fire fighters; it is constructed of treated fluorescent polyester and carries reflective striping.
- **Class 3.** This vest offers the highest level of visibility. It is worn in environments where the traffic is moving in excess of 55 mi/h (80 km/h), by roadway construction workers, utility workers, survey crews, and emergency response personnel.

law, each state is required to adopt the provisions in this manual. Section 6I, "The Control of Traffic Through Incident Management Areas," applies to all incidents that fire fighters might encounter on or near the roadway. It defines a **traffic incident** as an emergency traffic occurrence, a natural disaster, or other unplanned event that affects or impedes the normal flow of traffic. When traffic incidents occur, some form of **traffic control** must take place.

The goals of traffic control are fourfold:

- To improve responder safety while working at the incident
- To keep the traffic flowing as smoothly as possible around the incident
- To prevent the occurrence of secondary accidents at the scene
- To prevent unnecessary use of the surrounding road system

Within 15 minutes of arriving on the scene of a traffic incident, the IC should estimate the magnitude of the incident, the expected length of the queue of backed-up motorists on the highway or roadway, and the duration of the incident **FIGURE 7-16**. According to *MUTCD*, traffic incidents may be classified into one of three general classes of duration, each of which presents its own unique hazards and traffic control needs:

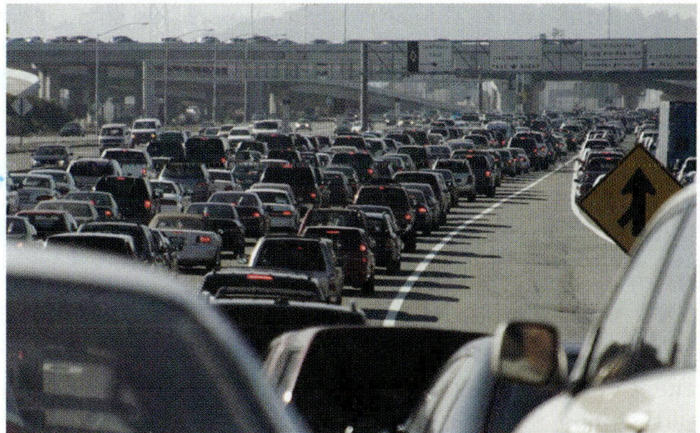

Figure 7-16 Traffic incident.
© Aaron Kohr/Shutterstock, Inc.

1. **Major traffic incidents** include fatal crashes involving multiple vehicles, hazardous materials incidents on the highway, and other disasters. They usually require closing all or part of the highway for a period exceeding 2 hours. When this type of incident occurs, fire personnel must request assistance from traffic engineering and law enforcement to divert traffic around and past the incident.
2. **Intermediate traffic incidents** are less severe in nature and usually affect the lanes of travel for 30 minutes to 2 hours. Traffic control is required to divert moving traffic around and past the incident. The highway may need to be closed for a short period to allow fire fighters to accomplish their task. Law enforcement personnel usually handle traffic control needs.
3. **Minor traffic incidents** may involve minor crashes and disabled vehicles. Lane closures are kept to a minimum and are less than 30 minutes in duration. Traffic control is needed only briefly, if at all. Fire personnel may handle any minor traffic control needs.

MUTCD defines a **traffic incident management area (TIMA)** as an area of highway where temporary traffic controls are imposed by authorized officials in response to a traffic incident, natural disaster, hazardous material spill, or other unplanned incident. This area is further subdivided into the following sections:

- The **advance warning area** is the section of highway where motorists are informed about the upcoming situation ahead. It may be identified by an emergency vehicle with its lights activated or by warning signs. On highways, the advance warning signs should be positioned farther ahead of the actual site because of the high speeds at which vehicles are traveling. When roadways are smaller and have lower speed limits, the distance can be shortened.
- The **transition area** is where the vehicle is redirected from its normal path and where lane changes and closures are made.
- The **activity area** is the section where the work activity takes place. It may be stationary or may move as work progresses.
- The **buffer space** is a lateral and/or longitudinal area that separates motorist flow from the work space or an

unsafe area. This area might also provide some recovery space for an errant vehicle.

- The **incident space** is the area where the actual incident is located.
- The **traffic space** is the portion of the highway in which traffic is routed through the activity area.
- The **termination area** is the area where the normal flow of traffic resumes.

By defining these areas, fire personnel gain a better understanding of where fire apparatus should be positioned at the scene. Communicating this information to incoming apparatus and describing their placement become easier when the scene is divided into separate areas.

Motor Vehicle Accidents

A **motor vehicle accident (MVA)** may involve one or more vehicles, either on or off the roadway. This type of emergency is a very common reason for calling out fire fighters. In metropolitan areas, the majority of these incidents tend to result in only very minor damage to both the vehicles and the passengers. By comparison, MVAs in rural areas and highways may have quite different outcomes; they are usually very serious and result in great damage to both the vehicles and the passengers.

As the fire apparatus approaches the accident scene, traffic is usually backed up behind the MVA. This makes the approach to the scene slower than normal and may be frustrating for the fire fighters, who are ready to go to work. As the driver/operator, you must not get impatient and allow your emotions to get the best of you. Proceed with caution and remain calm. In this situation, you must have a consistent approach to the incident site. Do not weave the fire apparatus in and out of traffic to gain access to the scene, as such maneuvers confuse other motorists about your intentions. Keep the fire apparatus in the far left lane while approaching the scene. If necessary, the fire officer can use the public address system on the fire apparatus to direct the backed-up traffic to the far right and allow the fire apparatus to reach the scene.

SAFETY TIP

On August 5, 1999, two career fire fighters of the Midwest City Fire Department (MCFD) were struck by a motor vehicle on a wet and busy interstate. MCFD Ladder Company 2 and Squad 2 had responded to a single motor vehicle accident on the interstate. The ladder apparatus was positioned approximately 150 ft (45 m) behind Squad 2, near the median wall, with its emergency lights left on.

A few minutes after arriving on scene, Ladder Company 2 was hit from behind by a passenger vehicle. Fire fighters began to attend to the injuries of this driver while other members began to flag traffic away. A fire fighter who was watching the oncoming traffic situation noticed a vehicle coming toward the rear of Ladder Company 2 and the fire fighters. Two warnings were yelled out over the radio. This car hit several fire fighters as they were attempting to flee its path. The vehicle collided with the median wall and wedged into the space between Ladder Company 2 and the wall. Several company members were able to avoid the impact of the vehicle, but two fire fighters and a civilian were not so fortunate. The impact knocked the three individuals approximately 47 ft (14 m), killing one fire fighter and severely injuring the other fire fighter and the civilian. While the fire fighters were attending to the injured people, yet another vehicle spun out of control on the interstate and struck the vehicle that had impacted the rear of Ladder Company 2.

Positioning at an Intersection

Based on Coaching the Emergency Vehicle Operator (CEVO) courses, motor vehicle accidents are more likely to occur at an intersection than anywhere else. These accidents usually involve more than one vehicle. A unique hazard that is present with an accident in an intersection is large groups of people attempting to help the accident victims. Traffic control should be the first priority once the fire apparatus arrives at the scene. If the moving traffic is not controlled, then the scene will not be safe for fire fighters. For most incidents, the fire apparatus itself can be positioned to shield the work area and to protect emergency responders from moving traffic.

Whenever possible, police should be called for assistance with traffic control. Police officers are specifically trained to carry out this type of operation. The initial fire apparatus must assess the parking needs of later-arriving units and specifically direct the parking and placement of these vehicles as they arrive to provide protective blocking of the scene. When parking the fire apparatus to protect the scene, be sure to protect the work area as well. Doing so ensures that victims can be extricated, treated, moved about the scene, and loaded into ambulances safely. Do not position the fire apparatus exhaust in the direction of the victims who are entrapped in motor vehicles.

At intersections or at sites where the incident is near the middle of the street, two or more sides of the incident may need

DRIVER/OPERATOR TIP

If the fire apparatus is equipped with a traffic control device, it may be tied into the emergency lighting system. In such a case, when the emergency lights are activated, so is the traffic control device. While the fire apparatus is positioned at an intersection for the response to an emergency and operating its emergency lights, this may pose a problem: The intersection lights will continue to cycle through at the request of the apparatus' traffic control device. To overcome this problem, the traffic control device is designed to shut off when the fire apparatus' parking brake is set. This system ensures that the fire apparatus can operate its emergency lights while parked and not disrupt the directional lights at an intersection.

Voice of Experience

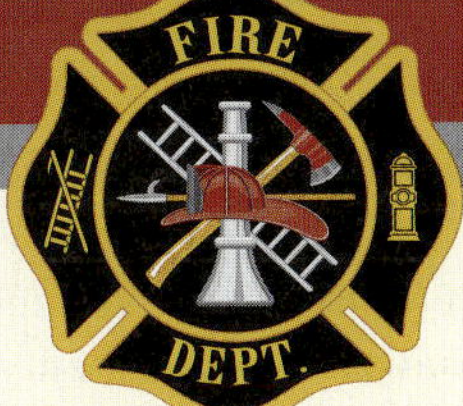

Because some incidents have a greater potential for violence than others, it may not always be a good idea to drive slowly past the address and stage a distance from the scene. All responses are department specific, but if you are dealing with a potentially violent scene, it is often safer to have the police secure a scene before making your presence known to those involved in the incident.

In our department, we have had numerous occasions where our personnel arrived before the police department but staged within sight of the scene. Passing or staging within sight of the scene often just creates more tension in a situation that requires more calm. We have had involved parties actually charge at our apparatus because they believe we should be administering care, even though our protocols require the police to secure such a scene for everyone's safety before we can move in.

At one particular incident several years ago, a subject at such a scene fired a rifle from a second-story window. The bullet traveled more than half a mile. Had our personnel been staged nearby, they would certainly have been in range of the bullet.

As a result of this incident, many of us choose to stage on a nearby side street, out of sight of the actual scene, until central dispatch advises us that the police have secured the scene. This prevents us from being sighted by the parties involved in the incident until the scene is secured. It also puts a buffer of structures between us and any possible gunfire, and we can quickly retreat from the area if involved parties approach.

Christopher Drake
Muskegon Fire Department
Muskegon, Michigan

to be protected. In such a case, fire apparatus should block all exposed sides. Where fire apparatus are limited in numbers, prioritize the blocking scheme from the most critical sides to the least critical. Once enough fire apparatus have blocked the scene, park or stage unneeded vehicles off the street whenever possible. When ambulances are positioned at a scene, always protect the victim loading areas.

Positioning on a Highway

Because speeds are higher, traffic volume is more significant, and civilian motorists have little opportunity to slow, stop, or change lanes, fire fighters must be constantly aware of moving vehicles on highways. Although at times the scene may seem safe, matters can change at a moment's notice.

When approaching an emergency scene on a highway, identify a position that will allow fire fighters to work in a safe area. Sometimes this may involve disrupting the normal flow of traffic or blocking it off completely. The safety of the fire fighters should always be the first priority—not the continuous flow of traffic. When doubt arises about the proper positioning of the fire apparatus, always err on the side of caution: Block the highway to provide a safe working area for fire fighters. For emergencies on a highway, continue to block the scene with the first-arriving fire apparatus to provide a safe working area. Other companies may then be used to provide additional blocking if needed. If possible, use the largest, heaviest fire apparatus (usually ladder apparatus) as the first blocker.

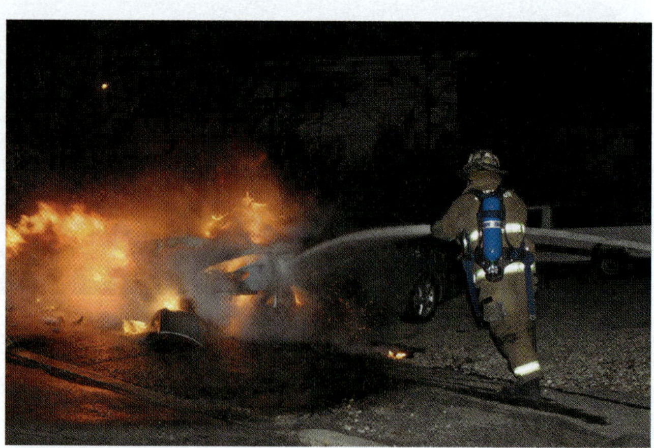

Figure 7-17 A vehicle fire.

Vehicle Fires

Fire departments respond to more vehicle fires than they do structure fires. In fact, approximately 25 percent of all reported fires in the United States involve vehicles. These types of fires should not be taken lightly. Given the various amounts of plastics, foams, and synthetic materials from which modern-day vehicles are constructed, a vehicle may be consumed quickly by an intense, fast-moving fire. Most often, the vehicle is so severely damaged before the fire department arrives on scene that it is a total loss. Indeed, the majority of vehicle fires result in a total loss.

When responding to a vehicle fire, do not position the fire apparatus where it will become an exposure hazard. FIGURE 7-17. Specifically, try to position the fire apparatus in a location that is uphill and upwind of the burning vehicle. While this may not always be the most advantageous position on the scene, you do not want smoke or flammable liquids to compromise the safe operation of the fire apparatus. If you have to position it downhill from the burning vehicle, create a dike in front of the fire apparatus to pool any flammable liquids. Be aware that the brakes on the burning vehicle may be compromised by the fire conditions, and the vehicle may roll downhill; do not place the fire apparatus in a position that might allow the burning vehicle to roll into it.

You should position the fire apparatus at a 45-degree angle to the burning vehicle to protect the area near the pump panel as well as the scene. Most fire apparatus have the fire pump mounted on the driver's side in the middle of the vehicle; this is the location where the driver/operator stands while operating the fire pump. Be aware of where the fire fighters are deploying hoselines at the scene. While the other members of the crew are extinguishing the fire, the driver/operator is responsible for providing adequate water from the pump and ensuring that the crew remains safe. This effort may involve positioning traffic cones or warning devices to alert oncoming traffic to the emergency scene.

Railroads

When positioning the fire apparatus near a railroad track, try to place it on the same side as the incident. This placement will ensure that fire fighters do not have to cross the tracks, thereby risking injury or death from oncoming trains. Every railroad track should be considered active. If possible, contact dispatch and request that the railroad tracks be shut down while on-scene operations continue. Whenever possible, the apparatus should not enter the railroad right-of-way until confirmation is received from the railroad that train traffic has been suspended. ***Never*** park the fire apparatus on top of the railroad tracks.

Positioning at the Emergency Medical Scene

An emergency medical scene can be just as dangerous as the other types of incidents to which fire fighters respond. Usually, the danger is not associated with the emergency scene itself but rather with the people involved. Every day, fire personnel somewhere are surprised by a scene that becomes violent when initially it appeared safe. At a moment's notice, what looks like a routine call can turn into a deadly encounter. Thus the first priority when arriving at an EMS scene is to provide a protected environment for fire fighters to work in. If the fire fighters are not safe, then they cannot provide adequate care. Ideally, the driver/operator should position the fire apparatus either 100 ft (30 m) before or after the address. This placement will allow the entire crew to size up the situation and recognize any potential hazards. Do not position the fire apparatus directly in front of the address, as such placement does not allow the entire crew adequate time to identify or react to any potential hazards.

Some incidents have a greater potential for violence than others, including assaults, fights, and domestic disputes. When fire companies are requested to respond to these types of calls, you should turn off the emergency lights and siren a few blocks away from the physical address of the incident. Fire personnel should enter the scene on their own terms and not rush into an unknown situation. For such calls, you should drive slowly past the address and park the fire apparatus at least 100 ft (30 m) from the building/location.

At EMS scenes, the fire apparatus should be positioned for a quick exit. If necessary, turn it around. This may involve backing the fire apparatus into an alley or side street. NFPA 1002, *Standard for Fire Apparatus Driver/Operator Professional Qualifications*, requires that all driver/operators complete an exercise—the alley dock exercise—that simulates the process of backing a fire apparatus into an alley or tight space. This exercise measures your ability to drive on a street past a simulated area and then back up the fire apparatus into the dock provided.

During the alley dock exercise, a street may be simulated by arranging marker cones 40 ft (12 m) from a boundary line. The marker cones should mark off an area 12 ft (4 m) wide and 20 ft (6 m) long, indicating the "dock" the fire apparatus will back into. As part of the exercise, you will pass the marker cones with the dock on the left and then back up the fire apparatus, using a left turn into the dock. This exercise should then be completed with the dock on the right side of the fire apparatus. The minimum depth of the apparatus bay is determined by the length of the fire apparatus. During the entire alley dock exercise, the fire apparatus must remain within the marked boundary and move in a continuous motion, except when required to change direction of travel. A spotter is necessary for this exercise.

To perform the alley dock exercise, follow the steps in SKILL DRILL 7-4.

Special Emergency Scene Positioning

Although some incidents occur with less frequency than others, the need for proper scene positioning is always paramount. Special emergency scenes may include anything from a building collapse to a hazardous materials incident. During these incidents, fire fighters should be very cautious and resist the urge to rush into the scene and mitigate the situation. These incidents often unfold slowly at first, until enough information has been gathered to determine the appropriate course of action.

When responding to these incidents and preparing to position the apparatus, the driver/operator must consider the **control zones**. These areas at an incident—which are labeled "hot," "warm," or "cold" based on the severity of the incident—surround the incident:

- **Hot zone.** The area for entry teams and rescue teams only. This zone immediately surrounds the dangers of the site (e.g., hazardous materials release) and is demarcated to protect personnel outside the zone.
- **Warm zone.** The area for properly trained and equipped personnel only. This zone is where personnel and equipment decontamination and hot zone support take place.
- **Cold zone.** The area for staging vehicles and equipment until requested by the IC. The command post is located in this zone. The public and the media should be kept clear of the cold zone at all times.

The following list identifies some ideas for proper apparatus positioning during these incidents:

- **Hazardous materials incident.** The first course of action at any hazardous materials incident is to isolate the area and prevent anyone from entering it. The first-arriving company may have to position its apparatus to block a highway to prevent anyone from entering the scene. The proper apparatus position for these incidents is uphill and upwind. The material should be identified; once the scene is deemed safe, and if needed, the apparatus may then be driven closer to the scene.
- **Building collapse.** During this type of incident, the primary danger to fire fighters and fire apparatus is secondary collapse. Position the apparatus out of the collapse zone. Heavy equipment such as bulldozers and cranes may be required for on-scene operations. Do not block this equipment from reaching the incident; always leave a path for its entrance and exit.
- **Trench collapse.** Once a trench fails, the probability of secondary collapse is quite high. For this reason, first-arriving units should be positioned no closer than 150 ft (45 m) to the trench. All other incoming nonessential apparatus should stage at least 200 ft (60 m) away from the trench. Only equipment that is needed for a rescue should be brought any closer than the first-arriving units.
- **Terrorism.** These types of incidents may present as an explosion, a building collapse, release of radioactive material, or any other potential hazard. Terrorist incidents have the potential to injure and kill large numbers of people. During a possible terrorist incident, fire fighters should position the apparatus based on the demands of the emergency. Be aware of the potential for future hazards and the possible need for rapid escape, but position the apparatus to best accomplish the tasks at hand.

SKILL DRILL 7-4

Performing the Alley Dock Exercise NFPA 1002, 4.3.4, 4.3.4(B)

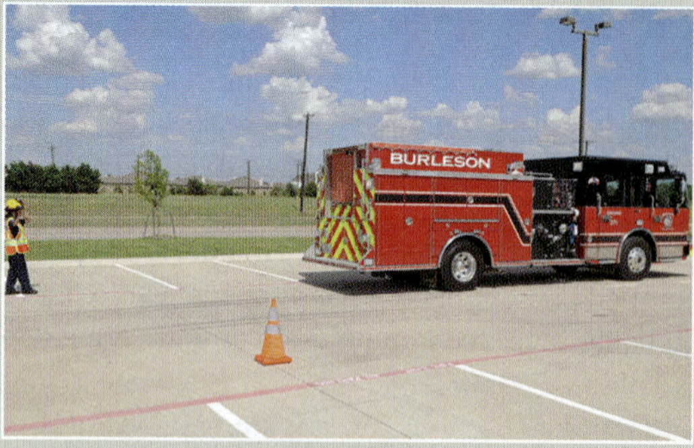

1 Position the rear of the fire apparatus past the dock's opening and at a 90-degree angle to the marker cones.

Ensure that a spotter is correctly positioned behind the fire apparatus.

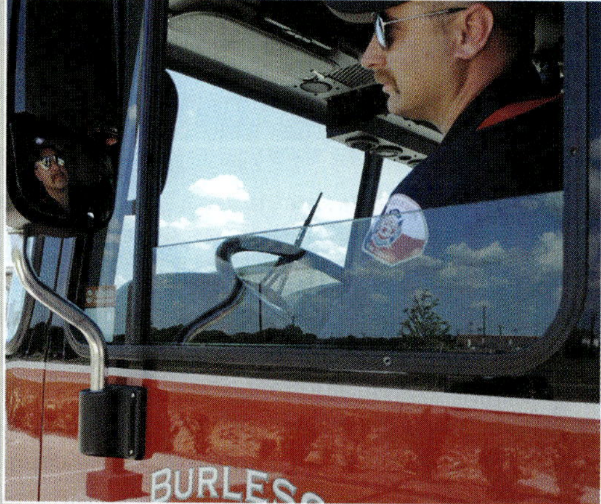

2 Activate the emergency lights.

Roll down the windows.

Turn off any mounted stereo equipment.

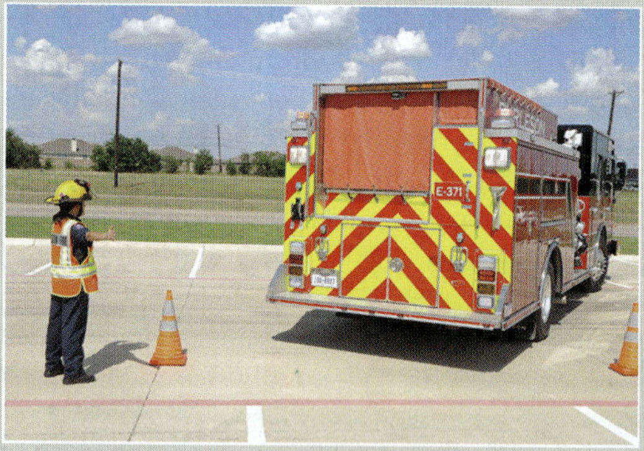

3 Disengage the parking brake, if set.

Shift the transmission into reverse.

Proceed in a reverse mode, and turn the fire apparatus to align it with the objective.

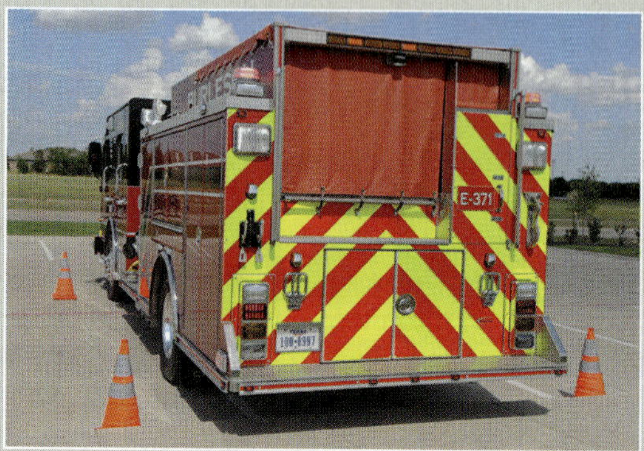

4 Continue backing the fire apparatus until it has reached the desired objective or the spotter signals "stop."

After-Action Review

IN SUMMARY

- The communications center gives the dispatch information to the responding fire apparatus.
- As the driver/operator, you must disseminate the dispatch information and identify which information will aid your crew in locating the emergency and responding to it.
- The response process begins when the alarm is received at the fire station. Dispatch messages will include the location of the incident, the type of emergency, and the units that are due to respond.
- A variety of maps may be used to locate the sites of emergency incidents.
- No member of any fire department should be allowed to drive an emergency vehicle or fire apparatus until he or she has completed a training course approved by the fire department.
- Fire fighters should always be cautious during the response. As the fire apparatus approaches the scene, the driver/operator should slow down, identify the correct address/location, and recognize any potential hazards.
- While approaching a fire scene, the driver/operator should attempt to view at least three sides of the structure.
- Operating at an emergency scene that is located either on or adjacent to a highway or an intersection is extremely dangerous.
- The first priority upon arrival at an EMS scene is to provide a protected environment for fire fighters to work in.
- Upon arrival at a scene, traffic safety should be a major concern. Always check for traffic before exiting the apparatus. Follow departmental SOPs to close streets quickly and block access for civilian vehicles to the incident.
- When responding to a special emergency scene, the driver/operator must consider the control zones (areas at the incident that are labeled "hot," "warm," or "cold" based on the severity of the incident) that surround the incident.

KEY TERMS

activity area The area of the incident scene where the work activity takes place; it may be stationary or may move as work progresses.

advance warning area The section of highway where drivers are informed about an upcoming situation ahead.

aerial device An aerial ladder, elevating platform, aerial ladder platform, or water tower that is designed to position personnel, handle materials, provide continuous egress, or discharge water.

ambulance A vehicle designed, equipped, and operated for the treatment and transport of ill and injured persons.

auxiliary appliance A standpipe and/or sprinkler system.

brake fade Reduction in stopping power that can occur after repeated application of the brakes, especially in high-load or high-speed conditions.

braking distance The distance that the fire apparatus travels from the time the brakes are activated until the fire apparatus makes a complete stop.

buffer space The lateral and/or longitudinal area that separates traffic flow from a work space or an unsafe area; it might also provide some recovery space for an errant vehicle.

centrifugal force The outward force that is exerted away from the center of rotation. Also, the tendency for objects to be pulled outward when rotating around a center.

Code 1 response Response in a fire apparatus in which no emergency lights or sirens are activated.

Code 2 response Response in a fire apparatus in which only the emergency lights are activated; no audible devices are activated.

Code 3 response Response in a fire apparatus in which both the emergency lights and the sirens are activated.

collapse zone An area encompassing a distance of 1½ times the height of a building. Fire fighters and fire apparatus must not be located in this area in case of a building collapse.

command vehicle A vehicle that the fire chief uses to respond to the fire scene.

communications center A building or portion of a building that is specifically configured for the primary purpose of providing emergency communications services or public safety answering point (PSAP) services to one or more public safety agencies under the authority or authorities having jurisdiction.

control zones A series of areas at hazardous materials incidents that are designated based on safety concerns and the degree of hazard present.

corner safe areas Areas outside a building where two walls intersect; these areas are less likely to receive any damage during a building collapse.

critical speed The maximum speed that a fire apparatus can safely travel around a curve.

dispatch To send out emergency response resources promptly to an address or incident location for a specific purpose.

emitter A device that emits a visible flashing light at a specified frequency, thereby activating the receiver on a traffic signal.

freelancing The dangerous practice of acting independently of command instructions.

global positioning system (GPS) A satellite-based radio navigation system consisting of three segments: space, control, and user.

incident space The area where the actual incident is located.

intermediate traffic incidents A traffic incident that affects the lanes of travel for 30 minutes to 2 hours.

Level I staging Initial staging of fire apparatus in which three or more units are dispatched to an emergency incident.

Level II staging Placement of all reserve resources in a central location until requested to the scene.

liquid surge The force imposed upon a fire apparatus by the contents of a partially filled water or foam concentrate tank when the vehicle is accelerated, decelerated, or turned.

major traffic incidents A traffic incident that involves a fatal crash, a multiple-vehicle incident, a hazardous materials incident on the highway, or other disaster.

minor traffic incidents A traffic incident that involves a minor crash and/or disabled vehicles.

mobile data terminals (MDTs) A computer that is located on the fire apparatus.

motor vehicle accident (MVA) An incident that involves one vehicle colliding with another vehicle or another object and that may result in injury, property damage, and possibly death.

parking brake The main brake that prevents a fire apparatus from moving even when it is turned off and there is no one operating it.

preincident plan A document developed by gathering general and detailed data, which are then used by responding personnel to determine the resources and actions necessary to mitigate anticipated emergencies at a specific facility.

reaction distance The distance that the fire apparatus travels after the driver/operator recognizes the hazard, removes his or her foot from the accelerator, and applies the brakes.

receiver A device placed on or near a traffic signal to recognize a signal from the emitter on an emergency vehicle and preempt the normal cycle of the traffic light.

response The deployment of an emergency service resource to an incident. (NFPA 901)

size-up The observation and evaluation of existing factors that are used to develop objectives, strategy, and tactics for fire suppression. (NFPA 1051)

staging A specific function whereby resources are assembled in an area at or near the incident scene to await instructions or assignments.

staging area A prearranged, strategically placed area, where support response personnel, vehicles, and other equipment can be held in an organized state of readiness for use during an emergency.

staging area manager The person responsible for maintaining the operations of the staging area.

termination area The area where the normal flow of traffic resumes after a traffic incident.

total stopping distance The distance that it takes for the driver/operator to recognize a hazard, process the need to stop the fire apparatus, apply the brakes, and then come to a complete stop.

traffic control The direction or management of vehicle traffic such that scene safety is maintained and rescue operations can proceed without interruption.

traffic incident A natural disaster or other unplanned event that affects or impedes the normal flow of traffic.

traffic incident management area (TIMA) An area of highway where temporary traffic controls are imposed by authorized officials in response to an accident, natural disaster, hazardous materials spill, or other unplanned incident.

traffic signal preemption system A system that allows the normal operation of a traffic signal to be changed so as to assist emergency vehicles in responding to an emergency.

traffic space The portion of the highway where traffic is routed through the activity area of a traffic incident.

transition area The area where vehicles are redirected from their normal path and where lane changes and closures are made in a traffic incident.

REFERENCES

Dunn, V. *Safety and Survival on the Fireground*. Tulsa, OK: Pennwell Books; 1992.

National Fire Protection Association (NFPA) 1001, *Standard for Fire Fighter Professional Qualifications*. 2013. https://www.nfpa.org/codes-and-standards/all-codes-and-standards/list-of-codes-and-standards/detail?code=1001. Accessed January 17, 2018.

National Fire Protection Association (NFPA) 1002, *Standard for Fire Apparatus Driver/Operator Professional Qualifications*. 2017. http://www.nfpa.org/codes-and-standards/all-codes-and-standards/list-of-codes-and-standards/detail?code=1002. Accessed January 17, 2018.

National Fire Protection Association (NFPA) 1500, *Standard on Fire Department Occupational Safety, Health, and*

Wellness Program. 2018. https://downloads.nfpa.org/codes-and-standards/all-codes-and-standards/list-of-codes-and-standards/detail?code=1500. Accessed January 17, 2018.

National Fire Protection Association (NFPA) 1561, *Standard on Emergency Services Incident Management System and Command Safety*. 2014. https://downloads.nfpa.org/codes-and-standards/all-codes-and-standards/list-of-codes-and-standards/detail?code=1561. Accessed January 17, 2018.

National Fire Protection Association (NFPA) 1620, *Standard for Pre-incident Planning*. 2015. https://downloads.nfpa.org/codes-and-standards/all-codes-and-standards/list-of-codes-and-standards/detail?code=1620. Accessed January 17, 2018.

National Fire Protection Association (NFPA) 1901, *Standard for Automotive Fire Apparatus*. 2016. https://downloads.nfpa.org/codes-and-standards/all-codes-and-standards/list-of-codes-and-standards/detail?code=1901. Accessed January 17, 2018.

National Fire Protection Association. *Fire Fighter Fatalities in the US, 2016*, Figure 2. http://www.nfpa.org/news-and-research/fire-statistics-and-reports/fire-statistics/the-fire-service/fatalities-and-injuries/firefighter-fatalities-in-the-united-states. Accessed August 22, 2017.

U.S. Department of Transportation, Federal Highway Administration. *Manual on Uniform Traffic Control Devices for Streets and Highways (MUTCD)*. Washington, DC: U.S. Department of Transportation; 2009.

On Scene

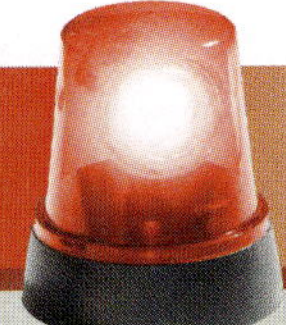

During the emergency response, you concentrate on getting the other members of the crew to the scene quickly and safely. While the officer and the pipeman are thinking of the tasks they may be assigned, you must stay focused on the road and drive in a defensive manner. As you approach the scene, the incident commander assigns your engine company to assist with exposure protection at the rear of the building. Now that you are on scene, it is up to you to assist the other members of the crew and ensure that they have the tools and equipment necessary to perform their job.

1. What is a Code 3 response?
- **A.** Responding to an emergency without lights and sirens
- **B.** Responding to a nonemergency with lights and sirens
- **C.** Responding to an emergency with lights and sirens
- **D.** Responding to an emergency with lights but not sirens

2. The movement of liquid inside a container as the container is moved is called:
- **A.** pressure.
- **B.** centrifugal force.
- **C.** liquid surge.
- **D.** critical speed.

3. If the apparatus begins to skid, you should do all of the following EXCEPT:
- **A.** stay off the brake.
- **B.** steer.
- **C.** continue to steer.
- **D.** engage the parking brake.

4. At the scene of a trench collapse, the first-arriving apparatus should be positioned no closer than ____ from the trench.
- **A.** 50 ft (15 m)
- **B.** 75 ft (25 m)
- **C.** 100 ft (30 m)
- **D.** 150 ft (45 m)

5. Which traffic safety vest is required for fire department personnel?
- **A.** Class 1
- **B.** Class 2
- **C.** Class 3
- **D.** Class 4

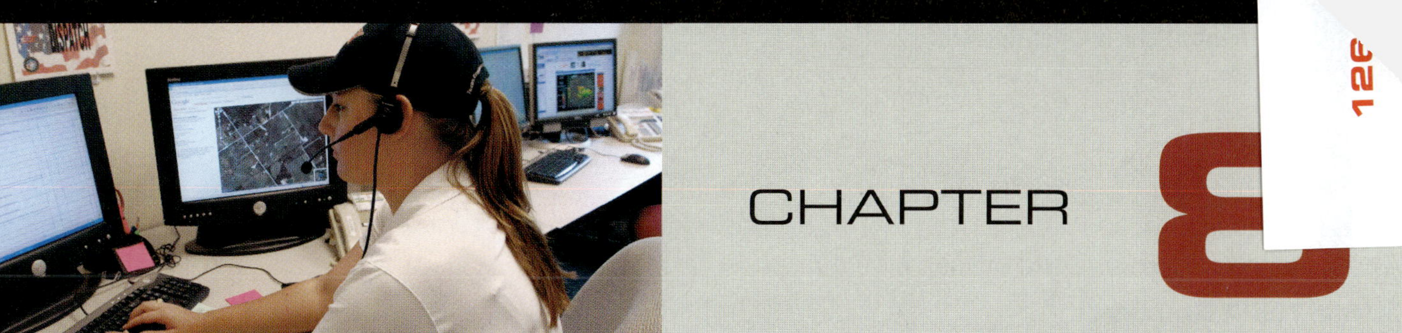

CHAPTER 8

Emergency Services Communications

KNOWLEDGE OBJECTIVES

After studying this chapter, you will be able to:

- Describe the role of the communications center in the fire service.
- Describe the role and responsibilities of a telecommunicator. (**NFPA 1002, 4.4.1**)
- List the requirements of a communications center. (p 588)
- Describe the equipment used in a communications center. (**NFPA 1002, 4.4.1**)
- Describe how computer-aided dispatch assists in dispatching the correct resources to an emergency incident. (**NFPA 1002, 4.4.1**)
- Describe the basic services provided by the communications center. (**NFPA 1002, 4.4.1**)
- List the five major steps in processing an emergency incident. (**NFPA 1002, 4.4.1(A)**)
- Describe how telecommunicators conduct a telephone interrogation. (**NFPA 1002, 4.4.1(A)**)
- Describe how location validation systems operate.
- Describe the three types of fire service radios. (**NFPA 1002, 4.4.3**)
- Describe how two-way radio systems operate. (**NFPA 1002, 4.4.3**)
- Explain how a repeater system works to enhance fire service communications. (**NFPA 1002, 4.4.3**)
- Explain how a trunking system works to enhance fire service communications. (**NFPA 1002, 4.4.3**)
- Describe the basic principles of effective radio communication. (**NFPA 1002, 4.4.3**)
- Describe when to use plain language and how ten-codes are implemented in fire service communications. (**NFPA 1002, 4.4.3(A)**)
- Describe fire department procedures for answering nonemergency business and personal telephone calls. (**NFPA 1002, 4.4.2, 4.4.2(A)**)

SKILLS OBJECTIVES

After studying this chapter, you will be able to:

- Receive a call and initiate a response to an emergency. (**NFPA 1002, 4.4.2(B)**)
- Observe the operation of a communications center.
- Demonstrate how to use a portable radio. (**NFPA 1002, 4.4.1(B)**)
- Operate and answer the fire station telephone. (**NFPA 1002, 4.4.2(A), 4.4.2(B)**)
- Define emergency traffic. (**NFPA 1002, 4.4.3(B)**)

- Explain how to initiate a mayday call. (**NFPA 1002, 4.4.4, 4.4.4(A), 4.4.4(B)**)
- Describe common evacuation signals. (**NFPA 1002, 4.4.3(A)**)

Additional NFPA Standards

- **NFPA 1001**, *Standard for Fire Fighter Professional Qualifications*
- **NFPA 1221**, *Standard for the Installation, Maintenance, and Use of Emergency Services Communications Systems*

Emergency Call

At 3:04 AM, you are dispatched to a report of a fire at 3256 West Madison. Your captain asks if any additional details are available, and the dispatcher reports that the caller said there was smoke coming from the eaves of the building and then hung up. You are getting excited about the prospect of a working fire—but then the dispatcher comes back and says that this may be a false report, because the caller used a cell phone from the east side of town. Your aggravation level rises at the prospect of being woken up for another false call—at least until the dispatcher comes back with a frantic sound in her voice and says that a home security company just reported a fire alarm at 3256 *East* Madison. Thoughts plow through your mind, and you wonder what is going on.

1. What is the process for receiving 911 calls in an emergency communications center?
2. How would the dispatcher know where the cell phone call originated?
3. How is the dispatcher able to communicate this information so quickly?

Introduction

Rapidly developing technology and advanced communications systems are having a tremendous effect on fire department communications. As a driver/operator, you must be familiar with the communications systems, equipment, and procedures used in your department. This chapter provides a basic guide to help you understand how fire department communications systems work and how commonly used systems are configured.

Every fire department depends on a functional communications system. When a citizen requests assistance or an alarm sounds, the communications center dispatches the appropriate units to the incident, and it continues to maintain communication with those units throughout the entire duration of the incident. The communications system is the link between fire personnel on the scene, the rest of the organization, and other agencies and people. The communications center monitors everything that happens at the incident scene and processes all requests for assistance or special resources.

At the scene, fire personnel need to communicate with one another so that the incident commander (IC) can manage the operation efficiently based on progress reports or requests for assistance from fire companies. The Incident Command System (ICS) depends on the presence of a functional on-site communications system. During incidents, fire personnel must be able to communicate not only with one another but also with other emergency response agencies.

The communications center does more than simply dispatch units and communicate with them during emergency operations. It also tracks the location and status of every other fire department unit. The communications center must always know which units can be dispatched to an incident, and it must be able to contact those units promptly. In addition, it is responsible for redeploying units to maintain adequate coverage for all areas.

Along with meeting these special communications requirements, a fire department must have a communications infrastructure that allows it to function as an effective organization. Basic administration and day-to-day management require an efficient communications network, including telephone and data links with every fire station and work site.

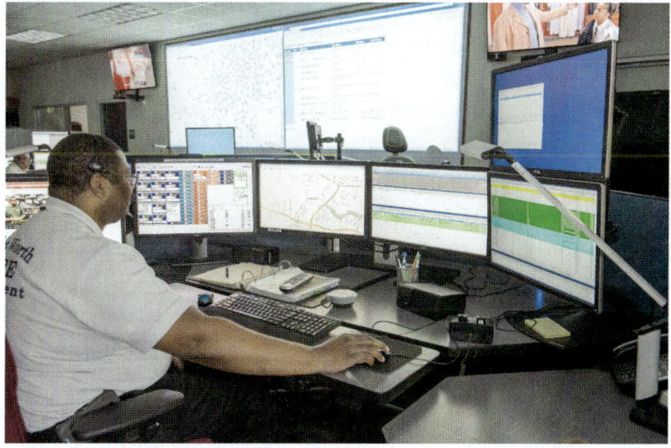

Figure 8-1 No matter what their size, all communications centers perform the same basic functions.

The Communications Center

Most requests for fire department response are made by either landline telephone or cellular (cell) phone. According to the National Emergency Number Association (NENA, 2017), more than 96 percent of the population in the United States has access to some type of 911 system to report an emergency. Emergency and nonemergency calls received via this system are then directed to a **public safety communications center** for that community or jurisdiction. The communications center may be a designated **public safety answering point (PSAP)**, which serves and dispatches multiple agencies (fire, emergency medical services [EMS], and law enforcement), or it may be a standalone communications center, which serves and dispatches only a single agency (e.g., the fire department). Some communications centers work with several fire departments or with all of the fire departments in a county or region.

A joint facility may house separate personnel and independent systems for each service delivery agency; alternatively, the entire operation may be integrated, with all employees being cross-trained to receive calls and dispatch responders to any type of emergency incident. When fire, EMS, and law enforcement communications are located in the same facility, the call can be answered, processed, and dispatched immediately. If these agencies operate in separate facilities, those calls must be transferred to the appropriate telecommunicator. Some agencies, on larger incidents, also have a mobile communications center that allows dispatchers to be on site and run communications for an incident. The call-taking process is described in more detail later in this chapter.

Regardless of how or where the call is transferred, the public safety communications center is the hub of the fire department's emergency response system. It serves as the central processing point for all information related to an emergency incident and all information related to the location, status, and activities of fire department units. It connects and controls all of the department's communications systems or serves as the PSAP. The communications center functions much like the human brain—that is, information comes in via the nerves, is processed, and is then sent back out to be acted upon by the various parts of the body.

The communications center is a physical location, whose size and complexity will vary depending on the needs of the department. The communications center for one department may be a small room in the fire station; another department may have a specially designed, highly sophisticated facility with advanced technological equipment. The fire department in a small community may need a simple system, whereas the public safety agencies in a metropolitan area may require complex capabilities. Some distinct differences between rural and urban dispatch centers are apparent—specifically, the number of dispatchers needed at any given time, the type of training required, and, to some extent, the type of equipment used. No matter what their size, however, all communications centers perform the same basic functions **FIGURE 8-1**.

Telecommunicators

The employees who staff a communications center are known as dispatchers or **telecommunicators**. The job of a telecommunicator can be complicated, demanding, and extremely stressful. Even in the face of these challenges, the successful telecommunicator is able to receive, process, or disseminate information, understand and follow complicated procedures, perform multiple tasks effectively, memorize information, and make decisions quickly. Just as special qualities can make an individual a good fire fighter, so a telecommunicator must possess certain qualities to meet all of the modern challenges and fill this role successfully. Telecommunicators who have been professionally trained to work in a public safety communications environment, and who have completed advanced training and professional certification programs, will be well prepared to be the skilled, competent individuals needed to fulfill this critical role in the public safety system.

One of the telecommunicator's most important skills is the ability to communicate effectively with citizens to obtain critical information, even when the caller is highly stressed or in extreme personal danger. Even if an emotional caller criticizes or insults the telecommunicator, the telecommunicator must respond professionally and focus on obtaining the essential information. Voice control and the ability to maintain one's composure under pressure are important qualities in this role; the telecommunicator must always be clear, calm, and in control.

A telecommunicator must be skilled in operating all of the systems and equipment in the communications center. He or she must understand and follow the fire department's operational procedures, particularly those relating to dispatch policies and protocols, radio communications, and incident management. The telecommunicator must keep track of the status and location of each unit at all times and monitor the overall deployment and availability of resources throughout the system. National Fire Protection Association (NFPA) 1061, *Standard for Public Safety Telecommunications Personnel Professional Qualifications*, contains a complete list of qualifications for telecommunicator candidates.

Communications Facility Requirements

The fire department communications center must be designed and operated to ensure that its critical mission can be performed with a very high degree of reliability. The performance requirements in NFPA 1221, *Standard for the Installation, Maintenance, and Use of Emergency Services Communications Systems*, govern the design and construction of a fire department or public safety communications center. These requirements apply whether the communications center serves a small community with only one or two fire stations or a metropolitan area with dozens of stations.

The communications center should be well protected against natural threats such as floods, and it should be able to withstand predictable damaging forces such as floods, earthquakes, snowstorms, tornados, hurricanes, and other severe storms. It should be located so that it can continue to function in times of civil unrest. In addition, this center should be able to operate at maximum capacity, without interruption, even when other community services are severely affected. The building should be equipped with emergency generators and other systems so that it can continue to operate for several days in even the most challenging conditions.

NFPA 1221 also requires backup systems for all of the critical equipment in a communications center so that the failure of a single component or system will not disable the entire operation. For example, there must be more than one way of transmitting a dispatch message from the communications center to each fire station. A backup radio transmitter should be available, and the telephone system must be able to receive calls even if part of the system is damaged. The design of the facility should minimize its vulnerability to a fire originating inside the building as well as to nearby fires. The building must also be physically secured to prevent unauthorized entry.

A backup communications center at a different location should be established as well. If some unanticipated situation makes it impossible to operate from the primary location, this backup location can be activated to ensure ongoing operation of the communications function.

Plans need to be in place for the reporting of emergencies in the event that the emergency communications center fails. Some communities have plans in place to locate fire department and law enforcement vehicles at strategic locations so citizens can report emergencies. Fire station personnel may also plan to staff a watch desk to report emergencies from citizens who walk into the fire station.

Computer-Aided Dispatch

Computers are used in almost all communications centers. Most large communications centers use sophisticated **computer-aided dispatch (CAD)** systems that perform many functions; many smaller centers have smaller-scale, less sophisticated versions of CAD systems.

A CAD system helps meet the most important objective in processing an emergency call—namely, sending the appropriate units to the correct location as quickly as possible. As the name suggests, a CAD system is a combination of hardware and software designed to assist a telecommunicator by performing specific functions more quickly and efficiently than they can be done manually.

Once the address is determined and the incident description is in the CAD system, the system quickly makes a recommendation on the appropriate units to dispatch. While all of the functions performed by a CAD system can be performed manually by trained and experienced telecommunicators, the system can make a recommendation on the appropriate units to dispatch in less than a second FIGURE 8-2. Data links that provide the location of the caller and automatically enter the address can also save time. If duplicate addresses might exist or if the address entered is not a valid location, the CAD system will prompt the telecommunicator to ask the caller for more information.

The most advanced type of CAD system utilizes **global positioning system (GPS)** data devices to confirm the location of the caller. The **geographic information system (GIS)** stores and integrates data gathered from GPS. The CAD system determines where each unit is located, which units are available to respond to a call, which units are assigned to incidents, which units are temporarily assigned to cover different areas, and what the closest fire stations are, in order of response, for any

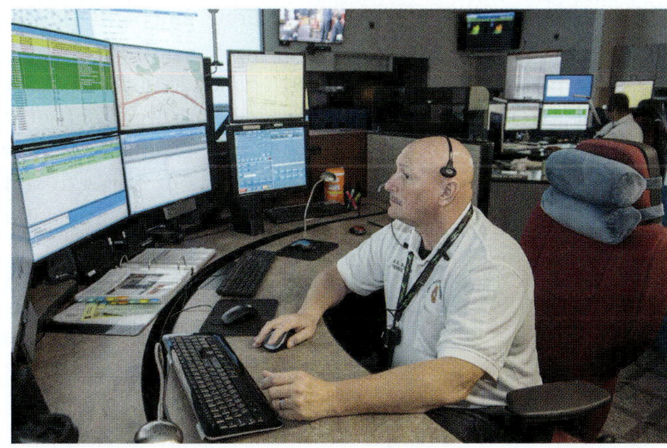

Figure 8-2 A CAD system enables a telecommunicator to work more quickly and efficiently.

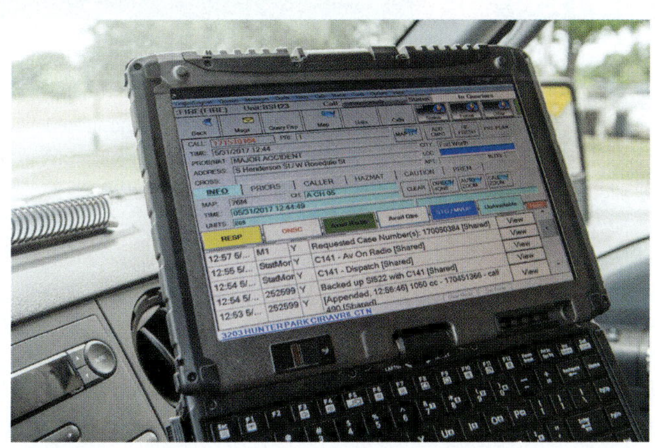

Figure 8-3 Some CAD systems transmit dispatch information directly to terminals in fire stations and mobile data terminals in the apparatus.

location. Using this information, it can identify which units can respond quickly to an alarm, even if some of the units that would normally respond to the call are currently unavailable. A major advantage of a CAD system is that it automatically captures and stores every event as it occurs. Before such systems were developed, someone had to write down and time-stamp every transaction, including every radio transmission; all of these hard-copy logs then had to be retained for future reference.

Some CAD systems transmit dispatch information directly to **mobile data terminals (MDTs)** or to computers that are located in the fire station or on the apparatus FIGURE 8-3. In addition, these systems can provide immediate access to information such as preincident plans, hazardous materials lists, lockbox locations, and information such as whether persons with limited mobility reside at the address of the emergency call. By linking the CAD system to other data files, fire personnel gain access to even more useful information such as travel route instructions, maps, and reference materials.

Voice Recorders and Activity Logs

Almost everything that happens in a communications center is recorded, either by a **voice recording system** or by an **activity logging system**. Most communications centers can automatically record everything that is said over the telephone or radio, 24 hours a day. In addition, most have an instant playback unit that allows the telecommunicator to replay conversations for the previous 10 to 15 minutes at the touch of a button. This feature is particularly valuable if the caller talks very quickly, has an unusual accent, hangs up, or is disconnected. The telecommunicator can replay the message several times, if necessary, to determine exactly what was said.

The logging system keeps a detailed record of every incident and activity that occurs. These records include every call that is entered, every unit that is dispatched, and every significant event that occurs in relation to an emergency incident. Times are recorded when a call is received, when the units are dispatched, when they report that they are en route, when they arrive at the scene, when the incident is under control, and when the last unit leaves the scene.

Voice recorders and activity logs are maintained for several reasons. First, they serve as legal records of the official delivery of a government service by a public agency (i.e., the fire department). These records may be required for legal proceedings, sometimes years after an incident occurred. They may be needed to defend the fire department's actions when questions are raised about an unfortunate outcome. The records provided by voice recorders and activity logs accurately document the events and can often demonstrate that the organization and its employees performed ethically, responsibly, and professionally. They also make it difficult to hide an error, if a mistake was made.

Second, records are valuable in reviewing and analyzing information about department operations. Good record keeping enables a fire department to examine what happened on a particular call as well as to measure workloads, system performance, activity trends, and other factors as part of its planning and budget preparation. For example, analysts and planners can use data from CAD systems to study deployment strategies and to make the most efficient use of fire department resources.

The telecommunicator's first responsibility is to obtain the information that is required to dispatch the appropriate units to the correct location FIGURE 8-4. At that point, the incident must be processed according to standard protocols. Using the CAD system information (if available), the telecommunicator must decide which agencies or units should respond and transmit the necessary information to them. The generally accepted performance objective is that the time from when a call reaches the communications center until the units are dispatched should be approximately 90 seconds (NFPA 1221, 2016).

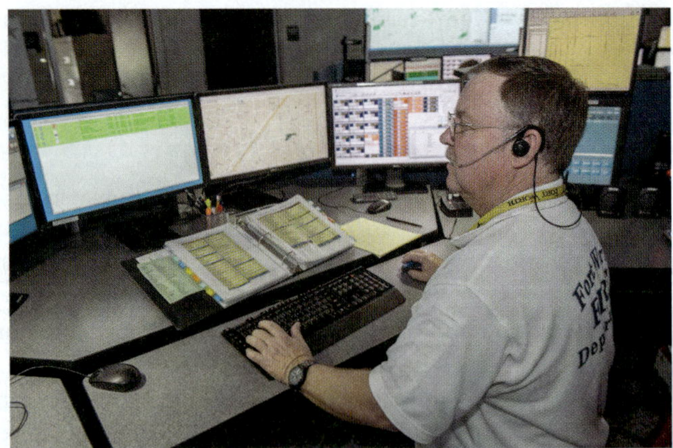

Figure 8-4 Telecommunicators must obtain information and relay it accurately to the appropriate responders.

Communications Center Operations

Several different functions are performed in a fire department or public safety communications center. All of these activities must be performed accurately and efficiently, even in the most challenging circumstances. For example, the activity level in a communications center can ratchet up from calm to extreme in less than a minute during an emergency, but the chaos outside must not affect the operations inside. If the communications center fails to perform its mission, the fire department will not be able to deliver much-needed emergency services.

A communications center performs the following basic functions:

- Receiving calls for emergency incidents and dispatching fire department units
- Supporting the operations of those fire department units delivering emergency services
- Coordinating fire department operations with other agencies
- Keeping track of the status of each fire department unit at all times
- Monitoring the level of coverage and managing the deployment of available units
- Notifying designated individuals and agencies of particular events and situations
- Maintaining records of all emergency-related activities
- Maintaining information required for dispatch purposes

Most fire department responses begin when a call comes in to the communications center, which then dispatches one or more units. Even if a citizen reports an emergency directly to a fire station or a crew discovers a situation, the communications center should also be immediately notified so that it can initiate the emergency response process.

As noted earlier, the communications center should have both a primary method and a backup method of transmitting alarms to stations. Although radio, telephone, and public address systems are often used to transmit information to fire stations, the use of fixed or mobile computer terminals and printers to transmit dispatch messages is increasing. Some fire departments still use a system of bells to transmit alarms. Although volunteer or rural departments may use outdoor sirens or horns to summon fire personnel to an emergency, most volunteer fire fighters receive dispatch messages over pagers or cell phones.

Processing an emergency incident includes the following steps:

1. Call receipt
2. Location validation
3. Classification and prioritization
4. Unit selection
5. Dispatch

LISTEN UP!

Dispatchers must be careful about which information is given to the public. Information such as availability of individual fire departments, apparatus placement, and available equipment should be monitored. Standard operating procedures (SOPs) should clarify which information is allowed to be broadcast and which information is not.

Call Receipt

Call receipt refers to the process of receiving an initial call and obtaining the necessary information to initiate a response. It includes telephone calls from the general public as well as other notification methods, such as automatic fire alarm systems, public fire alarm boxes, requests from other agencies, calls reported directly to fire stations, and calls initiated via radio from fire department units or other public safety agencies.

Telephones

The public generally uses landline telephones or cell phones to report emergency incidents. Today, most emergencies that occur outside a building are reported using a cell phone. In fact, some communities estimate that approximately 70 percent of their emergency calls are now reported with cell phones (Federal Communications Commission [FCC], 2016). In most communities, calls to 911 connect the caller with a PSAP. The PSAP can take the information immediately or transfer the call to the appropriate agency, based on the nature of the emergency. In some systems, calling 911 connects the caller directly with a telecommunicator, who obtains the required information.

In addition to receiving calls placed to 911, the communications center has a seven-digit nonemergency telephone number. Some people may use that number to report an emergency because they are not sure that their particular situation is serious enough to be considered a "true emergency."

DRIVER/OPERATOR TIP

Some communities have implemented a 311 system to handle nonemergency calls. This system is often used to link callers with health and human services or other community resources that can assist them with a problem that might not necessarily be life threatening in nature. The underlying premise of the 311 system is to reduce the number of nonemergency calls to 911.

Any number that is published as a fire department telephone number should be answered at all times, including nights and weekends. The 911 emergency number should always be pronounced as "nine-one-one," not "nine-eleven," since there is no "11" on a telephone.

The telecommunicator who takes the call must conduct a **telephone interrogation**, asking the caller questions to obtain the required information. Initially, the telecommunicator will need to know the location of the emergency and the nature of the situation. As discussed, many 911 systems can automatically provide the location of the telephone where a call originates. This information may be unavailable or inaccurate, however, if the call was made on a cell phone or from someplace other than the location of the emergency incident. The exact location must be obtained so that units can respond directly to the incident scene.

The telecommunicator must also interpret the nature of the problem from the caller's description. The caller may be distressed, excited, and unable to organize his or her thoughts. Sometimes, there may be language barriers; the caller might speak a different language or might not know the right words to explain the situation. Telecommunicators must follow SOPs and use active listening to interpret the information. Many communications centers specify a structured set of questions that telecommunicators should ask to obtain and classify information about the nature of the situation. The telecommunicator must remember that the caller thinks the situation is an emergency, and he or she must treat every call as such until it is determined that no emergency exists.

Telecommunicators cannot allow gaps of silence to occur while questioning the caller. If the caller suddenly becomes silent, something may have happened to him or her; the caller might be in personal danger or extremely upset. Conversely, if the telecommunicator is silent, the caller might think that the telecommunicator is no longer on the line or no longer listening.

Disconnects are another problem, because callers to 911 might hang up accidentally or be disconnected after initially reaching the communications center. If the caller's location is known, a telecommunicator who is unable to return the call and reach the original caller will usually dispatch a police officer to the location to determine whether more help is needed.

A telecommunicator should never argue with a caller. Although callers may raise their voices, scream, or shout, the telecommunicator must continue to speak calmly and remain professional at all times. He or she should remember that the caller is simply reacting to the emergency situation.

With just two critical pieces of information—the location and nature of the problem—the telecommunicator can initiate a response. Local SOPs, however, may require the telecommunicator to obtain additional information. Getting the caller's name and contact phone number is useful in case it is necessary to call back for additional information. If the caller is in danger or distress, the telecommunicator should try to keep the line open and remain in contact with the caller until help arrives. In many communities, telecommunicators are trained to provide self-help instructions for callers, advising them on what to do until the fire department arrives. For example, if a building fire is being reported, the telecommunicator will advise the occupants to evacuate and wait outside; if the caller is reporting a medical incident, the telecommunicator may provide first-aid instructions, based on the patient's symptoms.

TDD/TTY/Text Phones. Speech- and/or hearing-impaired citizens can communicate by telephone using special relay devices that display text rather than transmitting audio **FIGURE 8-5**. Such systems include the teletype (TTY), the telecommunications device for the deaf (TDD), and text devices. **TTY/TDD systems** and text devices have a screen and a keyboard for exchanging words. The Americans with Disabilities Act requires that communications centers be able to receive calls via TTYs/TDDs and computer modems, as well as by voice communication. Telecommunicators must know how to use this equipment to communicate with speech- and hearing-impaired persons. Many communications centers have a special telephone line with a seven-digit number set aside for such calls.

While not all communication centers accept text-to-911 messages at this time, text service providers continue to develop these capabilities, and the **Federal Communications Commission (FCC)** urges communications centers to start accepting text messages when the service becomes available in their locations (FCC, 2017). Check TTY/TDD/text devices for any incoming calls that do not have voice contact at the other end.

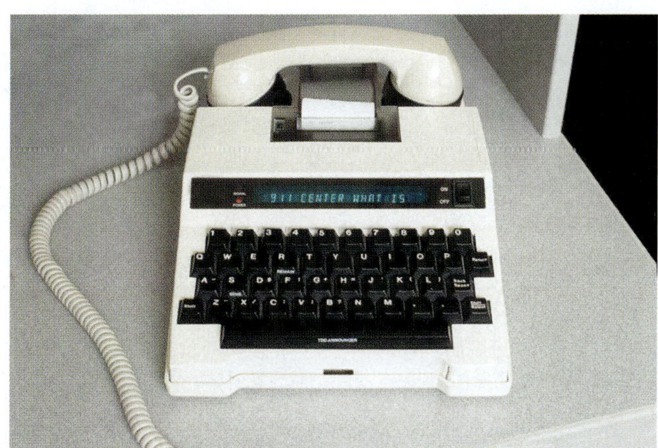

Figure 8-5 TTY/TDD/text devices enable speech- and/or hearing-impaired persons to communicate over telephone lines or wireless networks using text communication.

LISTEN UP!

Next-generation dispatch systems will permit communications centers to receive texts, video clips, and other communications from the general public.

Direct-Line Telephones. Even though cellular devices are often used for most communication functions, it is important to have a second means to communicate if the cellular system or radio system becomes inoperable. A **direct line** (or ring-down) telephone connects two predetermined points. Picking up the phone at one end causes an immediate ring at the other end. Direct-line connections often link police and fire communications centers or two fire communications centers that serve adjacent areas. Direct lines also may connect hospitals, private alarm companies, utility companies, airports, and similar facilities with the fire department communications center. These lines often operate in both directions so that the communications center can both receive calls for assistance and send notifications and requests for response.

The communications center may be connected by direct lines to each fire station in its jurisdiction. A direct line also can be linked to the station's public address speakers to announce dispatch messages.

Walk-ins

Although most emergencies are reported by telephone, some people actually come to a fire station seeking assistance **FIGURE 8-6**. When a walk-in occurs, the station should contact and advise the communications center of the situation immediately. The communications center will create an incident report and dispatch any additional assistance needed. Even if the units at the station can handle the situation, they should notify the communications center that they are occupied with an incident, as it affects their availability to respond to other calls.

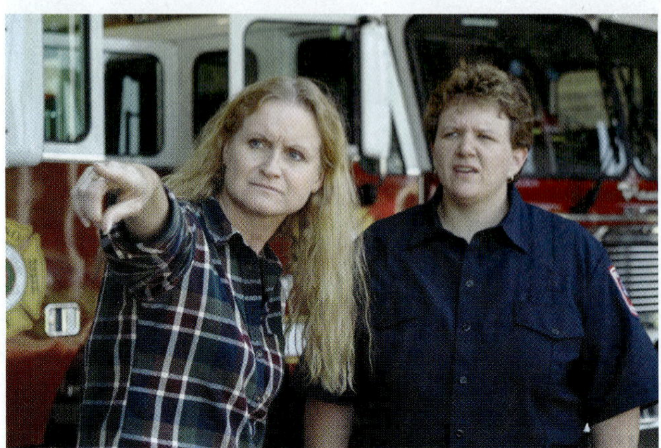

Figure 8-6 A citizen might walk into the fire station and report an emergency.

Citizens should be able to come to a fire station and report an emergency at all times, even when the station is unoccupied. Many departments install a direct-line telephone to the communications center just outside each fire station. These phones should be marked with a simple sign stating, "If the station is vacant, pick up the telephone in the red box to report an emergency." This enables citizens to quickly contact the dispatch center when the station is not occupied or when all units are out on emergency calls.

Location Validation

To process the request for service and before dispatching units, the telecommunicator must validate that the location information received is adequate. Potential duplicate addresses—such as two streets with the same or very similar names—must be eliminated from consideration. For example, it is important to differentiate 123 East Main Street from 123 West Main Street. This process of elimination is done through the geographic information system in CAD. The dispatch information must point to a valid location on a map or in a street index system, and that location must be within the geographic jurisdiction of the potential dispatch units. Without a valid address, a communications center will be unable to send units to the proper location.

Enhanced 911 Systems

Most 911 systems currently in operation are enhanced 911 systems, meaning that they have features that can help the telecommunicator obtain identifying information. For example, **automatic number identification (ANI)** shows the telephone number where the call originated. **Automatic location identification (ALI)** queries a database to show the location of the telephone, the subscriber's name, and other details **FIGURE 8-7**. Enhanced 911 is designed to improve dispatching time and accuracy. When combined with an accurate database, enhanced 911 generates a computer display listing all of the information when the call is received from a landline telephone. Another feature in an enhanced 911 system ensures that each call will be directed to the appropriate PSAP for that location.

The telecommunicator should always confirm that the information that is generated is correct and refers to the actual location of the emergency. If the caller has recently moved, the database may contain the old address. Also, sometimes a billing address for the telephone service is provided rather than the physical location of the telephone.

Although cell phones have certainly enhanced public access to emergency services, they have also created some challenges for dispatch operations. While efforts to provide location validation for calls received from cellular devices continue to advance, the locations of many 911 calls cannot be determined by the dispatcher, including a large number of calls made from cellular devices or those that use the Internet for phone transmission using **Voice over Internet Protocol (VoIP)**. VoIP technology

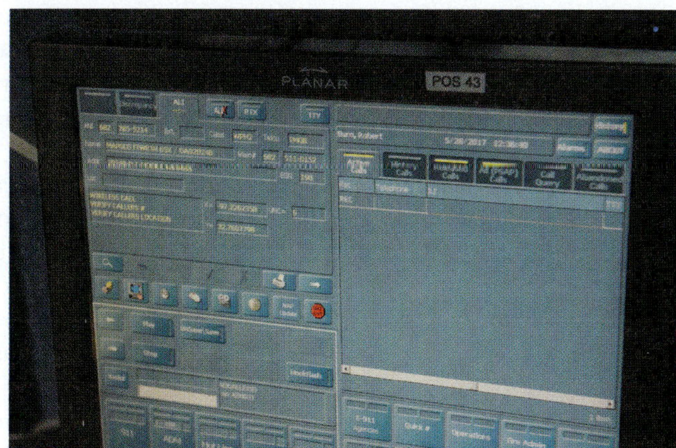

Figure 8-7 An automatic locator identification (ALI) system provides information about the origin of a 911 call.

converts a person's voice into a digital signal that can be sent via the Internet back to another computer, a VoIP phone, or a traditional phone with a specialized adapter.

The telecommunicator must also keep in mind that many people calling 911 may not know their exact location. In addition, the use of cell phones often results in numerous calls reporting the same incident, making it hard to determine the exact location of the emergency and overloading the dispatch center.

To address these challenges, next-generation 911 systems (NG911) allow digital information, including voice, photos, text messages, and video, to flow from any communications device through the network to a PSAP. They rely on high-quality mapping and the use of GIS to determine the location from which a call is being made. Although the technology to transition to NG911 is available, it is still evolving. PSAP technology is also advancing; in the near future, PSAPs may be able to receive data and alerts from safety devices, medical devices, and sensors and issue emergency alerts to wireless devices and highway alert systems.

Call Classification and Prioritization

Classification and prioritization is the process of assigning a response category to an incident, based on the nature of the reported problem. Most fire departments respond to many kinds of situations, ranging from outside ground cover fires and fires in high-rise buildings to heart attacks and multiple-casualty incidents. The nature of the call dictates the urgency of the call and its priority. Although most fire department calls are dispatched immediately, it is sometimes necessary to delay dispatch to a lower-priority call if a more urgent situation arises or if several calls come in at the same time. Some calls qualify for emergency response (red lights and siren); others are considered nonemergency events.

Call classification and prioritization is an important part of processing a request for service, because it will help the telecommunicator select the appropriate units to respond to the incident. The standard response to different incidents is established by the fire department's SOPs and can range from a single unit to an initial assignment of 10 or more units and dozens of fire personnel.

Unit Selection

Unit selection is the process of determining exactly which unit or units to dispatch, based on the location and classification of the incident. The usual policy is to dispatch the closest available unit that can provide the necessary assistance. When all units are available and in their fire stations, this determination can usually be made quickly based on preprogrammed information. Generally, the standard assignment to each type of incident in each geographic area is stored in a system of **run cards**. Run cards list units in the proper order of response, based on response distance or estimated response time, and often specify the units that would be dispatched through several levels of multiple alarms. They are prepared in advance and are usually entered into the CAD system. In years past, departments stored run cards in hard-copy form.

Unit selection becomes more complicated when some units are out of position or unavailable. This step of the dispatch often requires quick decision-making skills, even when the CAD system is programmed to follow set policies for various situations. Some dispatch centers are equipped with automatic vehicle locator systems that track apparatus by using GPS devices. These systems enable dispatchers to dispatch the closest units that are in service, thereby increasing the response efficiency. Many departments have entered into automatic mutual aid agreements that specify that the closest available units will be sent even if that requires dispatching units from several different jurisdictions.

DRIVER/OPERATOR TIP

On occasion, the communications center may receive calls about issues that cannot be handled by the fire department or other agencies participating in the communications system. In these cases, the telecommunicator should make every effort to accommodate the caller. If possible, transfer the caller to the proper agency. In addition, provide the caller with the proper contact information in case the call transfer fails. The caller will appreciate the assistance and retain a positive image of the department's service.

Most CAD systems are programmed to select the units for an incident automatically, based on the location, call classification, and actual status of all units. Such a system will recommend a dispatch assignment, which the telecommunicator can then accept or adjust, based on the circumstances or any special information. The same process is used to dispatch any additional units to an incident, whether it is a multiple alarm or a request for particular units or capabilities.

Dispatch

Dispatch is the important step of actually communicating the request for service by quickly and accurately alerting the selected units to respond and transmitting the necessary information to them. Fire departments use a variety of dispatch systems, ranging from telephone lines to radio systems. The communications center must have at least two separate methods of sending a dispatch message from the communications center to each fire station.

The primary connection can be a hard-wired circuit, a telephone line, a computer-based data link, a microwave transmission system, or a radio system. Most fire departments dispatch verbal messages to the appropriate fire stations. The dispatch message is broadcast over speakers in the fire station so that everyone immediately knows the location and nature of the incident and the units that should respond. Radio transmissions are used to contact a unit that is out of the station. The fire station or each vehicle must confirm that the message was received and the units are responding. If the communications center does not receive the confirmation within a set time period, it must dispatch substitute units.

A CAD system can be programmed to alert the appropriate fire stations automatically. Such a system can send the dispatch information to computer terminals or printers, sound distinctive tones, turn on lights and public address speakers, turn off the stove, and perform additional functions. The dispatch message also can go directly to each individual vehicle that has a computer terminal as well as to the station. The CAD notification often is accompanied by a verbal announcement over the radio and the fire station speakers.

Fire departments with volunteer responders must be able to reach them with a dispatch message. Some departments issue pagers to their individual volunteers or use cell phones for this purpose. These devices can receive vocal dispatch messages or text messages. Some CAD systems permit text messages to be sent to cell phones with incident information. Volunteer fire departments in some communities may also rely on outdoor sirens, horns, or whistles to notify their members of an emergency. These audible devices usually can be activated by remote control from the communications center. Volunteers then call the communications center by radio or telephone to receive specific instructions.

Operational Support and Coordination

After the communications center dispatches the units, it begins to provide incident support and coordination. Someone in the communications center must remain in contact with the responding units throughout the entirety of the incident. The telecommunicator must confirm that the dispatched units actually received the alarm, record their en route times, provide any additional or updated information, and record their on-scene arrival times.

Operational support and coordination encompass all communications between the units and the communications center during an entire incident. Two-way radios, laptop computers, mobile communications devices, telephones, and mobile computer terminals may all be used to exchange information.

Generally, the IC will communicate with a telecommunicator operating a radio in the communications center. Progress and incident status reports, requests for additional units or release of extra units, notifications, and requests for information or outside resources are examples of incident communications. The communications center closely monitors the radio and provides any needed support for the incident.

Each part of the public safety network—fire, EMS, and police—must be aware of what other agencies are doing at the incident. The communications center serves as the hub of the network that supports units operating at emergency incidents, and it coordinates the fire department's activities and requirements with other agencies and resources. For example, the telecommunicator might need to notify nonemergency resources such as gas, electric, or telephone companies of the incident and request that they take certain actions. The communications center should have accurate, current telephone numbers and contact information for every relevant agency.

Status Tracking and Deployment Management

The communications center must know the location and status of every fire department unit at all times. Units should never get "lost" in the system, whether they are available for dispatch, assigned to an incident, or in the repair shop. As previously stated, the communications center must always know which units are available and which units are not available for dispatch. The changing conditions at an incident may require frequent reassignment of units, including ambulances. In addition, units may be needed from outside the normal response area or from other districts.

Tracking the status of the various units is difficult if the telecommunicator must rely on radio reports and colored magnets or tags on a map or status board. CAD systems make this job much easier, because status changes can be entered through digital status units or computer terminals.

Communications centers must continually monitor the availability of units in each geographic area and redeploy units when an area has insufficient coverage. Many fire departments list both unit relocations and multiple response units on their run cards. This information is only valid, however, if major incidents occur one at a time and when all units are available. If a department has a large volume of routine incidents, it may need to redeploy units to balance coverage, even when no major incidents are in progress.

Usually, a supervisor in the communications center is responsible for determining when and where to redeploy units as well as for requesting coverage from surrounding jurisdictions. For example, units from many different jurisdictions may be

Voice of Experience

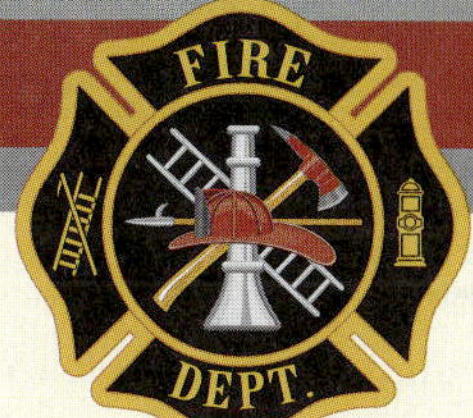

On an early fall evening, our dispatch center received a 911 emergency call from a frantic woman. The woman was overly excited, and the telecommunicator could tell that this was a real emergency by the sound of her voice. The woman was reporting that her daughter's house was on fire. Instead of the daughter calling the dispatch center directly, she called her mother on instinct. More than likely the daughter had more confidence in her mother "making the call" than if she would have made it herself. This shows how some people will react when they are under extreme pressure or, in this case, an emergency situation.

Once our dispatch center received the call, the standard operating procedure was to activate a general alarm for the department, bringing two engines, one ladder tower, and one straight stick to the scene. When the first engine and department chief arrived at the reported address, there were no visible signs of a fire or smoke in the area. They continued to investigate the address and surrounding area but came up with nothing. The chief notified dispatch of the situation and asked dispatch to verify the information with the initial caller. The telecommunicator once again restated that the call seemed legitimate due to the nature of the caller's message and the urgency in her voice.

It was then that chief decided to have all responding apparatus proceed with caution to the scene for further investigation and until verification with the caller could be completed. When the telecommunicator called the woman back for verification of the correct address, he was advised by the caller that the house that was on fire was her other daughter's home. She had provided the wrong address. The daughter's home was located two towns over and 15 miles away.

In this case, the telecommunicator asked all the right questions and was given an incorrect address from a third party; the caller's voice was legitimate, as was the nature of the incident and the homeowner's relationship to the caller. Unfortunately, this is an example of how misinformation can be given when someone is excited during an emergency situation.

Richard J. Kosmoski
Middlesex County Fire Academy
Sayreville, New Jersey

redeployed to respond to large-scale incidents under regional or statewide plans. These plans must include a system for tracking every unit and a designated communications center for maintaining contact with all units.

Taking Calls: Emergency, Nonemergency, and Personal Calls

One of the first things you should learn when assigned to a fire station is how to use the telephone and intercom/radio systems. You must be able to use them to answer a call or to announce a response. Keep your personal calls to a minimum, so incoming phone lines remain open to receive emergency calls.

A driver/operator who answers the telephone in a fire station, fire department facility, or communications center is a representative of the fire department. Use your department's standard greeting when you answer the phone: "Good afternoon, Pleasant Town Fire Department. Engineer Smith speaking. How may I help you?" Be prompt, polite, professional, and concise.

Detailed SOPs for obtaining information and processing calls should be provided to any fire personnel assigned to answer incoming emergency telephone lines. An emergency call can come in on any fire department telephone line. As mentioned earlier, someone may call your fire station directly instead of dialing 911 or another published emergency number. If this happens, you are responsible for ensuring that the caller receives the appropriate emergency assistance. Your department's SOPs should outline exactly which steps you should take in this situation, such as whether you should take the information yourself or connect the caller directly to the communications center, if possible.

Fire personnel should understand the steps followed by the personnel who staff the communications center as they receive calls, solicit needed information from a caller, and dispatch appropriate units to an emergency. Follow the steps in SKILL DRILL 8-1 to receive a call and obtain the essential information from a caller and to initiate a response to an emergency.

Touring the Communications Center

It is helpful to new driver/operators to tour the emergency communications center. Observing the actual operation of this center will give you a much better understanding of the telecommunicator's role. SKILL DRILL 8-2 lists the steps for touring your local communications center.

DRIVER/OPERATOR TIP

Vehicle locator systems and mobile tracking devices are valuable tools to accurately and effectively keep command staff and communication dispatchers up-to-date on the status of all units. These systems are especially useful in large departments and at large emergency incidents.

Radio Systems

Fire department communications systems depend on two-way radio systems. Radios link the communications center and individual units; they also link units at an incident scene. A radio system is an integral component of the ICS because it links all of the units on an incident, both up and down the chain of command and across the organization chart. Usually, every fire department vehicle has a mobile radio, and at least one—if not every—member of a team carries a portable radio during an emergency incident. A radio may be the team member's only link to the incident organization and the only means to call for help in a dangerous situation. Radios also are used to transmit dispatch information to fire stations, to page volunteer fire fighters, and to link mobile computer terminals.

Fire departments use many different types of radios and radio systems. Technological advances are rapidly adding new features and system configurations, making it impossible to describe all of the possible features, principles of operation, and systems here. Instead, this section describes common systems and operating features. As a driver/operator, you must know how to operate your assigned radio and learn your own department's radio procedures.

Radio Equipment

Three types of fire service radios are distinguished: the portable radio, the mobile radio, and the base station.

A **portable radio** is a hand-held two-way radio that is small enough for a driver/operator to carry at all times FIGURE 8-8. The radio body contains an integrated speaker and microphone, an on/off switch or knob, a volume control, channel select switch, and a "push-to-talk" (PTT) button.

A portable radio must have an antenna to receive and transmit signals. A popular optional attachment is an extension microphone/speaker unit that can be clipped to a collar or shoulder strap, while the radio remains in a pocket or pouch.

A portable radio is usually powered by a rechargeable battery, which should be checked at the beginning of each shift or prior to each use. Because the battery has a limited capacity, it must be recharged or replaced after extended operations. Battery-operated portable radios also have limited transmitting power. The signal can be heard only within a certain range and is easily blocked or overpowered by a stronger signal.

Mobile radios are more powerful two-way radios that are permanently mounted in vehicles and powered by the vehicle's electrical system FIGURE 8-9. Both mobile and portable radios share similar features, but mobile radios usually have a fixed speaker and an attached, hand-held microphone on a coiled cord. The PTT button is on the microphone, and the antenna is usually mounted on the exterior of the vehicle. Fire apparatus often include headsets with a combined intercom/radio system that enables crew members to talk to each other and hear the radio.

Pump/Water Supply Operator

SKILL DRILL 8-1

Receiving a Call and Initiating a Response to an Emergency

NFPA 1002, 4.4.2(A), 4.4.2(B)

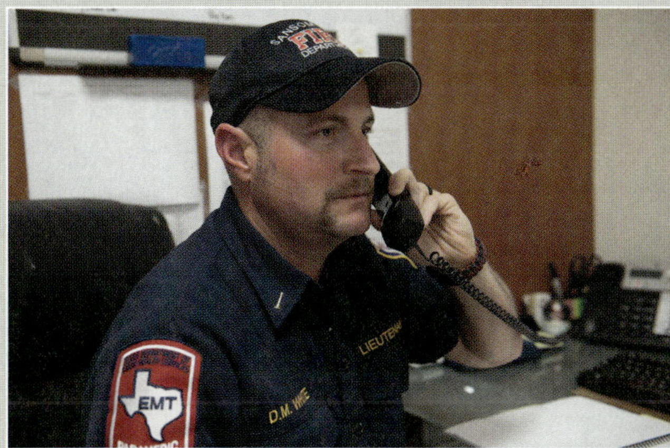

1 Answer promptly and professionally. Identify yourself, your agency, and your location. Determine immediately whether there is an emergency. If the call involves an emergency, follow your department SOPs. Organize your questions to get the following information:

- Incident location (including cross streets and identifying landmarks)
- Type of incident/situation
- Scene safety information
- When the incident occurred
- Caller's name
- Caller's location, if different from the incident location
- Caller's callback number

Always terminate the call in a courteous manner, and let the caller hang up first.

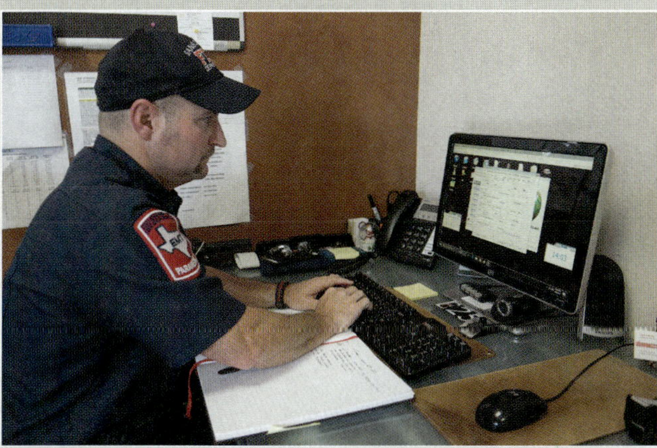

2 Record the information needed, including the date and time of the call. Initiate an alarm following the protocols of your communications center. The protocols in your department may vary from the steps listed here. Follow the protocols of the agency having jurisdiction for your department's communications.

LISTEN UP!

Stay professional, and remember that many citizens with scanners are listening to everything you say.

Base station radios are permanently mounted in a building, such as a fire station, communications center, or remote transmitter site FIGURE 8-10. These kinds of radios are more powerful than either portable or mobile radios. The antenna of the base station is often mounted on a radio tower so the transmissions

Pump/Water Supply Operator

SKILL DRILL 8-2

Touring the Communications Center

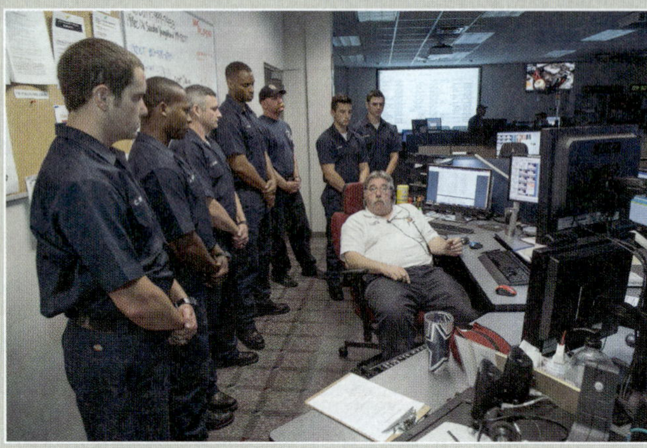

1. Arrange for a tour. Conduct yourself in a professional manner. Observe the use of equipment.

2. Observe the receipt of a reported emergency. Differentiate the needs of fire, police, and EMS personnel. Understand the telecommunicator's job.

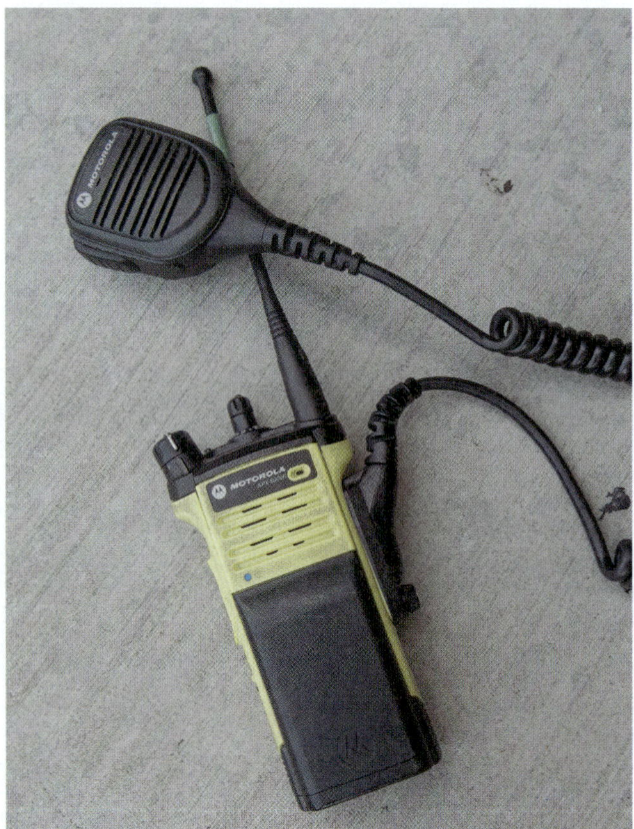

Figure 8-8 A portable radio should be carried by each individual driver/operator.

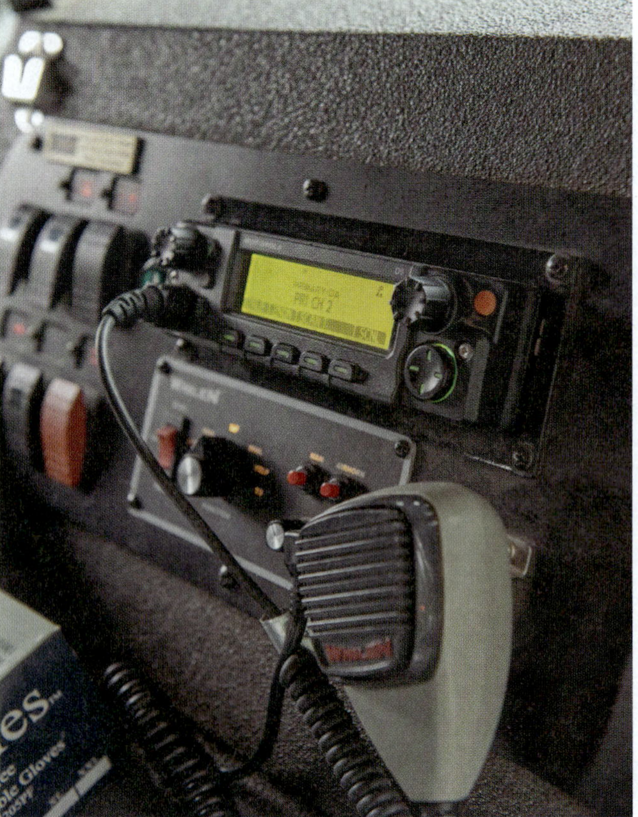

Figure 8-9 A mobile radio is permanently mounted in a vehicle.

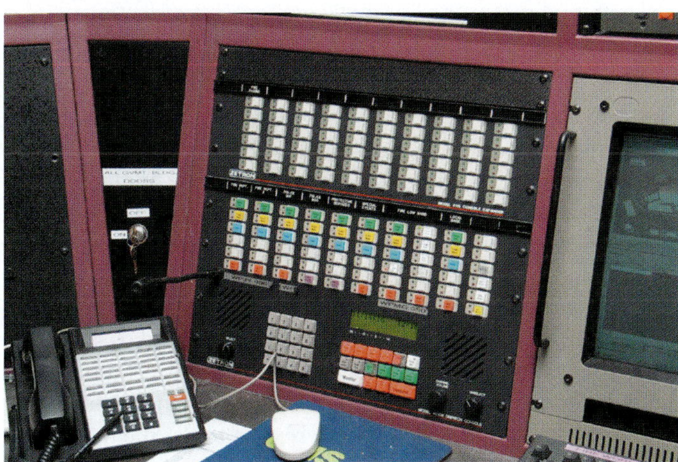

Figure 8-10 Base station radios are installed at fixed locations.

DRIVER/OPERATOR TIP

To enable fire personnel to communicate more effectively while wearing a self-contained breathing apparatus (SCBA) mask, several manufacturers have developed electronic communication systems that interface a portable radio with SCBA face pieces. These devices enable fire personnel to hear messages more clearly while wearing SCBA and to transmit information over their portable radios more easily, clearly, and simply. If your department uses this type of device, learn how to listen to messages transmitted through it.

have a wide coverage area FIGURE 8-11. Public safety radio systems often use multiple base stations at different locations to cover large geographic areas. The communications center operates these stations by remote control.

As discussed earlier, MDTs are computers that are located in the fire station or on the apparatus and that transmit data by radio or cellular signal. An MDT allows for greatly expanded communication capabilities. Instead of having to listen to the dispatcher and determine whether he said "11345 Main Street" or "11354 Main Street," you can look at the terminal where the address is displayed and obtain directions. An MDT may also allow for communication without the use of the radio. For example, driver/operators can press a button on the MDT that corresponds with *en route* or *on scene*, thereby communicating their acknowledgment of a message to dispatch. Satellite communications can track the apparatus' progress to the scene via GPS mapping and can provide important scene information. Some departments use MDTs to track unit status, transmit dispatch messages, and exchange different types of information.

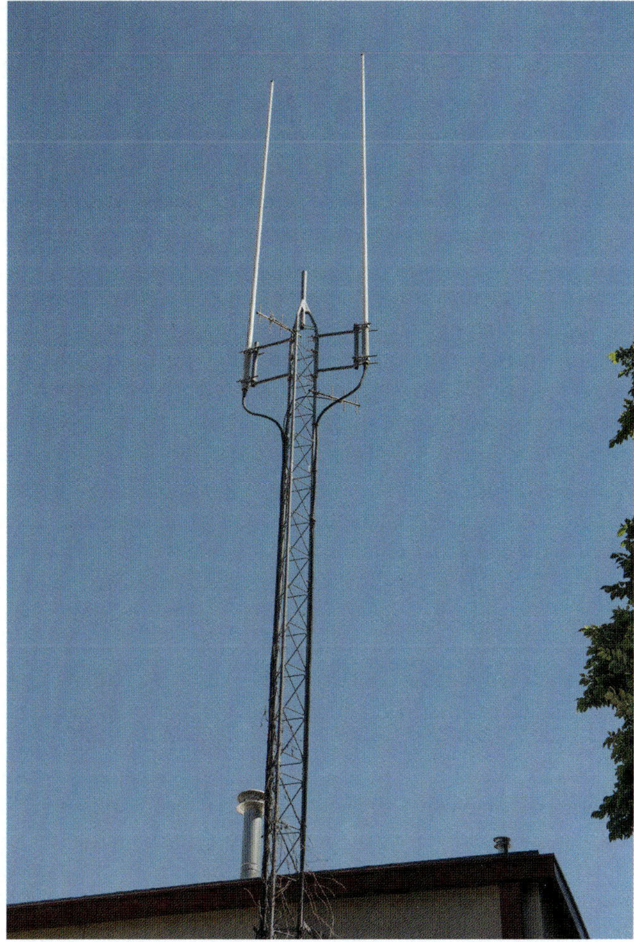

Figure 8-11 A base station radio antenna is often mounted on a radio tower to provide maximum coverage.

Radio Operation

In the United States, the design, installation, and operation of two-way radio systems are regulated by the FCC. The FCC has established strict limitations governing the assignment of frequencies to ensure that all users have adequate access. Every system must be licensed and operated within these guidelines.

Radios work by broadcasting electronic signals on certain frequencies, which are designated in units of megahertz (MHz). A **frequency** is the number of cycle (oscillations) per second of a radio signal; only those radios tuned to that specific frequency can hear the message. The FCC licenses an agency to operate on one or more specific frequencies. These frequencies are often programmed into the radio and can be adjusted only by a qualified technician.

A radio **channel** is one or more assigned frequencies used to carry voice and/or data communications. Assigned radio frequencies may be used in a variety of systems. With a **simplex channel** (push to talk, release to listen), each radio transmits signals and receives signals on the same frequency, so a message goes directly from one radio to every other radio that is set to receive that frequency. When one party transmits, the other can only receive. With a **duplex channel**, two different frequencies are used at the same time to permit simultaneous transmission (talk) and reception (listen)—analogous to how a telephone works. Duplex channels are used with repeater systems, which are described later in this chapter. **Multiplex channels** combine both analog and digital signals and can simultaneously transmit two or more different types of information, such as voice and telemetry, in either or both directions over the same frequency.

Frequency bands are portions of the radio frequency (RF) spectrum assigned for specific uses. The most commonly used bands for public safety communications are the **very high-frequency (VHF) band** and the **ultrahigh-frequency (UHF) band**. The VHF band, which extends from roughly 30 to 300 MHz, has been arbitrarily divided into a low band (30 to 50 MHz) and a high band (132 to 174 MHz).

U.S. fire service frequencies are located in several different ranges, including 33 to 46 MHz (VHF low band); 150 to 174 MHz (VHF high band); 450 to 460 MHz (UHF band); 700 MHz; and 800 to 900 MHz. Additional groups of frequencies are allocated in specific geographic areas with a high demand for public safety agency radio channels. Each band has certain advantages and disadvantages related to geographic coverage, topography (hills and valleys), and penetration into structures. Some bands have a large number of different users, which can cause interference problems, particularly in densely populated metropolitan areas.

Generally, one radio can be programmed to operate on several frequencies in a particular band. This limitation may become a problem if neighboring fire departments or police, fire, and EMS systems within the same jurisdiction operate on different bands. When different agencies working at the same incident communicate via different bands, they must make complicated arrangements with cross-band repeaters and multiple radios in command vehicles so that they can communicate with one another.

Currently, public safety frequencies are being reallocated and changed. These changes, which will result in many departments operating on new frequencies, are designed to improve the operation of public safety radios and data transmission.

Repeater Systems

Radio messages can be broadcast over only a limited distance, for two reasons: (1) The signal weakens as it travels farther from the source and (2) buildings, tunnels, and topography may create interference. These problems are most significant for hand-held portable radios, which have limited transmitting power. Mobile radios that operate in systems covering large geographic areas face similar problems. To compensate for these shortcomings, fire departments may use radio repeater systems FIGURE 8-12.

A **repeater** is a special base station that uses two separate frequencies—one to receive messages and one to transmit messages. It has a large antenna that is able to receive lower-power signals, such as those from a portable radio, from a long distance away. The signal is then rebroadcast to all of the radios set on the designated channel with all the power of the base station. Communications systems that use repeaters usually have outstanding systemwide communications and are able to get the best signal from portable radios. This approach enables the transmission to reach a wider coverage area.

Many public safety radio systems have multiple receivers, which are geographically distributed over the service area to capture weak signals. The individual receivers forward their signals to a device that selects the strongest signal and rebroadcasts it over the system's base station radio(s) and transmission tower(s). With this configuration, messages that originate from a mobile or hand-held portable radio have as strong a signal as a base station radio at the communications center. As long as the original signal is strong enough to reach one of the voter receivers, the system is effective. If the signal does not reach a repeater, however, no one will hear it.

Some fire departments switch from a duplex channel to a simplex channel for on-scene communications. This configuration is sometimes called a **talk-around channel**, because it bypasses the repeater system. In this case, the radios transmit and receive on the same frequency, and the signal is not repeated. A talk-around channel often works well for short-distance communications, such as from the command post to crews inside a house fire or from one unit to another inside a building. Conversations on a talk-around channel cannot be monitored by the communications center; instead, the IC must use a more powerful radio on a repeater channel to maintain contact with the communications center.

Mobile repeater systems also can boost signals at the incident scene by creating a localized, on-site repeater system. The mobile repeater can be permanently mounted in a vehicle or set up at the command post. It captures the weak signal from a

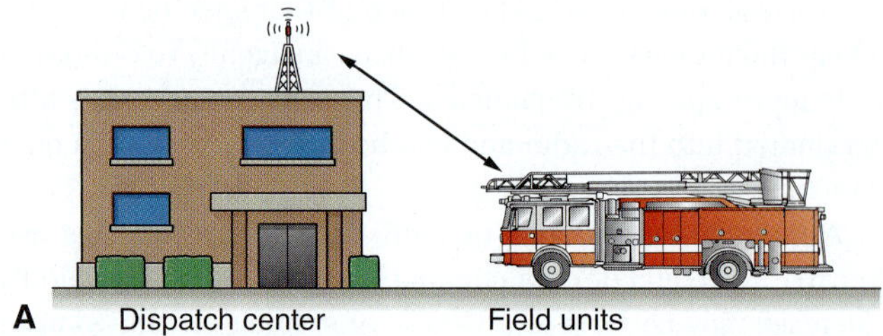

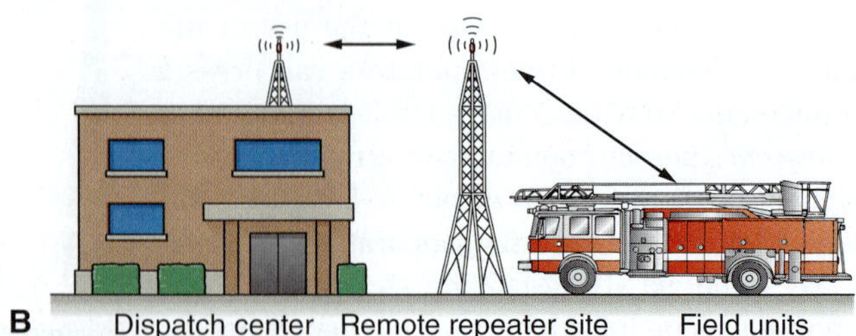

Figure 8-12 Direct and repeater channels send and receive transmissions in different ways. **A.** Direct channel (simplex). **B.** Repeater channel (duplex).

portable radio for rebroadcast. Some fire departments use cross-band repeaters, which boost the power of a weak signal and transmit it over a different radio band. In this way, a fire fighter using a UHF portable radio inside a building can communicate with the IC who is outside on a VHF radio. Similar systems may be used in large buildings or underground structures so crews working inside can communicate with units on the outside or with the communications center.

Trunking Systems

Radio systems based on newer technology and digital communications are being introduced to take advantage of the additional frequencies being allocated by the FCC for public safety use. Unfortunately, these new systems are generally incompatible with older radios and require expensive infrastructure changes.

Digital radio systems allow the transmission of digital signals (computer) or analog (voice) signals that have been digitized and compressed by a computer. With digital **trunked radios**, which are either 800- or 900-MHz systems, many frequencies—instead of just one or two—are assigned to a group. These groups can be thought of as virtual channels that appear and disappear as conversations occur. As a radio conversation begins, a computer selects or *scans* for the next open frequency and directs all of the radios in the talk group to receive the message on that frequency. As the conversation continues, participants will likely speak on different frequencies because the computer is constantly monitoring for frequency load and reassigning transmissions to unused frequencies. A trunking system makes more efficient use of available frequencies and can provide coverage over extensive networks. As a consequence, users do not need to worry about being able to transmit or receive. In a trunking system, the computer switches users to another channel without their knowledge, and users operate their radios as they normally do. Such systems also allow different radios to be tied together for a given incident. In addition, different agencies can be linked on the same trunking system. For instance, public works, the highway department, fire department, and the police department could all be linked for a specific incident if they needed to share radio communications.

Using digital technology also is more efficient than using analog technology and enables more users to communicate at the same time in a limited portion of the radio spectrum.

Using a Radio

As a driver/operator, you must learn how to operate any radio assigned to you and how to work with the particular radio systems used by your fire department. You must know when to use "Channel 3" or "Tac 5" or "Charlie 2," which buttons to press, and which knobs to turn. Study the training materials and SOPs provided by your department to learn this information.

When a radio is assigned to you, make sure you know how to operate and maintain it. Check the battery to confirm that it is fully charged. Learn the protocol for changing and recharging portable radio batteries. On the fireground, your radio is your link to the outside world. It must work properly—because your life may depend on it.

To use a radio, follow the steps in SKILL DRILL 8-3.

If you hold a portable radio perpendicular to the ground with the antenna pointing toward the sky, you will get better transmission and reception. Range and transmission quality also will improve if you remove the radio from the radio pocket or belt clip before you use it.

You should be familiar with all departmental SOPs governing the use of radios. All radio transmissions should be pertinent to the situation, with unnecessary radio traffic being avoided. Remember that radio communications are automatically recorded. They also may be heard by everyone with a radio scanner, including the news media and the general public. Given this fact, you should avoid saying anything of a sensitive nature or anything you might later regret. Voice recorders and radio tapes provide a complete record of everything that is said and can be admissible as evidence in a legal case.

Most fire departments use plain English for radio communications, but some use codes for standard messages. A few departments have developed intricate systems of radio codes to fit any situation. **Ten-codes**, a system of coded messages that begin with the number 10, were once widely used. They can be problematic when units from different jurisdictions have to communicate with one another. To be effective, codes must be understood by all parties and mean the same thing to all users. The National Incident Management System (NIMS) and NFPA standards recommend using plain English rather than codes. If your department uses radio codes, you must know all of the codes and understand how they are used. Even plain English may include some generally accepted terminology within a system, such as "code blue" for a cardiac arrest. The objective is to be clearly and easily understood, without having to explain every message in detail. If your department has a few codes or special words for special situations, they should be specified in the SOPs.

DRIVER/OPERATOR TIP

Verifying the information received over the radio is vital. Always restate an important message or instruction to confirm that it has been received and understood.

IC: Command to Engine 207. We need you to establish a water supply on the "C" side of the structure for defensive operations.

Engine 207: Engine 207 copies. We are going to the "C" side of the structure to establish a water supply for defensive operations.

LISTEN UP!

Ten-codes are not approved by NIMS. Using plain English is the preferred method of communication.

Pump/Water Supply Operator

SKILL DRILL 8-3

Using a Radio NFPA 1002, 4.4.1(B)

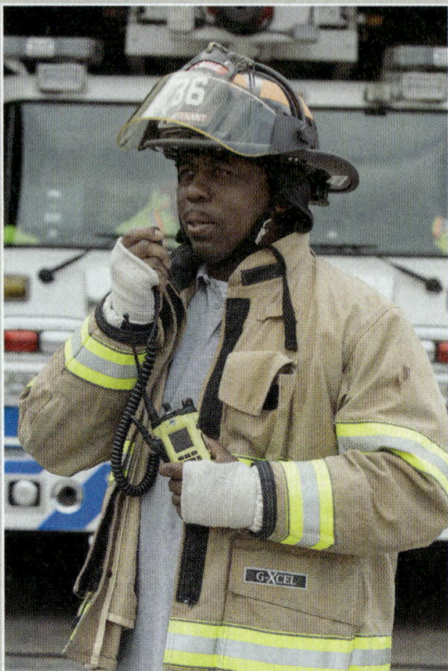

1. Listen to determine that the channel is clear of any other traffic. Press the "push-to-talk" (PTT) button, and wait at least 2 seconds before speaking. This delay enables the system to capture the channel without cutting off the first part of the message. Some systems sound a distinctive tone when the channel is ready.
2. Speak across the microphone at a 45-degree angle, and hold the microphone 1 to 2 inches (2.5 to 5 cm) from your mouth. Never speak on the radio if you have something in your mouth.
3. Know what you are going to say before you start talking. Speak clearly, and keep the message brief and to the point.
4. Release the PTT button only after you have finished speaking.

Emergency Messages

Sometimes the telecommunicator must interrupt normal radio transmissions for **emergency traffic**. Emergency traffic is an urgent message that takes priority over all other communications. When a unit needs to transmit emergency traffic, the telecommunicator generates a distinctive alert tone to notify everyone on the frequency to stand by, so the channel is available for the emergency communication. Once the emergency message is complete, the telecommunicator notifies all units to resume normal radio traffic.

Some radio systems also have emergency buttons located on portable and mobile units that allow fire personnel in trouble to push the button to transmit an emergency signal to the dispatcher. This button alerts the communications center that the ID assigned to that radio has an emergency need and, in some cases, identifies the location of the unit in trouble. If your radios are equipped with this feature, learn the procedure for using it.

The most important emergency traffic is a team member's call for help. Most departments use **mayday** to indicate that member is lost, is missing, or requires immediate assistance. If a mayday call is heard on the radio, all other radio traffic should stop immediately. The team member making the mayday call should describe the situation, location, and help needed. Fire personnel should study and practice the procedure for responding to a mayday call.

Some agencies utilize the acronym LUNAR to report a mayday. LUNAR stands for **Location**, your location in the building/incident; **Unit**, the unit you are assigned to; **Name**, who you are; **Air**, the amount of air you have in your cylinder; **Resources**, what you need to get out of the mayday situation.

An example of a mayday call follows:

Driver/Operator: MAYDAY . . . MAYDAY . . . MAYDAY.
[All radio traffic stops.]
IC: Unit calling MAYDAY, go ahead.
Driver/operator: This is Engine 403. We are on the "D" side of the building and have just been struck by a vehicle. Two fire fighters are injured. We need medical assistance and a replacement engine.
IC: Command copied. Engine 403, you've been struck by a vehicle on the "D" side of the structure and have two fire fighters injured. I'm sending two engines and two ambulances to your location.

The procedure for responding to a mayday call—which is used when fire personnel are in imminent danger—should be studied and practiced frequently.

Another emergency traffic message is "evacuate the building," which warns all units inside a structure to abandon the building immediately. Most fire departments have specified a standard **evacuation signal** to warn all personnel to pull back to a safe location. The evacuation signal that is commonly used is a sequence of three blasts on an apparatus air horn, repeated several times, or sirens sounded on "high-low" for 15 seconds. An evacuation warning should be announced at least three times to ensure that everyone hears it; the warning should also be announced on the radio by the IC. Because no universal evacuation signal has been established, driver/operators must learn their department's SOP for emergency evacuation.

After the evacuation, the radio airwaves should remain clear so the IC can do a roll call of all units. This step ensures that all personnel have safely exited the building. After the roll call, the IC will allow the resumption of normal radio traffic.

LISTEN UP!

Today most people carry a wide variety of personal communication devices. These cell phones and tablets are capable of transmitting and receiving voice messages, text, pictures, videos, and data. These devices are certainly of great help to us as we seek to assist others in emergency situations, but it is important to keep in mind that private and protected information, which can be transmitted using these devices, can cause great grief and harm to a citizen. Inappropriate use of personal devices violates the privacy rights of that person and can subject you and your department to serious legal action.

Become familiar with the policy of your department regarding the use of private cell phones for taking pictures of people in emergency situations. Do not ever consider posting any such pictures on the Internet.

After-Action Review

IN SUMMARY

- Every fire department depends on a functional communications system.
- The communications center is the central processing point for all information related to an emergency incident and all information related to the location, status, and activities of fire department units. Depending on the size of the fire department, the communications center may be a small room or a large building; it may serve one fire department or several public service agencies.
- Telecommunicators receive information from citizens and process that information to correctly dispatch resources to an emergency incident.
- Computer-aided dispatch (CAD) enables telecommunicators to work more effectively. Such a system tracks the status of units and assists the telecommunicator in quickly dispatching units to an emergency incident. Some CAD systems transmit dispatch information directly to mobile data terminals.
- Most communications centers automatically record everything that is said over the telephone or radio. This feature can prove valuable if the caller talks very quickly, has a strong accent, hangs up, or is disconnected. The recordings also serve as legal records for the fire department. They can assist in reviewing and analyzing information about department operations as well.
- A communications center performs the following basic functions:
  - Receiving calls for emergency incidents and dispatching fire department units
  - Supporting the operations of fire department units delivering emergency services
  - Coordinating fire department operations with other agencies
  - Keeping track of the status of each fire department unit at all times
  - Monitoring the level of coverage and managing the deployment of available units
  - Notifying designated individuals and agencies of particular events and situations
  - Maintaining records of all emergency-related activities
  - Maintaining information required for dispatch purposes
- There are five major steps in processing an emergency incident:
  - Call receipt—The process of receiving an initial call and gathering information.
  - Location validation—Ensuring that the address is valid.
  - Classification and prioritization—Assigning a response category based on the nature of the problem.
  - Unit selection—The process of determining exactly which unit or units to dispatch based on the location and classification of the incident.
  - Dispatch—The alerting of the selected units to respond and transmit information to them.
- Enhanced 911 systems are able to display information about where a landline call originated and even the name and address of the caller.
- The next generation of 911 systems are being designed to enable telecommunicators to pinpoint the location of an emergency call that is made with a cellular device.

- Fire department communications systems depend on two-way radio systems. A radio system is an integral component of the ICS because it links all of the units on an incident—both up and down the chain of command and across the organization chart.
- Three types of fire service radios may be used:
  - Portable radio—A hand-held two-way radio that the driver/operator carries at all times. The battery of such a radio should be checked at the beginning of each shift.
  - Mobile radio—A two-way radio permanently mounted in a vehicle and powered by the vehicle's electrical system.
  - Base station—A radio permanently mounted in a building, such as a fire station, communications center, or remote transmitter site. Public safety radio systems often use multiple base stations at different locations to cover large areas.
- Radios work by broadcasting electronic signals on certain frequencies. These frequencies are often programmed into the radio and can be adjusted only by a qualified technician.
- A radio channel uses either one frequency (simplex channel) or two frequencies (duplex channel). With a simplex channel, each radio transmits signals and receives signals on the same frequency, so a message goes directly from one radio to every other radio set to that frequency. With a duplex channel, each radio transmits signals on one frequency and receives messages on another frequency.
- In a repeater system, each radio channel uses two separate frequencies—one to transmit and the other to receive. When a low-power radio transmits over the first frequency, the signal is received by a repeater unit that automatically rebroadcasts it on the second frequency over a more powerful radio. All radios set on the designated channel receive the boosted signal on the second frequency. This approach enables the transmission to reach a wider coverage area.
- With a trunking system, a group of shared frequencies are controlled by a computer. The computer allocates the frequency for each transmission. The radio operator sets the radio on a talk group and communicates with the computer on a control frequency. When a user presses the transmit button, the computer assigns a frequency for that message and directs all of the radios in the talk group to receive the message on that frequency.
- Emergency traffic is an urgent message that takes priority over all other communications.
- When a unit needs to transmit emergency traffic, the telecommunicator generates a distinctive alert tone to notify everyone on the frequency to stand by, so the channel is available for the emergency communication. Once the emergency message is complete, the telecommunicator notifies all units to resume normal radio traffic.
- The most important emergency traffic is a team member's call for help. Most departments use "mayday" to indicate that a member is lost, is missing, or requires immediate assistance. If a mayday call is heard on the radio, all other radio traffic should stop immediately. The member making the mayday call should describe the situation, location, and help needed.
- A driver/operator who answers the telephone in a fire station, fire department facility, or communications center is a representative of the fire department. Use your department's standard greeting when you answer the phone. Be prompt, polite, professional, and concise.

KEY TERMS

activity logging system A device that keeps a detailed record of every incident and activity that occur.

automatic location identification (ALI) A series of data elements that inform the recipient of the location of the alarm. (NFPA 1221)

automatic number identification (ANI) A series of alphanumeric characters that informs the recipient of the source of the alarm. (NFPA 1221)

base station A stationary radio transceiver with an integral AC power supply. (NFPA 1221)

channel An assigned frequency or frequencies used to carry voice and/or data communications.

computer-aided dispatch (CAD) A combination of hardware and software that provides data entry, makes resource recommendations, and notifies and tracks those resources before, during, and after fire service alarms, preserving records of those alarms and status changes for later analysis. (NFPA 1221)

digital radio The transmission of information via radio waves using native digital (computer) data or analog (voice) signals that have been converted to a digital signal and compressed.

direct line A telephone that connects two predetermined points.

duplex channel The ability to transmit and receive simultaneously; a radio system that uses two frequencies per channel—one to transmit and the other to receive a message. Such a system uses a repeater site to transmit messages over a greater distance than is possible with a simplex system.

emergency traffic An urgent message, such as a call for help or evacuation, that is transmitted over a radio and that takes precedence over all normal radio traffic.

evacuation signal A distinctive signal intended to be recognized by the occupants as requiring evacuation of the building. (NFPA 72)

Federal Communications Commission (FCC) The federal regulatory authority that oversees radio communications in the United States.

frequency The number of cycles (oscillations) per second of a radio signal.

geographic information system (GIS) A system of computer software, hardware, data, and personnel that describes information tied to a spatial location. (NFPA 450)

global positioning system (GPS) A satellite-based radio navigation system composed of three segments: space, control, and user. (NFPA 414)

mayday A code indicating that a member is lost, missing, or trapped and requires immediate assistance.

mobile data terminals (MDTs) Technology that allows fire personnel to receive data while in the fire apparatus or at the station.

mobile radios A two-way radio that is permanently mounted in a fire apparatus.

multiplex channels Simultaneous transmission of multiple data streams, most often voice signals, in either or both directions over the same frequency on a radio.

portable radio A battery-operated, hand-held transceiver. (NFPA 1221)

public safety answering point (PSAP) A facility equipped and staffed to receive emergency and nonemergency calls requesting public safety services via telephone and other communication devices. (NFPA 1061)

public safety communications center A building or portion of a building that is specifically configured for the primary purpose of providing emergency communications services or public safety answering point (PSAP) services to one or more public safety agencies under the authority or authorities having jurisdiction. (NFPA 1061)

repeater A special base station radio that receives messages and signals on one frequency and then automatically retransmits them on a second frequency.

run cards Cards used to determine a predetermined response to an emergency.

simplex channel A radio system that uses one frequency to transmit and receive all messages. Transmissions can occur in either direction but not simultaneously in both; when one party transmits, the other can only receive, and the party that is transmitting is unable to receive.

talk-around channel A simplex channel used for on-site communications.

telecommunicators An individual whose primary responsibility is to receive, process, or disseminate information of a public safety nature via telecommunication devices. (NFPA 1061)

telephone interrogation The phase in a 911 call during which the telecommunicator asks questions to obtain vital information such as the location of the emergency.

ten-codes A system of predetermined coded messages, such as "What is your 10-20?", used by responders over the radio.

trunked radios A radio system that uses a computerized shared bank of frequencies to make the most efficient use of radio resources.

TTY/TDD systems User devices that allow speech- and/or hearing-impaired persons to communicate over a telephone system. TDD stands for telecommunications device for the deaf; TTY stands for teletype; text phones visually display text. The displayed text is the equivalent of a verbal conversation between two hearing persons.

ultrahigh-frequency (UHF) band Radio frequencies between 300 and 3000 MHz.

very high-frequency (VHF) band Radio frequencies between 30 and 300 MHz; the VHF spectrum is further divided into high and low bands.

Voice over Internet Protocol (VoIP) A technology that converts a person's voice into a digital signal that can be sent via the Internet back to another computer, VoIP phone, or a traditional phone with a specialized adapter.

voice recording system Recording devices or computer equipment connected to telephone lines and radio equipment in a communications center to record telephone calls and radio traffic.

REFERENCES

Americans with Disabilities Act. Title II Regulations (35.162). *Part 35 Nondiscrimination on the Basis of Disability in State and Local Government Services*. 2016. https://www.ada.gov/regs2010/titleII_2010/titleII_2010_regulations.htm#a35162. Accessed January 17, 2018.

Federal Communications Commission (FCC). *911 Wireless Services*. 2016. https://www.fcc.gov/consumers/guides/911-wireless-services. Accessed January 17, 2018.

Federal Communications Commission (FCC). *Text to 911: What You Need to Know*. 2017. https://www.fcc.gov/consumers/guides/what-you-need-know-about-text-911. Accessed January 17, 2018.

National Emergency Number Association (NENA). *9-1-1 Facts*. https://web.archive.org/web/20080804001221/http://www.nena.org/pages/ContentList.asp?CTID=22. Accessed January 17, 2018.

National Fire Protection Association (NFPA) 1001, *Standard for Fire Fighter Professional Qualifications*. 2013. https://www.nfpa.org/codes-and-standards/all-codes-and-standards/list-of-codes-and-standards/detail?code=1001. Accessed January 17, 2018.

National Fire Protection Association (NFPA) 1002, *Standard for Fire Apparatus Driver/Operator Professional Qualifications*. 2017. http://www.nfpa.org/codes-and-standards

/all-codes-and-standards/list-of-codes-and-standards /detail?code=1002. Accessed January 17, 2018.

National Fire Protection Association (NFPA) 1061, *Standard for Public Safety Telecommunications Personnel Professional Qualifications*. 2018. https://www.nfpa.org/codes-and-standards/all-codes-and-standards/list-of-codes-and-standards/detail?code=1061. Accessed January 17, 2018.

National Fire Protection Association (NFPA) 1221, *Standard for the Installation, Maintenance, and Use of Emergency Services Communications Systems*. 2016. https://www.nfpa.org/codes-and-standards/all-codes-and-standards/list-of-codes-and-standards/detail?code=1221. Accessed January 17, 2018.

On Scene

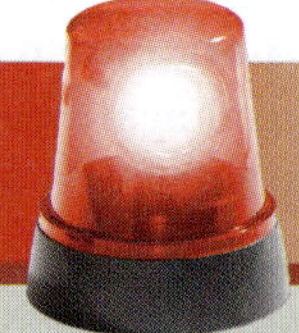

Today is the day you study dispatching in your training class. You see that 4 hours is allocated for this topic. You wonder how it can take 4 hours to describe how a dispatcher answers a phone, asks some questions, and then pushes a button to dispatch the fire units.

The director of the emergency communications center arrives and tells the class that you will be visiting the communications center. You are asked to sit next to a man with a headset on and five computer screens in front of him. He hands you a headset so you can listen in. Within minutes, you are amazed at how hard this job really is.

1. ____________ is an enhanced 911 service feature that displays where the call originated or where the phone service is billed.

A. Automatic location identification (ALI)

B. Automatic number identification (ANI)

C. A call box

D. A TDD/TTY/text phone system

2. A ____________ is a radio system that uses a shared bank of frequencies to make the most efficient use of radio resources.

A. trunked system

B. simplex system

C. radio repeater system

D. mobile data system

3. A ____________ is a radio system that uses one frequency to transmit and receive all messages.

A. trunked system

B. simplex system

C. radio repeater system

D. mobile data system

4. A(n) ____________ is a code indicating that a team member is lost, missing, or trapped and requires immediate assistance.

A. emergency evacuation signal

B. ten-code

C. box call

D. mayday

5. Two-way radios that are permanently mounted in vehicles and powered by the vehicle's electrical system are called:

A. portable radios.

B. mobile radios.

C. base radios.

D. simplex radios.

6. Which step comes first in the processing of an emergency incident in a communications center?

A. Classification and prioritization

B. Unit selection

C. Location validation

D. Dispatch

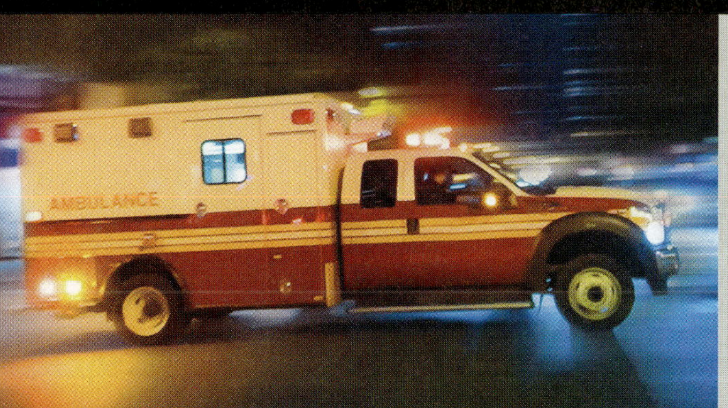

CHAPTER 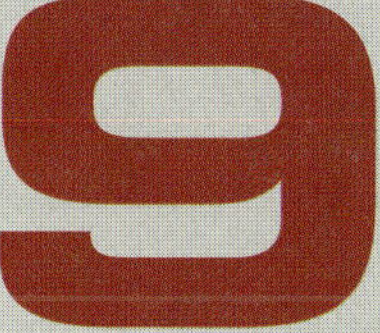

Technological Aids

OBJECTIVES

9.1 Identify various technological aids that may be used in emergency response.

9.2 Explain how to use a global positioning system in emergency vehicle operations.

9.3 Outline how traffic preemption systems work to assist in emergency response.

9.4 Discuss how mobile data terminals can be used to assist in communication efforts.

9.5 Describe how driver behavior monitoring systems can be used to improve emergency vehicle operation.

9.6 Identify the benefits and potential hazards involved in using technological aids.

9.7 Discuss the value of new and future developments in EMS technology.

SCENARIO

Your ambulance is transporting an unstable 68-year-old female patient to the stroke center. You approach an intersection with a red light. As you enter the intersection, you slow down and begin to make eye contact with the other drivers. A car comes barreling into the intersection from your right. You do everything you can to brake and try to steer away, but the car hits your vehicle's rear right quarter panel. Your vehicle is turned onto its side. Both vehicles come to a stop in the intersection.

Your initial concern is for any possible injuries. Fortunately, everyone in your ambulance was wearing their safety restraints, including shoulder restraints on the patient, so no one was hurt. You inform the dispatcher of the need for police, the fire department, and additional ambulances to transport your stroke patient and to check on the other vehicle's occupants. You follow all the steps in your service's policy on what to do if involved in a crash. Your ambulance will be out of service until it can be repaired, and the car that struck you had significant damage to its front end. The vehicle's driver did not sustain any injuries.

The local media station ran the story on the evening news as the headliner, implying that you were at fault. Fortunately for you, the entire incident was recorded by a driver monitoring device that has been installed in your ambulance for the past two years. It shows that you were traveling at an appropriate speed, made eye contact with the other motorists in the intersection, and had attempted to navigate the intersection lane by lane when suddenly a driver using her cell phone went around the right of a line of stopped vehicles and ran right into the rear quarter panel of your vehicle.

1. How is technology improving ambulance and driving safety?
2. How is technology making emergency driving less safe?
3. In a perfect world, what technologies would you want your area to implement?

Introduction

Technological devices can be extremely useful in emergency vehicle operations. The modern technological aids discussed in this chapter are used to help emergency vehicle operators find the best route, preempt traffic lights, communicate with dispatch and other EMS providers, and monitor driver performance. As technology continues to develop, it will be the responsibility of your agency's management to evaluate new products and decide if they are cost effective and will help reduce the probability of crashes while making response safer for emergency vehicle operators, patients, providers, and the general public. It will be your responsibility as the emergency vehicle operator to be trained in and fully understand the operations of all technologies that become incorporated into the operation of the emergency vehicle.

However, technological devices are not perfect solutions. We will discuss the dangers of emergency vehicle operators becoming distracted by or over-reliant upon these devices. For example, just because your vehicle has an automatic backup alarm does not mean you do not have to be aware of who or what is behind the vehicle when backing up. Indeed many ambulances today have a camera to the rear of the vehicle, yet a small object or child could be missed if you are not careful and do not always use a spotter.

Global Positioning Systems

A **global positioning system (GPS)** device can be used to accurately identify an object's location. GPS was originally developed in the 1970s by the U.S. Department of Defense for locating ballistic missile submarines, and the same technology is now used to help locate many different objects, such as cellular phones and commercial and private vehicles. This technology relies upon 24 satellites orbiting the earth in precise locations and 5 ground stations that are used to triangulate the GPS device's location FIGURE 9-1.

In EMS, GPS technology has been combined with global system for mobile communications (GSM) wireless coverage to enable an agency to do the following:

- Track an ambulance's location
- Allow dispatchers to identify which vehicle is closest to an assignment location to reduce response times
- Provide quick, efficient directions and rerouting
- Save money by decreasing fuel costs
- Use resources more efficiently

In some agencies without integrated GPS systems, personal navigation devices or smartphone applications may be used

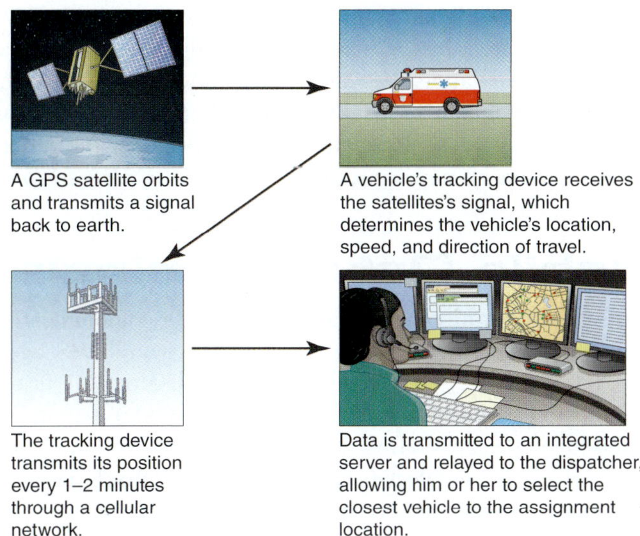

Figure 9-1 A GPS device enables an EMS agency to track its vehicles and helps crews locate addresses efficiently.

FIGURE 9-2. There are some possible risks to using personal GPS devices for navigation. First, they may be a distraction to the emergency vehicle operator. Just as you should not be driving and reading the map, the GPS unit can be a distraction, moving your eyes away from the road and mirrors. If possible, your partner should serve as the navigator and guide you based on the GPS or map; this approach will allow you to keep your attention on the road. Typically the GPS programs in a smartphone involve a very small screen, and they can be a major distraction. Driving while using a cell phone may not even be legal in your state. It is your responsibility as the emergency vehicle operator to understand your state laws. If you have questions, ask police in your jurisdiction.

SAFETY POINTER

Never attempt to program a GPS device while operating the vehicle.

GPS units, computers, and similar devices, depending on their placement in the vehicle, may block a section of the windshield and limit your view. When deciding to use a GPS unit, seriously consider the policies of your service, the size of the GPS

SAFETY POINTER

Always follow your agency's standard operating procedures (SOPs) regarding the use of GPS devices.

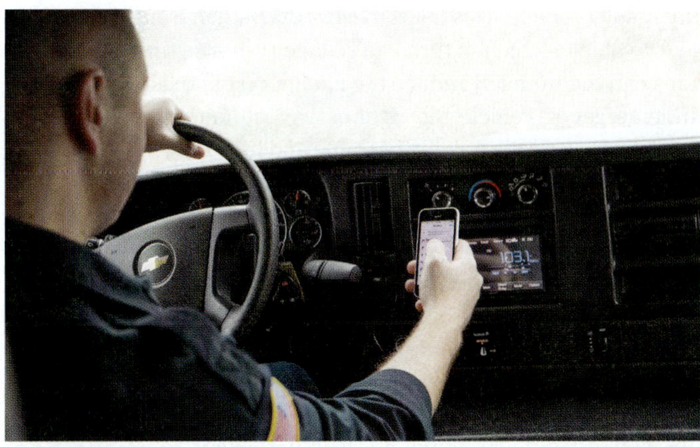

A

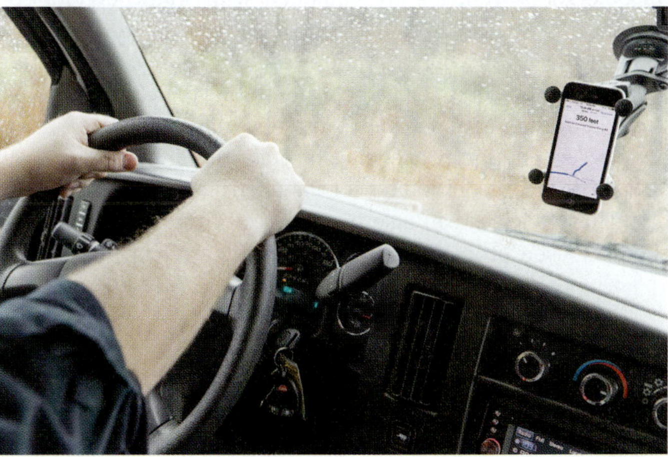

B

Figure 9-2 Personal GPS devices may be permitted by some agencies to assist with navigation. **A.** Unmounted they are a distraction, and **B.** mounted they are less distracting.

screen, and the location of the screen so that it does not interfere with your view of the road, traffic, and mirrors. It should also be easy to hear the directions over the other noises in the cab, such as the siren and communications radios.

Traffic Preemption Systems

Traffic preemption systems are a valuable technological aid to EMS response. These systems allow emergency responders to change traffic signals to allow them to clear an intersection and gain right-of-way. They rely on a series of receivers purchased by the municipality and installed at intersections with traffic lights, and emitters that are installed on the emergency vehicle FIGURE 9-3. When an emergency vehicle is responding to an assignment and approaches an intersection equipped with a traffic preemption system, the traffic light is preempted from its regular pattern. It will cycle through the caution (yellow) and red lights for all other directions, giving the green light and exclusive right-of-way to the emergency vehicle. This helps to clear the path in front of the emergency vehicle, which in turn can reduce response time. These systems can theoretically reduce the likelihood of collisions by giving the emergency vehicle the right-of-way, although their effectiveness depends on the volume of traffic and how long the emergency vehicle will be on the pathway being cleared by a series of green lights instead of the occasional red light.

Preemption priority is set so that if more than one emergency vehicle is approaching the intersection from different directions at the same time, only one will have the green light to proceed. Some systems include a flood light that notifies the public and other emergency vehicles of the direction of the emergency vehicle's approach as well as to confirm that the device has been activated. It is important to note that not all emergency vehicles are equipped with traffic preemption emitters. Therefore, it could happen that even if you have the right-of-way from your traffic preemption device, there could be another non-equipped vehicle attempting to proceed through the same intersection from a different direction. You should always use caution proceeding through the intersection, even with a traffic preemption device installed.

These devices can also be beneficial to patient care when they are used properly. Some services allow them to function independently of the emergency warning devices for transporting patients who are experiencing a time-critical event such as a stroke or heart attack. Using preemption devices allows the transporting ambulance to move efficiently through traffic but decreases the risk associated and the stress response the patient may have to emergency transport.

SAFETY POINTER

Traffic preemption systems are useful, but they do not remove your responsibility to ensure that the intersection is clear.

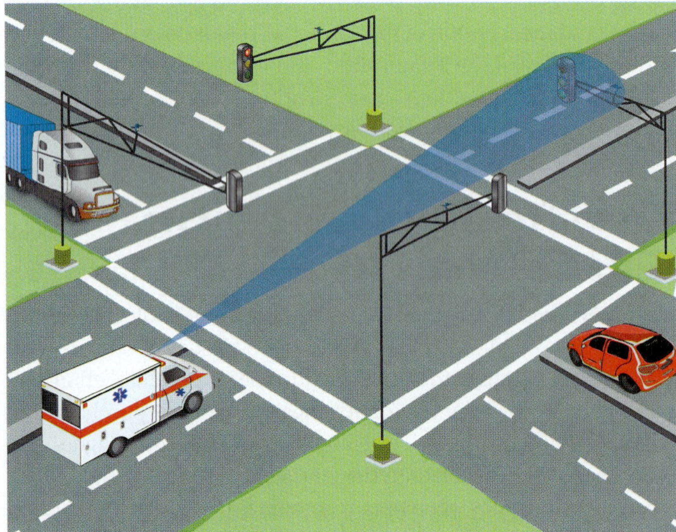

Figure 9-3 Traffic preemption systems work using infrared beams to trigger traffic lights to change, giving the emergency vehicle the exclusive right-of-way.

Mobile Data Terminals

Mobile data terminals (MDTs) are in-vehicle communication devices that have become the standard for many EMS agencies and emergency responders **FIGURE 9-4**. Most MDTs are an extension of the computer-aided dispatch (CAD) system and extend the CAD capabilities. Some services utilize an in-vehicle laptop computer (mobile data computer, or MDC) that is mounted in the cab of the ambulance. These terminals or laptops can provide extensive response mapping, locate other units, and secure real-time access to public databases. MDTs increase information sharing and facilitate delivery of mission-critical information to the field (i.e., location of hazardous materials, building plans, and emergency plans). Many of the newer systems can provide electronic patient care report (e-PCR) capabilities and billing information, and can even be used for continuing education while the unit is posted at a location between calls. Some also use buttons to mark status changes to limit radio traffic, especially in larger systems.

MDTs are typically mounted in the cab between the seats on a swivel system, providing easy access to both the passenger and the emergency vehicle operator. Placement of the devices must not interfere with the vehicle's air bag system. MDTs should never be used by the emergency vehicle operator during vehicle operation, as doing so would distract the operator from driving duties. Also, depending on where they are mounted, they may create a blind spot or vision issues at night due to their bright screens. Always follow your agency's SOPs regarding MDT use.

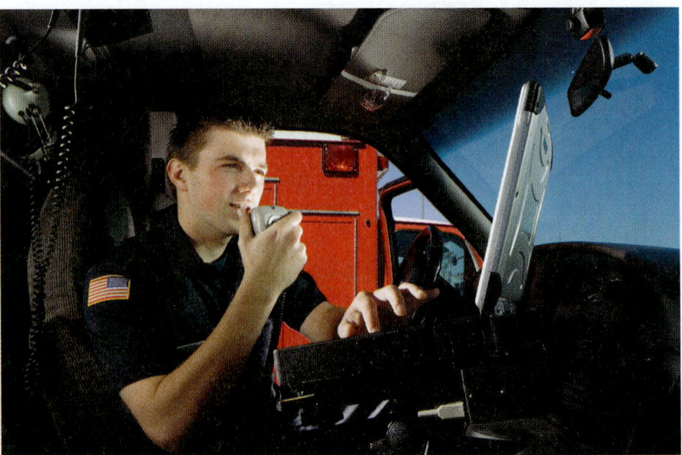

Figure 9-4 Mobile data terminals are a great resource for communication, planning, and reporting.

Driver Behavior Monitoring Systems

In the past, supervisors would have to accompany crews on the road to monitor driver performance or rely on observations and anecdotal evidence from other personnel to determine if emergency vehicle operators were using safe driving techniques. Unfortunately, this process of evaluation was inefficient, subjective, and unpredictable. Now, electronic **driver monitoring devices** can be used to monitor driver performance and help prevent collisions. These devices are also referred to as driver behavior monitoring systems (DBMS).

Driver monitoring devices record the driver's behavior, provide immediate feedback to the driver, and analyze the data to let the organization know the driver's overall compliance to driving standards. Electronic driver monitoring devices are valuable resources for evaluating and addressing any problems in driver performance. Using these monitoring devices, management may be able to determine which drivers need additional guidance and training before problems occur. In many cases, electronic monitoring can be used as evidence of a driver's innocence in the event of a collision.

Several different types of monitoring systems are available for EMS vehicles, including DriveCam™, envisionCAM™, Safety Vision™, and Road Safety™ FIGURE 9-5. While there are some differences in how the specific devices work, the general concept is the same. They use data recording devices such as video cameras and/or sensors to record the vehicle's location, forward and lateral movement, and driver activities FIGURE 9-6. In the event of any unexpected movement, such as a collision, quick acceleration, or sharp turn, the device will record information about the event, including use of turn signals, vehicle position and speed, and vehicle mechanical states (e.g., brake pressure). The data may be provided as real-time feedback to the driver and/or supervisors or may be analyzed by the manufacturer, with feedback later provided to the agency. The driver may be notified that an event has been recorded by a light on the device or an audible tone.

Management can review the recorded data with the emergency vehicle operator to provide further information or training regarding the event. Quality assurance personnel can maintain database files that track and cross check different types of events, frequency of events, and event details such as certain time of day and weather conditions. Your service's driving instructor may share with members/employees in their emergency vehicle operator course some clips taken from these recording devices, noting specific lessons to learn from.

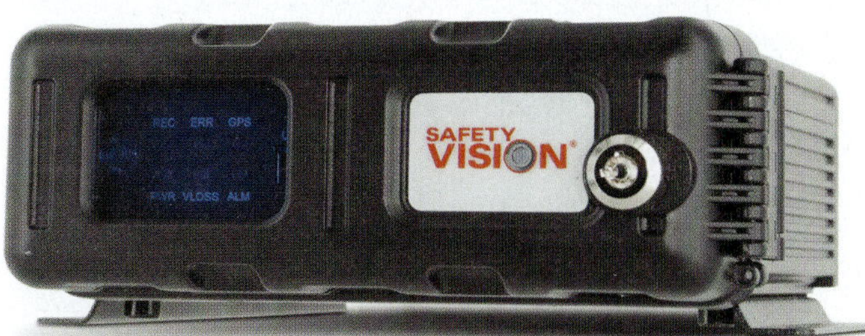

Figure 9-5 Sample driver behavior monitoring system.
© Safety Vision, LLC.

It is important to note that data from monitoring devices can serve as evidence to support the emergency vehicle operator in the event of a collision, and that the devices may also be used to provide safe drivers with positive feedback. Management can recognize personnel who are not involved in events that trigger the system and reward them for their safe driving habits FIGURE 9-7.

These devices may be cost prohibitive for some services. Before implementing one of these types of system, administrators should check whether they can receive an insurance discount for these devices. It is believed that being monitored and recorded decreases bad driving habits, which can decrease collisions and costs to the insurance companies. Also, because the evidence can show that companies were operating safely, legal costs associated with liability issues may be decreased.

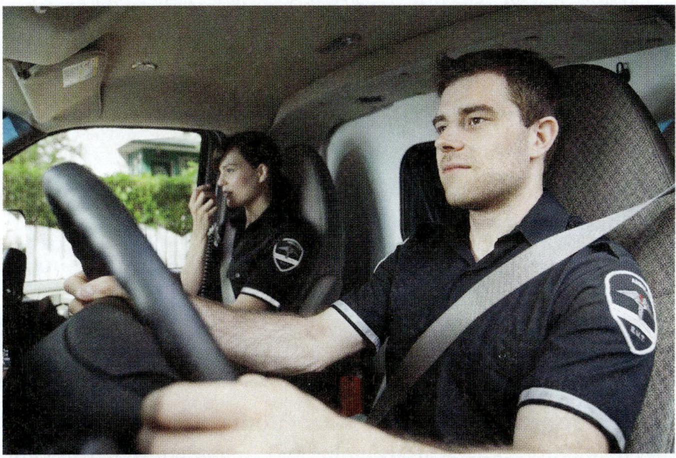

Figure 9-6 Monitoring devices can record drivers' actions.
© leaf/iStock/Getty.

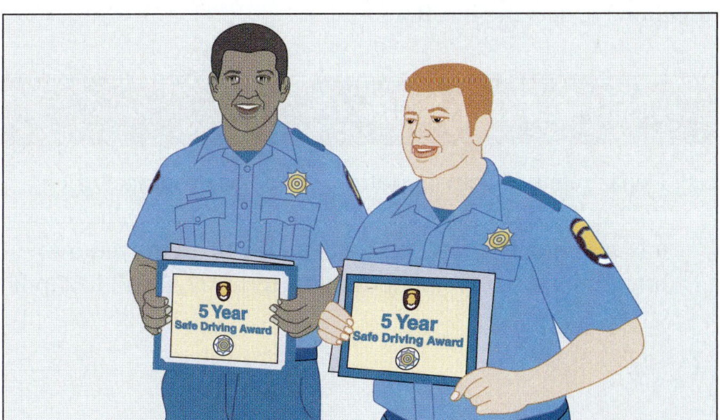

Figure 9-7 Rewarding personnel is one way to reinforce good driving habits.
© Jones & Bartlett Learning.

The Next Generation of EMS Technology

Since the new products in development are usually significant investments by the developing manufacturers, there is little "intel" on what devices are currently in development. One can only speculate that the systems in the ambulance will give us more computer-monitored feedback on the condition of the vehicle, its lights and compartments, and its handling. Just look at the advances in automobiles. There are guidance systems available in cars today that warn drivers when they are approaching danger and begin to slow their vehicle before a crash occurs. There are even systems that will parallel park an automobile! In the large trucks, adaptive cruise control will maintain a safe following distance behind the vehicle in front of the truck, and collision mitigation systems will slow the vehicle when there is danger of a collision.

More sophisticated GPS systems will be able to tell us where the traffic backups are and advise alternate routes to our calls. As health care moves to a paperless world, the use of e-PCRs and linkage to hospital patient data systems will become more prominent, eliminating duplication of documentation and arming the EMS provider in the field with historical data on the patient's medical record.

WRAP-UP

SUMMARY

- Technology can be useful and improve response and safety, but it also has its limitations. Improvements such as backup cameras cannot replace an actual spotter.
- Global positioning system (GPS) units, mobile data terminals/computers (MDTs/MDCs), and other mapping devices have made responding easier, but they also can be distractions for the driver and should not be used when driving.
- Traffic preemption systems work to assist in emergency response by giving emergency vehicles the right-of-way at intersections.
- MDTs or MDCs can provide valuable run information on the location of and hazards involved in a call and can even track ambulances' status without use of the radio.
- Driver monitoring systems can give feedback to drivers and agencies that can be used to correct risky and dangerous behaviors as well as reward safe driving habits.
- Each new type of technology should be evaluated for both its potential benefits and its limitations.

GLOSSARY

driver monitoring system A monitoring system that tracks driver actions, vehicle movement, and immediate environment around the vehicle using video cameras and sensors.

global positioning system (GPS) A satellite-based location and navigation system used to locate vehicles and provide directions to specific locations.

mobile data terminal (MDT) A computerized device similar to a laptop computer that is used to communicate with a central dispatch office.

traffic preemption system A system used to preempt traffic lights, giving emergency vehicles the right-of-way.

REFERENCE

U.S. Department of Transportation, ITS Joint Program Office (2006). *Traffic signal preemption for emergency vehicles: a cross-cutting study*. FHWA-JPO-05-010. Retrieved from http://ntl.bts.gov/lib/jpodocs/repts_te/14097_files/14097.pdf

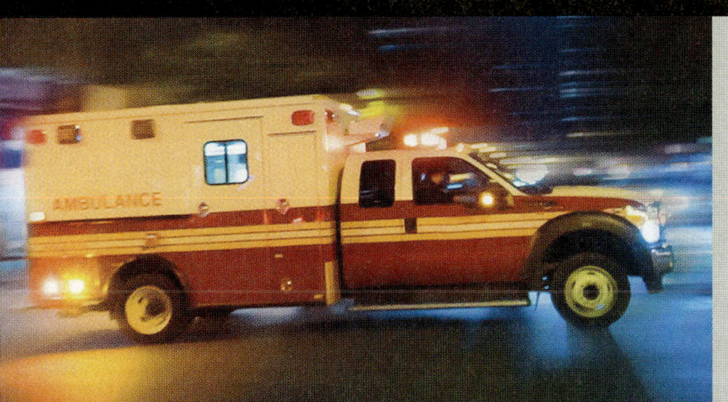

CHAPTER 10

Standard Operating Procedures

OBJECTIVES

10.1 Explain the general process used to develop a standard operating procedure (SOP).

10.2 Describe the key concepts to incorporate in an SOP for backing the EMS vehicle.

10.3 Discuss the key concepts to incorporate in an SOP for the use of safety restraints.

10.4 Describe the key concepts to incorporate in an SOP for driving range safety.

10.5 Describe the key concepts to incorporate in an SOP for a crash involving an EMS vehicle.

10.6 Discuss the key concepts to incorporate in an SOP for visibility at the scene of an emergency call.

10.7 Describe the key concepts to incorporate in a sample SOP on qualifications for new emergency vehicle operators.

10.8 Describe the key concepts to incorporate in an SOP for the avoidance of distractions while driving.

10.9 Describe the key concepts to incorporate in an SOP for alcohol and drug use.

SCENARIO

You and your partner are dispatched to an unconscious patient on the opposite side of town, on a street with which neither of you is familiar. You race out of the station urgently, without checking the map, since your agency recently installed a new global positioning system (GPS) navigation device in your unit. It is late afternoon, the sky is clear, the sun is bright and shining, and the roads are dry. Once in the ambulance, you engage your lights and siren and start down Main Street. It is a two-way street with cars parallel parked on both sides, so you keep a lookout for pedestrians.

You now need to use the new GPS unit and reach over to turn it on. You have one hand on the wheel as you are entering the address into the GPS unit, when suddenly you look up at the road and notice the ambulance has veered about 2 feet to the right and is approaching a parked flatbed truck. You see it and apply the brakes, but it is too late.

The collision happens with such force that it tears off the right doors and sidewalls of the ambulance. The windshield breaks, shattering glass all over the front cab. Your partner is unconscious, and there is blood all over the inside of the front cab of the ambulance.

You shut off the motor of the ambulance and immediately call the dispatcher to request the police, reassignment of your original call to another unit, and an ambulance for your partner. You exit the vehicle and go over to care for your partner whose right arm appears to be severely torn from the shoulder and is bleeding profusely. You can hear sirens in the background from the approaching ambulance.

1. When new technology is introduced in your department, what type of training should take place?
2. Can a GPS or navigation system replace sound knowledge of your response zone and preplanning a route?
3. How accurate and efficient are GPS maps and routes?

Introduction

Each state has its own set of motor vehicle laws, and local municipalities and departments often have their own, more specific, regulations as well. In addition to these rules, an EMS agency should have its own guidelines, known as **standard operating procedures (SOPs)**. An SOP is a very specific guideline designed to clarify or enhance state and local laws as well as describe the step-by-step procedures that management expects all personnel to follow to safely accomplish a specific job. These policies in many cases will carry the weight of the law.

For example, state law may allow the driver of an emergency vehicle to be exempt from following the posted speed limit when operating an emergency vehicle during an emergency operation. The local law may have a posted speed limit of 30 mph. However, if the state does not limit the speed of an emergency vehicle during a response, then there is no cap on the rate of travel according to the state. Beyond expecting the emergency vehicle operators to take full responsibility for all of their actions, an agency may wish to create an SOP on this issue. Some agencies have developed SOPs designed to cap or limit the speed of their vehicles (i.e., no more than 20 mph over the posted speed limit). SOPs can be legally binding, and it is your responsibility to be familiar with your agency's SOPs and follow them.

In this chapter we will discuss how SOPs are developed and their importance to every member of the organization. We will provide some key features of effective SOPs that every agency should seriously consider implementing if they do not already have an SOP on the specific topic.

SAFETY POINTER

Emergency vehicle operators must be compliant with the laws in their state and local jurisdictions as well as all agency SOPs.

How SOPs Are Developed

Since the emergency vehicle operator will need to follow SOPs in his or her agency, it is helpful to understand how they are developed. First there needs to be a topic or issue needing direction and/or clarification in which an SOP could be helpful. The officer, committee, or members who are empowered to develop the SOP should clearly define the problem or subject that needs to be addressed. (In our discussion here, we will pretend that you are the person charged with creating the new SOP.) Next, consider why the SOP is being developed and the need for its development. It takes time to develop a new policy, and it should not be an overreaction to an issue involving a single member or employee that could be better dealt with by meeting directly with the individual. Unfortunately, there are many policies in many organizations that were developed in this manner rather than dealing with the specific person who caused the problem. Remember, once it becomes the policy of your agency, everyone will need to become familiar with the SOP and follow it.

SAFETY POINTER

When developing a policy, you should first define the **SMART objectives** of the policy. The acronym SMART is used to describe the key characteristics of meaningful objectives: *s*pecific, *m*easureable, *a*chievable, *r*ealistic, and *t*ime-bound.

Next do some research on the topic. Usually a problem identified in your agency has been identified in other agencies, so it is helpful to ask around and see samples of how other organizations chose to resolve the issue. Obtain copies of other agencies' SOPs on the specific topic to see how they dealt with the problem. You are not bound to solve your agency's problems in the same manner as agencies that are different than yours. After defining the problem and analyzing the other available SOPs, it is time to write a first draft. It will be helpful to circulate the draft (clearly marked as "draft") to a representative group of your members and management to ask them for their feedback on the clarity of the SOP and suggestions for improvements. If your agency has a legal counsel, you should ask for input to make sure the new SOP does not violate any laws and will be enforceable. Most agencies have a numbering system for their SOPs so they can be easily indexed by subject and located in a manual quickly. The SOP should clearly state who it is issued by and the date it becomes effective.

It is always helpful to get the input of the members or employees so the final version of the SOP can have ownership, buy-in, and a commitment from them to learn and follow the new SOP. Take the time to issue all members or employees a copy of the SOP and provide training as needed. After an SOP has been implemented, consider a review of all SOPs on a regular (e.g., annual) basis to see if they are still relevant, warranted, and effective.

Be Familiar With Your Agency's SOPs

Emergency vehicle operators must learn and fully comply with their agencies' SOPs just as they are expected to follow the rules of the road. Some services have a limited number of SOPs, which they train in and have come to believe in as the accepted standard of behavior for their service. Other agencies have volumes of SOPs, which most of their members or employees do not remember. Since all will be held up to the policy should there be a legal action, it is best to have fewer policies that everyone fully understands and complies with. Just as all EMS providers have to learn and follow the treatment protocols, all emergency vehicle operators should be required to learn and follow the service's vehicle operation SOPs. If you must refer to a pocket guide version until you commit them to memory, then do it that way. At the very least, bring a copy with you to work and review them until you are familiar with them. Employers need to make sure the most updated SOPs are available to all personnel and that everyone receives updates if they are changed.

Recommendations for Policies

The remainder of this chapter provides recommendations to incorporate into the development of specific SOPs on the following topics:

- Backing of the emergency vehicle
- Seatbelts and restraints in the emergency vehicle
- Safety procedures on the driving range
- Post-collision guidelines
- Visibility at the scene
- Qualifications for new emergency vehicle operators
- Avoidance of distractions while driving
- Alcohol and drug use

Most of these recommendations come from SOPs that have already been developed and are in place in organizations across the United States today. Rather than including specific agencies' SOPs as models, since there are so many excellent ones available, we have highlighted the key concepts that should be addressed in each policy area.

Other topics your agency should consider developing into an SOP include the following:

- Use of emergency warning devices
- Parking and securing a vehicle
- Basic defensive driving
- Service animal transportation
- Nonemergency driving
- Emergency driving
- Education and training requirements for your service

Backing of the EMS Vehicle

It is estimated that 25% of all emergency vehicle crashes occur while the emergency vehicle is operating in reverse. The average emergency vehicle operator may travel thousands of miles going forward. This same emergency vehicle operator will back up only 1 or 2 miles per year. The ratio of time or miles spent driving in reverse to the percentage of collisions is very concerning. We have a serious problem when we shift into reverse. Therefore, considerations in developing a backing policy should include the following:

- Backing should be avoided whenever possible. Where backing is unavoidable, a spotter or an assistant outside the vehicle should be used even when backup cameras are present. Only emergency services personnel should be used to do this. If a patient is on board and a spotter is not outside, then the EMS member with the patient should get out and spot the vehicle, provided that he or she is not actively engaged in patient care.
- When placing the vehicle in reverse, the horn should be tapped twice to let your spotter and everyone else around know you are about to back up. In addition, the reverse alarm should be functional every time the vehicle is placed in reverse.
- If no qualified spotter is available, whenever possible, the emergency vehicle operator should park the vehicle, get out, and make a complete 360-degree survey of the space cushion around all four sides of the vehicle to locate any obstructions or hazards present before backing the emergency vehicle.
- Spotters are never permitted to ride the tailgates or running boards, or hang off the rear of any emergency vehicle in motion. Spotters should be located to the driver's side rear of the emergency vehicle in a safe position so they can be observed in the operator's mirror.
- Spotters should use the proper hand signals when the emergency vehicle is being backed. Uniform hand signals should be established as part of the backing policy.
- The emergency vehicle should not be backed until the spotter is in the proper safe position and communicates via voice or visible signal to the operator. The spotter should always be visible to the emergency vehicle operator in the safe zone. If the emergency vehicle operator loses sight of the spotter, the vehicle should be stopped immediately. When the spotter is in the proper/safe position, the emergency vehicle can continue to back up.
- Backing should be done very slowly and with great caution. The vehicle's speed should be controlled with the brake and not the accelerator.

There are some general rules for the emergency vehicle operators and spotters to always consider when backing the vehicle:

- Never be in a rush when backing or parking.
- Do not start to back or park when unsure of the area.
- Do not put the emergency vehicle into reverse gear until it has come to a complete stop.
- When it is dark, use the side and rear spotlights when backing.
- If the emergency vehicle has a backup alarm and/or backup camera that can be disengaged, they should be in the on position at all times, especially when backing the emergency vehicle.
- When turning while backing, check front fender swing to avoid front-end collisions.

Finally, all emergency vehicle operators should practice backing the vehicle during their training. Start with backing between cones into a simulated garage. Try backing around the serpentine cone setup, and then practice backing into the garage at the EMS station.

Use of Seatbelts and Restraints

As EMS providers, we know better than the general public the traumatic and often fatal effects of automobile crashes. The lifesaving impact of seatbelts and restraints has been well researched and proven by the National Highway Traffic Safety Administration. Most states have passed laws requiring drivers and the occupants of vehicles to be belted when the vehicle is in motion. Some states have included an emergency vehicle waiver in their seatbelt law.

In regard to the front compartment of an ambulance, there is no acceptable reason for the emergency vehicle operator to waive the seatbelt requirement. If a family member is allowed to ride along to the hospital, it should be the vehicle operator's responsibility to make sure the person is properly belted. If the individual refuses to wear a seatbelt, it is best to not allow him or her to ride in the ambulance, as the individual could be seriously injured if the ambulance should be involved in a collision.

SAFETY POINTER

To ensure that any friend or family member of the patient is safely restrained, the emergency vehicle operator should assist the individual in buckling up prior to driving to the hospital.

When there are EMS providers or any family members in the patient compartment of the ambulance and the vehicle is in motion, they should be seatbelted. Even though it is often legal for the crew to be unrestrained in the patient compartment, it is never recommended. Some would argue that it is not always possible to be belted in when providing care to the patient. In reality, this is a very rare occurrence, and the manufacturers of ambulances are working on developing seats in tracks that can restrain the EMS provider while providing care FIGURE 10-1.

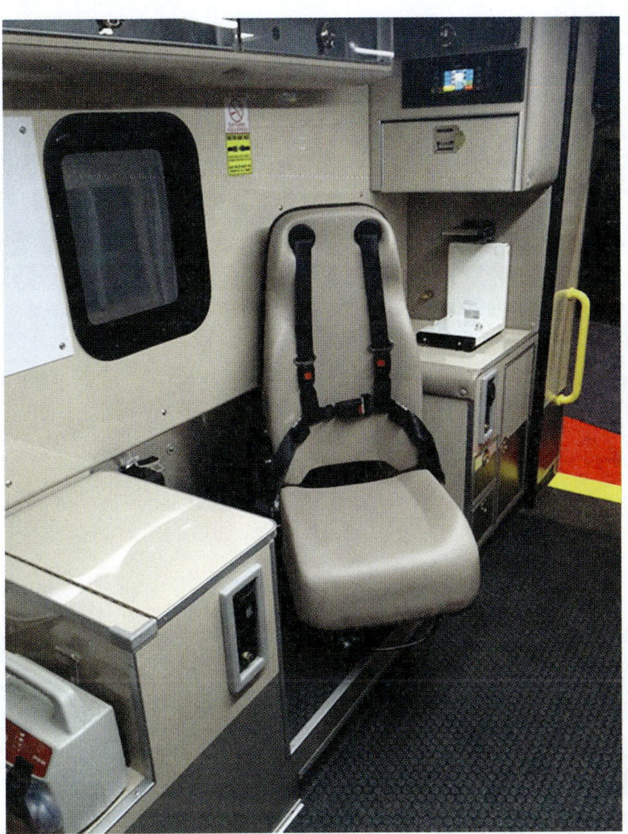

Figure 10-1 Safety seat with full harness belting.
Courtesy of Bob Elling.

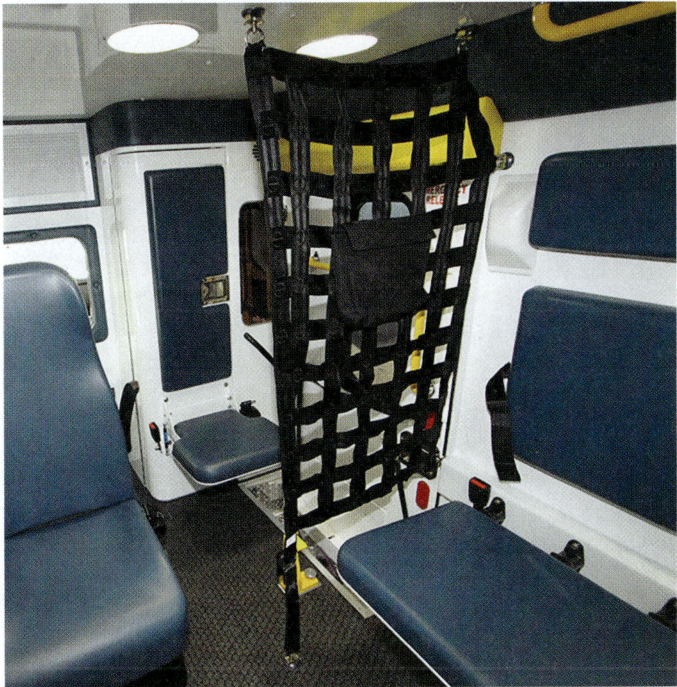

Figure 10-2 The cargo net is not an effective restraint device.
Courtesy of Crestline Coach Ltd.

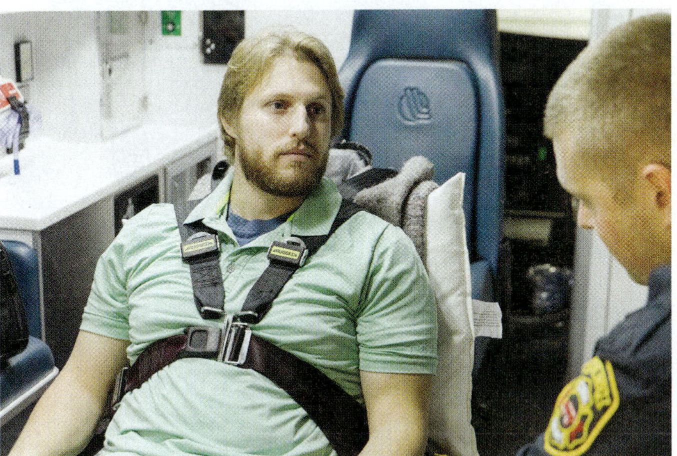

Figure 10-3 A patient with shoulder straps properly applied.
© Jones & Bartlett Learning.

Many EMS providers believe that the cargo net hanging at the end of the bench seat is a restraint device. There are some who even refer to it as the "medic catcher," since they believe it will hang intact and protect the provider from coming off the bench seat and hitting the cabinets that are normally across the doorway from the bench seat. Some providers also use the cargo net as a storage device, from which to hang cleaning sprays, quick-access packs, stethoscopes, and other items. Hanging objects from the cargo net makes it unsafe as a restraint device, and its ability to hold a provider in place during a collision is doubtful since, as some collision videos depict, the force of the provider's impact can cause the netting to come free. The cargo net should neither be considered a restraint device nor used as a storage device FIGURE 10-2.

The patient should always be properly restrained in the seatbelts on the stretcher, including the over-the-shoulder restraint FIGURE 10-3. If a pediatric patient is transported in the ambulance, he or she should be restrained in a properly sized car seat or in appropriate strapping on the stretcher FIGURE 10-4. Car seats are not made or rated to be placed in lateral positions, such as on the bench seat or in the CPR seat; they need to be on the cot or in the airway seat (at the head of the stretcher). With an integrated child restraint system, the airway seat opens into a child safety seat, which can be used to transport a child who is uninjured or who does not require continuous and/or intensive medical monitoring and/or interventions FIGURE 10-5.

Safety on the Driving Range

When a skills course is set up to complement the didactic component of the emergency vehicle operator course, it is imperative that this exercise be treated as a potentially dangerous event and that all care is taken when one or more vehicles are on the driving range. Do not assume that any emergency vehicle operator, regardless of experience level, is watching the other students at the range. Exercises should be clearly explained and demonstrated by the driver trainer. The emergency vehicle operator should then be allowed to practice the specific exercise (e.g., backing into a cone garage, serpentine maneuvers forward

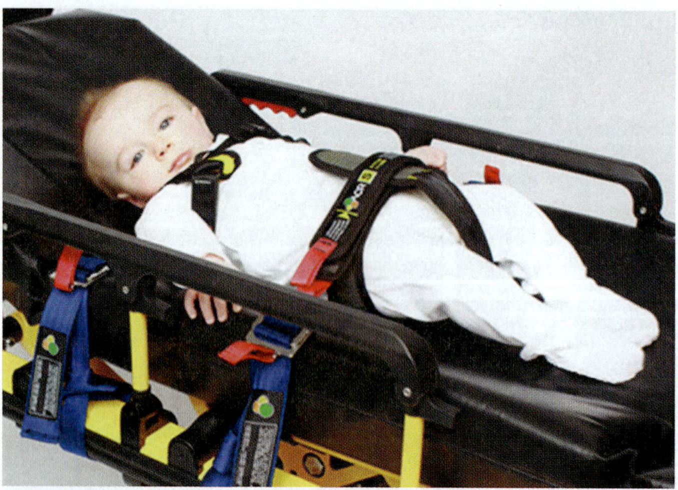

Figure 10-4 An injured child should be transported in an appropriately sized child restraint system on the stretcher.
Courtesy of Evac+Chair International Ltd.

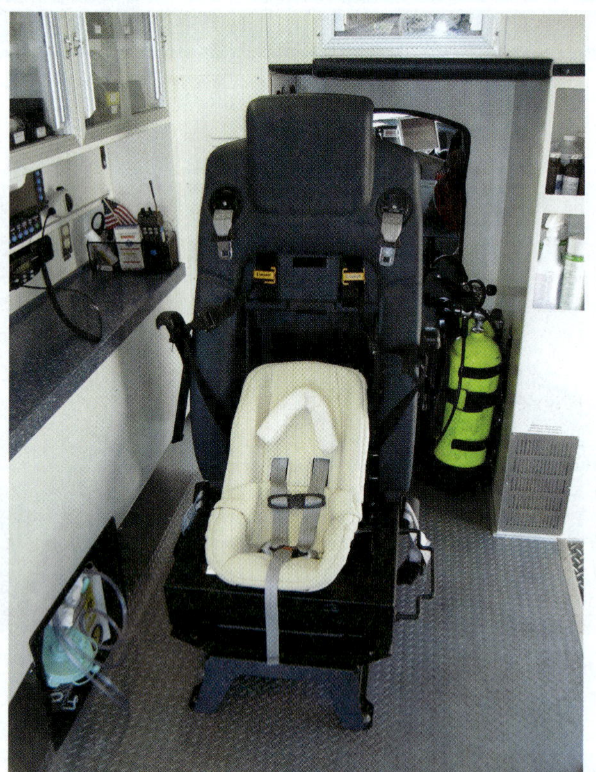

Figure 10-5 An integrated child restraint system.
Courtesy of Serenity Safety Products.

and backward, parallel parking the vehicle) without any other students on the driving range. It is not necessary to practice with a spotter in the backing exercises FIGURE 10-6.

There should be a clearly marked safety zone for other students in the class to stay within while awaiting their turn. Emergency vehicle operators who are driving the vehicles should stay away from the safety zones.

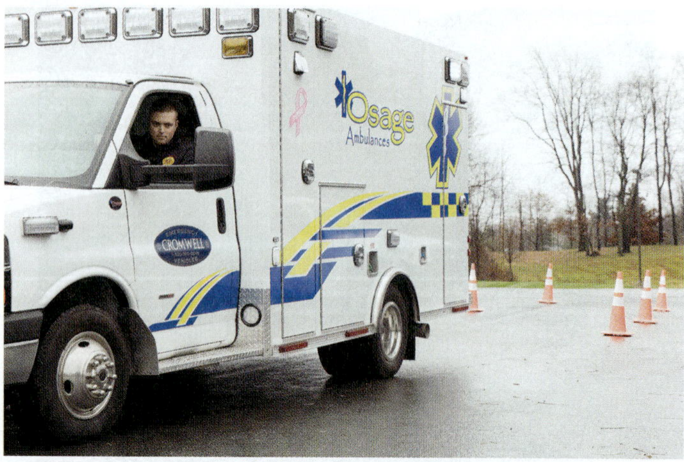

Figure 10-6 An EMS provider backing the ambulance on the range into some cones.
© Jones & Bartlett Learning.

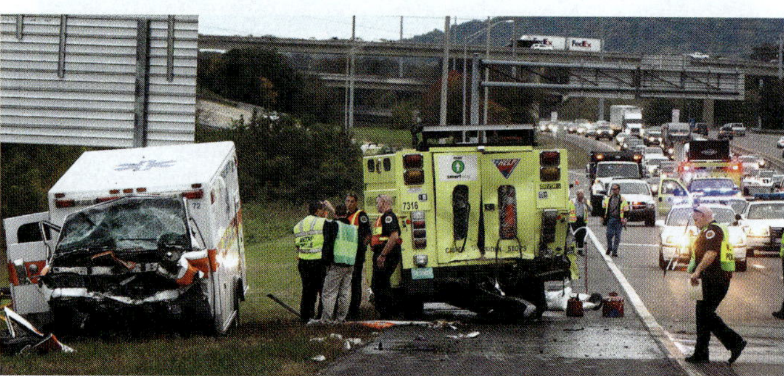

Figure 10-7 An ambulance crash scene.
© Larry McCormack/The Tennessean/AP Photo.

The training area should be large enough and free of obstacles to allow students to make mistakes without any consequences and without placing themselves or others in danger. As a rule, the range should be a minimum of 10 times the vehicle's length, and the width of the maneuver should include the total turning radius and the safe zone. The safe zone should be calculated as turning radius (TR) × $\frac{2}{3}$ × 2. The purpose of multiplying by 2 is to account for each side of the maneuver. For example, if working with a vehicle that is 25 feet long, we would determine the minimum length of our field by multiplying 25 feet by 10, which is 250 feet. The proper minimum safe zone for a vehicle with a 30-foot turning radius would be calculated as 30 feet × .66 × 2, which is 40 feet (20 feet for each side of the maneuver). The total width of the training area would then be 70 feet (30 feet + 40 feet).

Procedures Following a Crash

Unfortunately, at some point, each service will experience an ambulance collision FIGURE 10-7. An emergency vehicle collision can present a major problem for an agency, but that problem can be greatly intensified if providers do not know how to regain control of the situation or are not aware of any plans to deal with a collision. A policy for responding to crashes should include the following steps:

1. Notify the dispatcher right away and have the police, your supervisor, and other emergency services respond as necessary.
2. Determine whether there are injuries and whether an ambulance will be needed at the scene to treat and transport the injured, including your patient if you are carrying one.
3. Notify the dispatcher if the call you were responding to will require another unit to be sent in your place.
4. In most cases, it makes the most sense not to move the vehicles until the police have had the opportunity to document the scene. Moving the vehicles could have a detrimental effect on the investigation. Some states may have laws requiring vehicles to be moved out of traffic and not impede the traffic if there were no injuries involved. Follow your state and local laws as well as your department SOPs closely. If vehicles must be moved, take photos of the scene (not the damage) from a relative distance; try to include any road signs or markings and any geographic factors (e.g., hills, curves) that may have contributed to the collision. Also, mark the roadway at each point of the tires using the "T" method of a line alongside the tire and a line protruding out from the center hub. This helps in identifying the vehicles' positions.
5. Assign someone to deal with traffic appropriately until the police can take over that duty. Set up the proper flare or cone configuration that will assist motorists in identifying the collision and clearly move them away from the immediate area.
6. If the ambulance will need to be towed to a garage or body shop, make sure the drug box, HIPAA-protected documentation, and expensive equipment are removed and secured.
7. Services should have a policy that no personnel, except a designated public information officer, may talk to the media. Statements made while under duress could be inappropriate and come back at you or your service in a negative way.
8. If there is any injury, regardless of how minor, it should be evaluated at the time of the collision and not left until the following day. A worker's compensation package should be completed no matter how minuscule the injury.
9. All pertinent insurance information should be gathered as it would if the collision happened in a personal vehicle.
10. If law enforcement or department policies require a breathalyzer or field sobriety tests, make sure they are done out of the view of the public and news teams. Many times these are standard practices that can reflect poorly on the agency if shown in the media.

Visibility at the Scene

Traffic is a serious threat to the health and safety of the EMS providers and the emergency vehicle operator when working at the scene on a roadway. Whenever possible, law enforcement personnel will take responsibility for rerouting, stopping, or diverting traffic away from the EMS personnel and patients. All personnel must wear highly visible apparel, provided by the agency/department, when working in traffic on the roadway.

Qualifications for New Emergency Vehicle Operators

Your agency/department should clearly spell out what type of individual it is looking for as an applicant to become trained as an emergency vehicle operator. Considerations should include minimum age, years driving and clean record, maturity and good sense of responsibility, physical fitness, and dedication to improving driving skills.

The minimum duration and the specific objectives of the training program should be clearly spelled out. All emergency vehicle operator candidates need to understand the commitment they are making to become qualified.

It should be written in the SOP that the service will be conducting background checks of employees'/members' driver's licenses at the time of their initial application and/or qualification as an emergency vehicle operator as well as on a regular basis. It is the responsibility of the emergency vehicle operator to make the leadership of the agency aware of any serious infractions (points, moving violations, suspensions, crashes with injuries, DWIs/DWAIs) that occur while not at work at the agency. Many departments and states will require vehicle operators to carry their own automobile insurance even though they are covered by the department while working.

No Distractions While Driving Policy

Some states have already passed laws prohibiting talking on a cell phone and texting while driving because they take the driver's attention and hands away from vehicle operation. Yet, it is fairly common to drive down the highway and notice an emergency vehicle operator talking on a cell phone, talking on the radio, or in some instances texting or playing with the computer in the front of the ambulance. These are all distractions and can lead to a very serious crash. If you must use the phone, pull the vehicle over to a safe spot and use your cell phone to check in with your family or friends; do not do so while you are cruising down the highway.

As much as possible, eliminating the distractions to the emergency vehicle operator will help improve the safety of the ride to and from the call. Some services make it the responsibility of the crew member in the cab, who is not the driver, to deal with the radio transmissions and the maps or GPS devices while en route to the scene. Other distractions you may want to consider would include eating, drinking, and grooming while driving.

The bottom line here is that your SOP should be written in such a way as to minimize the distraction and create a sterile cab for the emergency vehicle operator.

Zero Tolerance for Alcohol and Drugs

The majority of the EMS and fire service agencies stand firmly behind EMS agencies strictly prohibiting any members or employees from responding to a call if they have been drinking. According to the International Association of Fire Chiefs' (IAFC) policy statement #3.04, Zero-Tolerance for Alcohol and Drinking in the Fire and Emergency Service (2003), "No member of a fire and emergency services agency/organization shall participate in any aspect of the organization and operation of the fire or emergency agency/organization under the influence of alcohol, including but not limited to any fire and emergency operations, fire-police, training, etc." The statement recommends that agencies develop written policies and have procedures in place for testing the blood alcohol levels of any individual involved in an incident that results in "measurable damage to apparatus or property, or injury/death of agency/organization personnel or civilians." The IAFC also suggests that any employee with an alcohol level of 0.02 or higher should be considered under the influence of alcohol. Both its 2003 policy statement and a subsequent position statement, "Drug and Alcohol-Free Awareness" (2012), recommend that members do not consume alcohol within eight hours of performing any emergency services duties. The 2012 position statement additionally recommends that agencies obtain legal advice and create policies that take into account the use of social halls for both department and non-department functions.

The IAFC's 2012 position statement also incorporates prescription and illicit drugs into its recommendations. Its position is that drug abuse should not be tolerated regardless of the type of drug, that there should also be zero tolerance of illegal drugs, and that agencies should have policies in place to test and suspend personnel during internal or external investigations. Prescription or over-the-counter drugs used while on duty should be approved by a healthcare professional and reported to a supervisor, who should verify that over-the-counter medications are allowed by the department physician and the safe use with the prescribing physician in the case of prescription drugs. The IAFC also suggests that Employee Assistance Programs be made available to members who are dealing with drug and alcohol abuse.

Each service's medical director, leadership and representatives from human resources, safety and risk department, and employee association or union should come to an agreement on a reasonable policy in reference to drugs, including prescription and over-the-counter medications, which can impair the emergency vehicle operator's driving abilities.

WRAP-UP

SUMMARY

- Emergency vehicle operators must understand how and why agencies develop SOPs.
- Emergency services should develop a clear policy for backing the emergency vehicle.
- Emergency services should clearly define requirements for the use of seatbelts and restraints in the emergency vehicle.
- Safety precautions must be in place whenever driving skills are being practiced at the driving range.
- Emergency services should clearly state the specifics that emergency vehicle operators should follow if involved in a collision while operating the emergency vehicle.
- A department policy should exist in regard to visibility on the scene of an emergency call.
- Emergency services should clearly define the requirements for providers to become qualified as emergency vehicle operators.
- A clear policy should be in place for eliminating distractions to the emergency vehicle operator while operating the emergency vehicle.
- All EMS agencies must have a zero-tolerance policy in place for substances that affect emergency vehicle operators' coordination and judgment when operating an emergency vehicle.

GLOSSARY

SMART objectives An acronym that describes the key characteristics of meaningful objectives: *s*pecific, *m*easureable, *a*chievable, *r*ealistic, and *t*ime-bound.

standard operating procedure (SOP) A policy issued by an agency's leadership to spell out how the employees or members are expected to perform in a specific instance or circumstance.

zero tolerance A policy that makes a given behavior absolutely unacceptable; it does not allow for "three strikes and you're out."

REFERENCES

International Association of Fire Chiefs. (n.d.). Guide to IAFC model policies and procedures for emergency vehicle safety. Retrieved from https://www.iafc.org/files/1SAFEhealthSHS/VehclSafety_IAFCpolAndProceds.pdf

International Association of Fire Chiefs. (2012). Position statement: drug and alcohol-free awareness. Retrieved from http://www.iafc.org/files/1ASSOC/IAFCposition_DrugAlcoholFree Awareness.pdf

International Association of Fire Chiefs. (2003). Zero-tolerance for alcohol and drinking in the fire and emergency service. Policy Number 03.04. Retrieved from http://www.iafc.org/files/downloads/ABOUT/POLICY_STATES/IAFCpol_Alcohol_inFireEmergServ.pdf

U.S. Department of Transportation, National Highway Traffic Safety Administration (2012). Working group best-practice recommendations for the safe transportation of children in emergency ground ambulances. DOT HS 811 677. Retrieved from http://www.nhtsa.gov/staticfiles/nti/pdf/811677.pdf

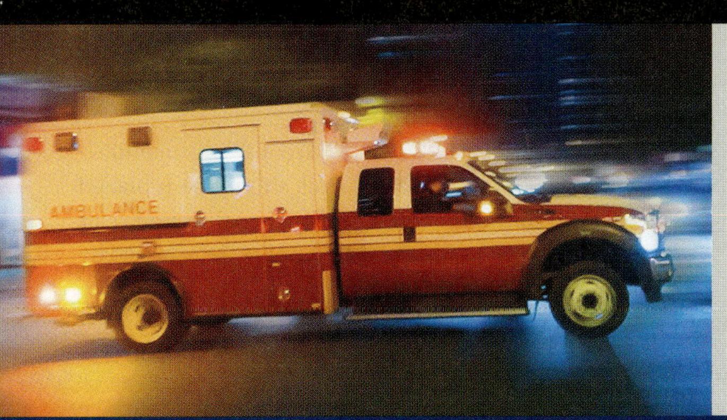

Appendix A

Daily/Weekly Inspection Check Sheet

You should first become familiar with all the information on the daily/weekly check sheet. Fill in the required information at the top of the worksheet.

The first section to work on with the daily/weekly form may be the engine. On some vehicles, you may have to raise the cab to inspect the engine. Follow the manufacturer's instructions.

1. Check the engine oil and transmission level.
   a. Make sure the engine is "off." Locate the dipstick, which is typically found on the right or left side of the engine. Wipe the top of the dipstick and tube off to ensure that no dirt will fall into the dipstick tube when the stick is raised. Remove the dipstick and visually inspect the current oil level as marked on the stick. Most dipsticks will have a "Low" mark and a "Full" mark. The oil level should be noted and the condition of the oil inspected.
   b. Look for any discoloration, moisture, or milky look, indicating possible coolant contamination or water intrusion. Is the oil thinned out, indicating a possible fuel oil dilution challenge? Are there any shiny metal particles, indicating a possible internal engine challenge?
2. Note whether you have to add any oil, and do a visual inspection to identify any leaks. The National Fire Protection Association (NFPA) classifies leaks into three categories. According to NFPA 1911, *Standard for the Inspection, Maintenance, Testing, and Retirement of In-Service Automotive Fire Apparatus*, chapter 3.3.72, *leakage* is the escape of a gas or fluid from its intended containment, generally at a connection. Class 1 Liquid Leakage is the presence of liquid, as indicated by wetness or discoloration, that is not great enough to form drops. Class 2 Liquid Leakage is leakage of liquid great enough to form drops but not enough to cause drops to fall from the item being inspected. Class 3 Liquid Leakage is leakage of liquid great enough to cause drops to fall from the item being inspected.
   a. Any Class 3 leakage should be noted and the vehicle taken out of service until it is remedied.
   b. Any Class 2 leakage in the fuel system should also cause the vehicle to be taken out of service.
3. Inspect the transmission fluid level by following the vehicle manufacturer's instructions. Most of today's emergency vehicles have an Allison automatic transmission, which is typically equipped with an electronic oil level sensor. It is recommended that these apparatus be inspected with the engine running, in neutral, at operating temperature on level ground, and at idle speed. Push the up and down arrow button on the shift pad the required number of times as described in the Allison operator's manual (either once or twice, depending on model year); the shift selector should display "OL." It will then go into a countdown mode to allow the fluid to drain into the sump. After the countdown is complete, the shift selector will display "OL OK" or "OL LO" for a low fluid level or "OL HI" for a high fluid level, followed by the amount low or high in quarts or liters.

   The electronic oil level inspection procedure is preferred over the dipstick. The dipstick method is not as accurate, because it does not take into account the fluid temperature and expansion that occurs with increasing temperature. It may be preferable to perform the transmission fluid level inspection after driving the vehicle, when it is up to operating temperature.
4. Check the engine coolant level. The engine should be cool during this inspection, and the level should be noted if it is low. Any Class 3 leakage or oil or fuel contamination should be noted and the vehicle taken out of service in such a case.
   a. Note the color of the coolant. Conventional-type ethylene glycol is typically a green, blue, or purple color; extended-life coolants, such as nitric organic acid technology (NOAT), typically have an orange or reddish color.
   b. If necessary, add more coolant. Most coolants today are permanent antifreeze types. Several types of coolants are available, however, and the correct type must be used for coolant top-off. Automotive antifreeze is generally *not* recommended for heavy-duty diesel engines. Do not mix different types of coolants in a cooling system, and do not use tap water in this system.
5. Check for integrity of the frame and suspension. Follow the vehicle manufacturer's instructions, and visually

inspect the frame and suspension for any rust, loose bolts, or attaching hardware, cracks, or deformations. Note any defects found and check NFPA 1911, chapter 6, for "out of service" conditions and reporting requirements.

6. Check the power steering fluid. Follow the vehicle manufacturer's instructions. Check for proper level and visually inspect condition for discoloration and or unusual odors such as a burnt smell. Inspect for leakage. Any Class 3 leakage requires that the vehicle be taken out of service.
7. Outside the engine:
   - **a.** Check for fluid leaks under the vehicle.
     - **i.** Identify the fluid, color, and location of the leaks, as they are keys to what may be leaking.
     - **ii.** Brown or dark fluid under the engine area may indicate a Class 3 leakage in the engine, placing the apparatus out of service.
     - **iii.** Red coloration under the transmission may indicate a Class 3 leakage in the transmission, placing the apparatus out of service.
     - **iv.** Brown or red fluid under the pump may indicate a Class 3 leakage in the pump transmission, placing the apparatus out of service.
     - **v.** Dark, heavy-consistency fluid under the rear axle may indicate a differential leak, which is also a Class 3 leakage, placing the apparatus out of service.
   - **b.** Check steering shafts and linkages.
     - **i.** Do good visual inspections on the steering column slip joints and U-joints.
     - **ii.** Do a visual inspection of the linkage under the vehicle. Are all pinch bolts, attaching nuts, and cotter keys in place and properly secured? Are the dust cover boots in good shape?
   - **c.** Check wheels and lug nuts.
     - **i.** Look at lug nuts for signs that they may be loose. Rust streaks may be a sign of loose lug retaining nuts.
   - **d.** Check tire condition.
     - **i.** Do good visual inspections looking for bulges, irregular wear, and tread depth. Note any unusual wear. Measure tread depth with a tire depth gauge. When inserted into the tire tread, the amount of tread left is indicated in increments of 1⁄32 inch (0.8 mm). The NFPA 1911 and DOT out of service criteria specify a minimum depth on steer axles of 4⁄32 inch (3.2 mm) and a minimum tread depth on drive axles of 2⁄32 inch (1.6 mm).
     - **ii.** Check tire date. Tire age can be determined by checking the DOT code found on either the inside or outside sidewall of each tire. The code begins with "DOT" and ends with a three-digit (through 1999) or four-digit (2000 and beyond) date code. The first two digits of the date code indicate the week of the year in which the tire was manufactured, and the last one or two digits identify the year of manufacture. For example, "DOT GJ HU234319" was manufactured in week 31 of 1999; "DOT BT FR872501" was manufactured in week 25 of 2001. Tires should be replaced every 7 years or more frequently when the tread wear exceeds state or federal standards as determined by measurement with a tread depth gauge.
   - **e.** Check tire air pressure.
     - **i.** Tires should be at room temperature. Let them rest at this temperature for at least 30 minutes.
     - **ii.** Use an accurate tire pressure gauge.
     - **iii.** Inflate the tires to the proper pressure. Tire pressure needs to be the tire manufacturer's suggested pressure for the weight on the tire. The vehicle should be weighed every year to get accurate weight data. The tire pressure recommended by the apparatus manufacturer may be found on a label in the cab; however, this pressure was determined when the vehicle was manufactured and based on the weight of the vehicle when new.
     - **iv.** The tire pressure on the sidewall of the tire is a maximum cold inflation pressure for that type of tire. Note the correct pressure for future daily/weekly checks. It is very important for safety reasons that the tire pressure be within 10 psi (70 kPa) of the recommended value. Low or high tire pressure can cause the vehicle to sway or maneuver dangerously.
     - **v.** Check the tire manufacturer's date document, the DOT code, the 7 years' maximum, and the out of service criteria.
   - **f.** Cab components:
     - **i.** Check the seats and seat belts.
       - **1)** Check for tears and frayed belts.
       - **2)** Check latching mechanisms.
       - **3)** If the cab is equipped with a seat belt warning system, check for its proper operation.
       - **4)** If a seat belt is torn or has melted webbing, missing or broken buckles, or loose mountings, the following shall apply:
         - **a)** If it is a seat other than the driver's seat, that seat shall be taken out of service.
         - **b)** If it is at the driver's seat, the entire apparatus shall be taken out of service.
     - **ii.** Start the engine, and check all gauges.
       - **1)** Do all gauges work properly? Does the volt and amp gauge indicate the alternator is charging properly? Do the air pressure gauges operate correctly?
       - **2)** Check for proper operation of the ABS brake indicator.
         - **a)** Does the ABS indicator illuminate on startup while it does a self-check and then go out?
     - **iii.** Check the windshield wipers.
       - **1)** Check for broken or missing windshield wipers.
       - **2)** Check the condition of the windshield wiper blades.

- **iv.** Check the rear-view mirror adjustment and operation.
  - **1)** Missing or broken rear-view mirrors that obstruct the driver/operator's view shall cause the apparatus to be taken out of service.
- **v.** Check the horn.
- **vi.** Check the steering shafts.
  - **1)** Inspect all steering system components for structural integrity, security of mounting, leakage, and condition.
- **vii.** Check the cab glass and mirrors.
  - **1)** A cracked or broken windshield that obstructs the driver/operator's view shall cause the apparatus to be taken out of service.

g. Electrical components:

- **i.** Check battery voltage and charging system voltage.
  - **1)** Test the batteries for storage and performance capabilities in accordance with the manufacturer's recommendation.
  - **2)** Before testing them, carefully inspect the batteries.
  - **3)** Clean the batteries of any accumulated dirt or corrosion, and check the connections to ensure that they are clean and tight.
  - **4)** Inspect the batteries for cracks, swelling, deformation, or other physical defects.
  - **5)** If the batteries are not sealed, verify that the cells have the proper electrolyte level, and add distilled water if necessary.
  - **6)** If the batteries are sealed, verify that any electrolyte level indicator indicates sufficient electrolyte is present.
  - **7)** With the shore power plugged in, check the battery charging system indicator light (if so equipped).
  - **8)** In the operator's seat with the shore power disconnected (if so equipped) and power or ignition switch in the "on" position, check the volt gauge to make sure that it reads 12 volts (on 12-volt systems) or slightly higher.
  - **9)** Start the vehicle and make sure the volt gauge goes up to 13 to 14 volts (on 12-volt systems).
  - **10)** With the vehicle running, visually check the amp gauge. It should show a positive number, indicating that the alternator is charging. You may increase engine rpms slightly to help verify this operation if necessary.
- **ii.** Check the line voltage system (if so equipped).
  - **1)** Inspect all power sources for security of mounting, condition, and fluid leakage.
  - **2)** Inspect all line voltage appliances and controls, including but not limited to the following appliances and controls, for security of mounting and condition:
    - **a)** Cord reels
    - **b)** Extension cords
    - **c)** Scene lights
    - **d)** Circuit breaker boxes
    - **e)** Switches
    - **f)** Relays
    - **g)** Receptacles
    - **h)** Inlet devices
    - **i)** Light towers
    - **j)** Other line voltage devices on the apparatus not otherwise specified
- **iii.** Check all lights (ICC and warning).
  - **1)** Inspect all fire apparatus lighting, including but not limited to the following, for security of mounting and deformation and for correct operation:
    - **a)** Headlights
    - **b)** Marker lights
    - **c)** Clearance lights
    - **d)** Turn signals and hazard lights
    - **e)** Brake lights
    - **f)** Dash lights
    - **g)** Other fire apparatus lighting equipment on the apparatus not otherwise specified

h. Brakes:

- **i.** Check the air system for proper air pressure.
  - **1)** Check the air pressure gauges on the dashboard. Most gauges today are electric, so you may need to have the battery switch and the ignition switch be in the "on" positions for the gauge to register the correct pressure.
  - **2)** Inspect the "Low Air" warning system to ensure that it activates at the manufacturer's suggested pressure. With the engine power off and the ignition on, pump the brakes several times to use up the air in the system. Note when the "Low Air" alarm activates.
- **ii.** Check the parking brake.
  - **1)** Inspect the parking brake for structural integrity, security of mounting, missing or broken parts, and wear.
  - **2)** Inspect the parking brake controls and activating mechanism for structural integrity, security of mounting, and missing or broken parts.
  - **3)** Operate the parking brake (air, hydraulic, or manual) to ensure that it holds the vehicle from movement. Use caution when performing this procedure; make sure that no one is around the vehicle in case it moves.
- **iii.** Check the hydraulic brake fluid level (if so equipped).
  - **1)** If the fire apparatus has a hydraulic brake system, the components to be inspected and maintained shall include, but are not be limited to, the following:
    - **a)** Pedal and linkage: Visual inspection to ensure that all linkage and attaching hardware is tight and in place.

b) Brake switches: Visual inspection to ensure that all switches are in place and wires are intact.
c) Master cylinder: Visual inspection to ensure there is no leakage. Class 2 leakage of hydraulic brake fluid is cause to take the apparatus out of service. Check the brake fluid level. If the master cylinder level is low, it suggests there is a leak somewhere in the system. This should be documented and further inspected by a qualified EVT.
d) Brake booster: Visual inspection to ensure that all attaching hardware is intact and tight.
e) Hydraulic lines: Visual inspection to ensure that all hydraulic lines are in place, clamps are in place, and no leakage is present. Class 2 leakage is cause to take the apparatus out of service.
f) Valves: Visual inspection of any brake valve that is visible to ensure that all attaching hardware is in place and tight and that no leaks are present. Class 2 leakage is cause to take the apparatus out of service.
g) Wheel cylinders or calipers: Visual inspection, if possible, to ensure that attaching hardware is in place and tight and no leaks are present. Class 2 leaks are cause to take the apparatus out of service. In most cases, the wheel cylinders and calipers will not be visible unless there is an inspection location on the braking system. In those cases, you should be aware of dampness or droplets of brake fluid dripping from the backing plate or brake assembly.
h) Brake shoes or disc brake pads: Visual inspection to ensure adequate thickness. This thickness must meet the manufacturer's minimum requirement. Note that the brake shoes or pads may not be visible without removing wheels or other parts. Some systems, however, have an inspection slot location for visual inspection.
i) Brake drums or rotors: Visual inspection should not find any cracks or bluing. Any deficiencies noted in the brake system should be noted and reported to the AHJ or the department's officer.
j) Warning devices: Visual inspection to ensure that they illuminate properly. Most systems will illuminate when the system is powered on and then will go off.
k) Mounting hardware: Visual inspection to ensure that all attaching hardware and/or clamps are in place and tight.
l) Fluid level and contamination: Fluid level and condition of fluid should be noted. A low fluid level indicates a leak. Note the color of the fluid and any discoloration. The fluid should not look burnt or milky. Any discoloration should be inspected by a qualified EVT.

i. Pump (if so equipped):
- **i.** Operate the pump; check the pump panel engine gauges.
- **ii.** Check the pump for pressure operation.
- **iii.** Check the discharge relief or pressure governor operation.
- **iv.** Check all pump drains.
- **v.** Check all discharge and intake valve operation.
- **vi.** Check the pump and tank for water leaks.
- **vii.** Check all valve bleeder/drain operations.
- **viii.** Check the primer pump operation.
- **ix.** Check the system vacuum for hold (leakage).
- **x.** Check the water tank level indicator.
- **xi.** Check the primer oil level (if applicable).
- **xii.** Check the transfer valve operation (if applicable).
- **xiii.** Check the booster reel operation (if applicable).
- **xiv.** Check all pump pressure gauge operations.
- **xv.** Check all cooler valves.
- **xvi.** Check for oil leaks in the pump area.

j. Aerial (if so equipped):
- **i.** Operate the aerial hydraulics.
- **ii.** Check the aerial outrigger operation.
- **iii.** Check the aerial operation.
- **iv.** Check the aerial hydraulic fluid level.
- **v.** Visually inspect the aerial structure.

Comments:

1. The driver/operator should document all deficiencies found and report them to the AHJ or the specific person taking care of such deficiencies in the fire department. Further evaluation may need to be performed by a qualified EVT. Most fire departments have a specific policy or procedure to follow for deficiencies or when taking an apparatus out of service.
2. The driver/operator should also inspect the following items and functionally test them for proper service in accordance with NFPA 1002, *Standard for Fire Apparatus Driver/Operator Professional Qualifications*, 5.1.1:

a. Water tank and other extinguishing agent levels (if applicable):
- **i.** Do a visual inspection of the water tank and extinguishing agent tank.
- **ii.** Check for any leakage.
- **iii.** Check the tank levels. Standard practice is to keep tanks full. Check your fire department's standard operating procedure.
- **iv.** Check the tank level-indicating devices for proper operation. Note whether the level-indicating device

is not functioning properly. An inspection should be performed to determine the cause, and an "out of service" determination needs to be made and put in writing to the AHJ.

b. Pumping systems:

i. The driver/operator needs to understand the "out of service" criteria for the pumping system. The following deficiencies of the fire pump shall cause the pumping system to be taken out of service:

1) Pump that will not engage

2) Pump shift indicators in the cab and on the operator's panel that do not function properly

3) Pressure control system that is not operational

4) Pump transmission components that have a Class 3 leakage of fluid

5) Pump operator's panel throttle that is not operational

6) Pump operator's engine speed advancement interlock that is not operational

c. Foam systems:

i. If the apparatus is equipped with a foam proportioning system, inspect and maintain that system in accordance with the recommendations of the foam system manufacturer.

ii. Inspect all components of the foam proportioning system for security of mounting, structural integrity, and leakage.

Glossary

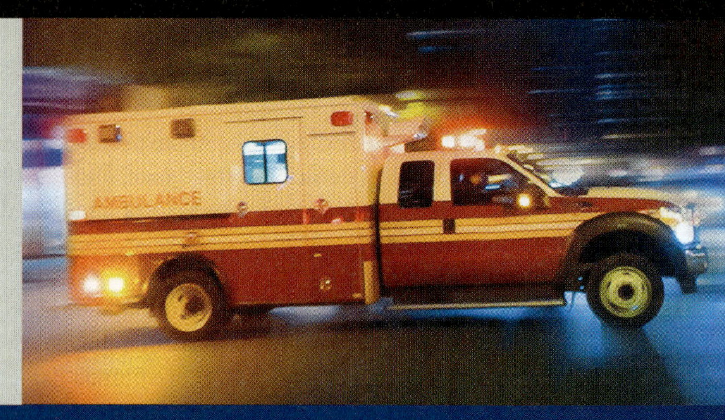

activity area The area of the incident scene where the work activity takes place; it may be stationary or may move as work progresses.

activity logging system A device that keeps a detailed record of every incident and activity that occur.

advance warning area The section of highway where drivers are informed about an upcoming situation ahead.

aerial device An aerial ladder, elevating platform, aerial ladder platform, or water tower that is designed to position personnel, handle materials, provide continuous egress, or discharge water.

air brakes A braking system that uses air as a medium for applying the brakes.

air pressure gauges Gauges that identify the air pressure stored in the tanks or reservoirs of an apparatus equipped with a pneumatic braking system.

alternator An electromechanical device that converts mechanical energy to electrical energy in the form of alternating current; automotive alternators use a set of rectifiers to convert alternating current to direct current to charge the vehicle batteries.

ambulance A vehicle designed, equipped, and operated for the treatment and transport of ill and injured persons.

antilock brakes A computerized braking system that prevents wheel lockup, helping the vehicle maintain directional control.

assessment center A series of simulation exercises for a promotional examination.

automatic location identification (ALI) A series of data elements that inform the recipient of the location of the alarm. (NFPA 1221)

automatic number identification (ANI) A series of alphanumeric characters that inform the recipient of the source of the alarm. (NFPA 1221)

auxiliary appliance A standpipe and/or sprinkler system.

base station A stationary radio transceiver with an integral AC power supply. (NFPA 1221)

battery A device that chemically stores electrical energy; it is generally used for starting the vehicle and short-term electrical use.

battery selector switch A switch used to disconnect all electrical power to the vehicle, thereby preventing discharge of the battery while the vehicle is not in use.

blind spots Areas around the fire apparatus that are not visible to the driver/operator.

brake fade Reduction in stopping power that can occur after repeated application of the brakes, especially in high-load or high-speed conditions.

braking distance The distance that the fire apparatus travels from the time that the brakes are activated until the fire apparatus makes a complete stop.

braking system The entire system that allows the vehicle operator to stop the vehicle by applying pressure to the vehicle's brake pedal.

buffer space The lateral and/or longitudinal area that separates traffic flow from a work space or an unsafe area; it might also provide some recovery space for an errant vehicle.

centrifugal force The outward force that is exerted away from the center of rotation. Also, the tendency for objects to be pulled outward when rotating around a center.

channel An assigned frequency or frequencies used to carry voice and/or data communications.

civil law The type of law that pertains to determining responsibility for a wrongful act and imposing monetary penalties (with or without criminal charges) if the defendant is found guilty.

Code 1 response Response in a fire apparatus in which no emergency lights or sirens are activated.

Code 2 response Response in a fire apparatus in which only the emergency lights are activated; no audible devices are activated.

Code 3 response Response in a fire apparatus in which both the emergency lights and the sirens are activated.

Code of Federal Regulations (CFR) A collection of permanent rules published in the *Federal Register* by the executive departments and agencies of the U.S. federal government. Its 50 titles represent broad areas of interest that are governed by federal regulation. Each volume of the CFR is updated annually and issued on a quarterly basis.

collapse zone An area encompassing a distance of 1½ times the height of a building. Fire fighters and fire apparatus must not be located in this area in case of a building collapse.

command vehicle A vehicle that the fire chief uses to respond to the fire scene.

commercial driver's license (CDL) A government-issued license that ensures the driver has met the requirements to operate certain types of commercial vehicles depending on the weight of the vehicle, the number of passengers, and the presence (or not) of any hazardous materials.

communications center A building or portion of a building that is specifically configured for the primary purpose of providing emergency communications services or public safety answering point (PSAP) services to one or more public safety agencies under the authority or authorities having jurisdiction.

computer-aided dispatch (CAD) A combination of hardware and software that provides data entry, makes resource recommendations, and notifies and tracks those resources before, during, and after fire service alarms, preserving records of those alarms and status changes for later analysis. (NFPA 1221)

control zones A series of areas at hazardous materials incidents that are designated based on safety concerns and the degree of hazard present.

corner safe areas Areas outside a building where two walls intersect; these areas are less likely to receive any damage during a building collapse.

criminal law The type of law that pertains to determining whether a statute has been violated and, if so, imposing a punishment (fine and/or imprisonment) on the guilty party.

critical incident stress debriefing (CISD) A postincident meeting designed to assist rescue personnel in dealing with psychological trauma as the result of an emergency. (NFPA 1006)

critical incident stress management (CISM) A program designed to reduce acute and chronic effects of stress related to job functions. (NFPA 450)

critical speed The maximum speed that a fire apparatus can safely travel around a curve.

defendant The person or party in a lawsuit who is charged with breaking the law and harming the plaintiff.

digital radio The transmission of information via radio waves using native digital (computer) data or analog (voice) signals that have been converted to a digital signal and compressed.

direct line A telephone that connects two predetermined points.

disc brakes A braking system designed with a disc and a brake caliper installed over the disc.

dispatch To send out emergency response resources promptly to an address or incident location for a specific purpose.

driver monitoring system A monitoring system that tracks driver actions, vehicle movement, and immediate environment around the vehicle using video cameras and sensors.

driver/operator A person who has satisfactorily completed the requirements of driver/operator as specified in NFPA 1002, *Standard for Fire Apparatus Driver/Operator Professional Qualifications*, and who is authorized by the authority having jurisdiction to drive, operate, or both drive and operate fire department vehicles. (NFPA 1451)

drum brakes A braking system that has a circular wheel hub with two semicircular brake shoes installed inside.

due regard The care exercised by a reasonably prudent person under the same circumstances.

duplex channel The ability to transmit and receive simultaneously; a radio system that uses two frequencies per channel—one to transmit and the other to receive a message. Such a system uses a repeater site to transmit messages over a greater distance than is possible with a simplex system.

electrical system The system that generates and maintains electrical energy required for vehicle operation as well as for patient care activities.

emergency traffic An urgent message, such as a call for help or evacuation, that is transmitted over a radio and that takes precedence over all normal radio traffic.

emitter A device that emits a visible flashing light at a specified frequency, thereby activating the receiver on a traffic signal.

employee assistance programs (EAPs) An employee-sponsored service designed for personal or family problems, including mental health, substance abuse, various addictions, marital problems, parenting problems, emotional problems, or financial or legal concerns. (NFPA 450)

engine A device that provides the mechanical motive force for propelling a vehicle and powering its subsystems.

evacuation signal A distinctive signal intended to be recognized by the occupants as requiring evacuation of the building. (NFPA 72)

exhaust system The system for removing dangerous exhaust gases from the engine.

Federal Communications Commission (FCC) The federal regulatory authority that oversees radio communications in the United States.

fire department vehicle Any vehicle, including fire apparatus, operated by a fire department.

freelancing The dangerous practice of acting independently of command instructions.

frequency The number of cycles (oscillations) per second of a radio signal.

fuel gauge A gauge that indicates the amount of fuel in the fire apparatus' fuel tank.

geographic information system (GIS) A system of computer software, hardware, data, and personnel that describes information tied to a spatial location. (NFPA 450)

global positioning system (GPS) A satellite-based location and navigation system used to locate vehicles and provide directions to specific locations.

gross negligence A more serious form of negligence that implies reckless conduct and a blatant disregard for the safety and lives of others. The line between negligence and gross negligence may need to be determined by a court.

hydraulic brakes A braking system that uses fluid to charge and activate the brakes.

ignition switch A switch that engages operational power to the chassis of a motor vehicle.

incident space The area where the actual incident is located.

intermediate traffic incidents A traffic incident that affects the lanes of travel for 30 minutes to 2 hours.

inverter An electrical device that converts direct current to alternating current; it provides 110-volt current.

job aids A tool, device, or system used to assist a person with executing specific tasks.

Level I staging Initial staging of fire apparatus in which three or more units are dispatched to an emergency incident.

Level II staging Placement of all reserve resources in a central location until requested to the scene.

liability Legal accountability or obligation.

liquid surge The force imposed upon a fire apparatus by the contents of a partially filled water or foam concentrate tank when the vehicle is accelerated, decelerated, or turned.

major traffic incidents A traffic incident that involves a fatal crash, a multiple-vehicle incident, a hazardous materials incident on the highway, or other disaster.

mayday A code indicating that a member is lost, missing, or trapped and requires immediate assistance.

microsleeping A brief break with consciousness in which a person loses awareness of his or her surroundings and momentarily enters a state of sleep.

minor traffic incidents A traffic incident that involves a minor crash and/or disabled vehicles.

mobile data terminal (MDT) A computerized device similar to a laptop computer that is used to communicate with a central dispatch office.

mobile data terminals (MDTs) Technology that allows fire personnel to receive data while in the fire apparatus or at the station.

mobile radios A two-way radio that is permanently mounted in a fire apparatus.

morbidity Illness or harm; a diseased state.

mortality Death; the quality of being mortal.

motor vehicle accident (MVA) An incident that involves one vehicle colliding with another vehicle or another object and that may result in injury, property damage, and possibly death.

multiplex channels Simultaneous transmission of multiple data streams, most often voice signals, in either or both directions over the same frequency on a radio.

negligence Failure to exercise due caution.

Occupational Safety and Health Administration (OSHA) The U.S. federal agency that regulates worker safety and, in some cases, responder safety. OSHA is part of the U.S. Department of Labor.

oil pressure gauge A gauge that identifies the pressure of the lubricating oil in the fire apparatus engine.

parking brake The main brake that prevents a fire apparatus from moving even when it is turned off and there is no one operating it.

plaintiff The person or party who files a complaint in a lawsuit claiming to have been harmed by the defendant.

portable radio A battery-operated, hand-held transceiver. (NFPA 1221)

preincident plan A document developed by gathering general and detailed data, which are then used by responding personnel to determine the resources and actions necessary to mitigate anticipated emergencies at a specific facility.

preponderance of the evidence A requirement in determining the guilt of a defendant that the majority of evidence presented in a case favor the plaintiff's argument.

preventable collision A collision in which the driver failed to do everything reasonable to prevent its occurrence.

preventive maintenance Scheduled servicing, inspection, or replacement of specific items in the vehicle to reduce potential problems.

public safety answering point (PSAP) A facility equipped and staffed to receive emergency and nonemergency calls requesting public safety services via telephone and other communication devices. (NFPA 1061)

public safety communications center A building or portion of a building that is specifically configured for the primary purpose of providing emergency communications services or public safety answering point (PSAP) services to one or more public safety agencies under the authority or authorities having jurisdiction. (NFPA 1061)

reaction distance The distance that the fire apparatus travels after the driver/operator recognizes the hazard, removes his or her foot from the accelerator, and applies the brakes.

reasonable doubt The lack of certainty that a person may justifiably feel based on the evidence at hand regarding the alleged guilt of a defendant.

receiver A device placed on or near a traffic signal to recognize a signal from the emitter on an emergency vehicle and preempt the normal cycle of the traffic light.

repeater A special base station radio that receives messages and signals on one frequency and then automatically retransmits them on a second frequency.

response The deployment of an emergency service resource to an incident. (NFPA 901)

road rage Aggressive or angry behavior by a driver of a motor vehicle that may include rude gestures, verbal insults or threats, or unsafe driving.

run cards Cards used to determine a predetermined response to an emergency.

simplex channel A radio system that uses one frequency to transmit and receive all messages. Transmissions can occur in either direction but not simultaneously in both; when one party transmits, the other can only receive, and the party that is transmitting is unable to receive.

size-up The observation and evaluation of existing factors that are used to develop objectives, strategy, and tactics for fire suppression. (NFPA 1051)

sleep deprivation The state of having insufficient sleep.

SMART objectives An acronym that describes the key characteristics of meaningful objectives: *s*pecific, *m*easureable, *a*chievable, *r*ealistic, and *t*ime-bound.

spotter A person who guides the driver/operator into the appropriate position while operating in a confined space or in reverse mode.

staging A specific function whereby resources are assembled in an area at or near the incident scene to await instructions or assignments.

staging area A prearranged, strategically placed area, where support response personnel, vehicles, and other equipment can be held in an organized state of readiness for use during an emergency.

staging area manager The person responsible for maintaining the operations of the staging area.

standard operating procedure (SOP) A policy issued by an agency's leadership to spell out how the employees or members are expected to perform in a specific instance or circumstance.

starter switch The switch that engages the starter motor for cranking.

stressors Conditions that create excessive physical and mental pressures on a person's body; any type of stimulus that causes stress.

suspension system The system that supports the vehicle and allows it to absorb the impact from bumpy roads without affecting the ride inside the cab and patient compartment.

system check sequence A series of checks that an electrical system completes to ensure that all of the systems are functioning properly before the fire apparatus is started.

tactical benchmarks Objectives that are required to be completed during the operational phase of an incident.

talk-around channel A simplex channel used for on-site communications.

telecommunicators An individual whose primary responsibility is to receive, process, or disseminate information of a public safety nature via telecommunication devices. (NFPA 1061)

telephone interrogation The phase in a 911 call during which the telecommunicator asks questions to obtain vital information such as the location of the emergency.

ten-codes A system of predetermined coded messages, such as "What is your 10-20?", used by responders over the radio.

termination area The area where the normal flow of traffic resumes after a traffic incident.

total stopping distance The distance that it takes for the driver/operator to recognize a hazard, process the need to stop the fire apparatus, apply the brakes, and then come to a complete stop.

traffic control The direction or management of vehicle traffic such that scene safety is maintained and rescue operations can proceed without interruption.

traffic incident A natural disaster or other unplanned event that affects or impedes the normal flow of traffic.

traffic incident management area (TIMA) An area of highway where temporary traffic controls are imposed by authorized officials in response to an accident, natural disaster, hazardous materials spill, or other unplanned incident.

traffic preemption system A system used to preempt traffic lights, giving emergency vehicles the right-of-way.

traffic signal preemption system A system that allows the normal operation of a traffic signal to be changed so as to assist emergency vehicles in responding to an emergency.

traffic space The portion of the highway where traffic is routed through the activity area of a traffic incident.

transition area The area where vehicles are redirected from their normal path and where lane changes and closures are made in a traffic incident.

transmission A device that provides speed and torque conversions from the engine to the wheels using gear ratios; it reduces the higher engine speed to the slower wheel speed, increasing torque in the process.

true emergency A situation in which there is a high probability of death or serious injury to an individual or of significant property loss.

trunked radios A radio system that uses a computerized shared bank of frequencies to make the most efficient use of radio resources.

TTY/TDD systems User devices that allow speech- and/or hearing-impaired persons to communicate over a telephone system. TDD stands for telecommunications device for the deaf; TTY stands for teletype; text phones visually display text. The displayed text is the equivalent of a verbal conversation between two hearing persons.

ultrahigh-frequency (UHF) band Radio frequencies between 300 and 3000 MHz.

valve stem An opening to the valve that admits air to a tire and automatically closes to seal in pressure.

vehicle dynamics Vehicle construction and mechanical design characteristics that directly affect the handling, stability, maneuverability, functionality, and safety of a vehicle.

vehicle intercom system A communication system that is permanently mounted inside the cab of the fire apparatus and allows fire fighters to communicate more effectively.

very high-frequency (VHF) band Radio frequencies between 30 and 300 MHz; the VHF spectrum is further divided into high and low bands.

Voice over Internet Protocol (VoIP) A technology that converts a person's voice into a digital signal that can be sent via the Internet back to another computer, VoIP phone, or a traditional phone with a specialized adapter.

voice recording system Recording devices or computer equipment connected to telephone lines and radio equipment in a communications center to record telephone calls and radio traffic.

voltmeter A device that measures the voltage across a battery's terminals and gives an indication of the electrical condition of the battery.

zero tolerance A policy that makes a given behavior absolutely unacceptable; it does not allow for "three strikes and you're out."

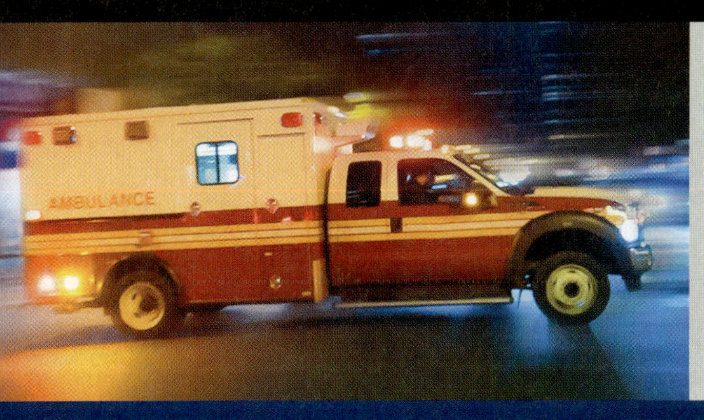

Index

Note: Page numbers followed by *f* or *t* indicate material in figures or tables.

A

ABCDE mnemonics, 15
activity area, 115
activity logging system, 129, 130*f*
advance warning area, 115
adverse weather conditions, 42
  collisions and, 53
aerial device, 108
aggressive driving, 42
air brakes, 64
  leakage test, 64
air compressor cutoff test, 65
air-conditioning system, vehicle inspection, 66
air horns, noise from, 97
air pressure gauges, 72
airbags, 31–32
alcohol use, 12, 47, 160
ALI. *See* automatic location identification
alley dock exercise, performing, 119, 120
ALSAPS method, 64–65
alternators, 63
ambulances. *See also* vehicle inspection and maintenance
  airbags in, 31–32
  backing on range into cones, 158, 158*f*
  crash scene, 158–159, 158*f*
  equipment security in, 32
  helmets in, 32
  inspection checklist, 58, 59*f*
  noise levels within, 43
  passenger safety in, 33–34
  patient safety in, 32–33, 33*f*
  positioning, 111–112
  safe work zone, 34–35, 34*f*
  seatbelts in, 31
  vehicle positioning, 35, 111–112
Americans with Disabilities Act, 131
ANI. *See* automatic number identification
antennas, external, 60
anti-slide airbags, 31
antilock brakes, 64
ASE. *See* Automotive Service Excellence
assessment center, 23
attitude, personal, 30–31, 42
audible warning devices, 44
automatic location identification (ALI), 132, 133*f*
automatic number identification (ANI), 132
automatic tire pressure gauges, 66
Automotive Service Excellence (ASE), 67
auxiliary appliances, 111
auxiliary braking systems, 102

B

backing collisions, 53
backing policy, 156
  ambulance, 158, 158*f*
  EMS vehicle, 156
backup communications center, 128
base station radios, 137, 139, 139*f*
batteries, 63
  selector switch, 72
blind spots, 5
brake fade, 100
braking distance, 100
braking system, inspection, 63–65, 64*f*
bridges, fire apparatus on, 102
buffer space, 115
building collapse, 119

C

CAD. *See* computer-aided dispatch
Cal-OSHA, 8
call classification and prioritization, 133
call for help, by team member, 142
call receipt
  defined, 130
  telephones, 130–132, 131*f*
  walk-ins, 132, 132*f*
call-taking process, 127, 136, 137
Canadian Ministry of Transportation (MOT), 20
cancer, 11
cargo net, 157, 157*f*
carpet airbags, 31
CDL. *See* commercial driver's license
cell phones, 130–134
  use of as distraction, 41
Centers for Disease Control and Prevention, 29
centrifugal force, 101
certified emergency vehicle technicians, 18, 18*f*
CEVO. *See* Coaching the Emergency Vehicle Operator
CFR. *See* Code of Federal Regulations
channel, radio, 139
children
  as passenger, 33–34
  safety seat, 157, 158*f*
CISD. *See* critical incident stress debriefing

CISM. *See* critical incident stress management
civil law, 50
  legal entanglements, avoiding, 54, 54*f*
  liability in cases of collisions, 54
Coaching the Emergency Vehicle Operator (CEVO), 116
Code 1 response, 99
Code 2 response, 98
Code 3 response, 98
Code of Federal Regulations (CFR), 8
cold zone, 119
cold/flu, 30, 45
collapse zone, 109
collisions, 6, 7*f*. *See also specific types*
  with fixed objects, 53
  liability in cases of, 54
  types of, 53–54, 54*f*
command vehicles, 111
command/chief's vehicle, 20, 20*f*
commercial driver's license (CDL), 20
communications
  facility requirements, 128
  fire fighters, 5
communications center, 93, 127*f*
  communications facility requirements, 128
  computer-aided dispatch, 128–129, 129*f*
  operations
    call classification and prioritization, 133
    call receipt, 130–132, 131*f*, 132*f*
    dispatch, 134
    emergency, nonemergency, and personal calls, 136, 137
    location validation, 132–133, 133*f*
    operational support and coordination, 134
    status tracking and deployment management, 134, 136
    touring the communications center, 136, 138
    unit selection, 133
  telecommunicators, 127–128, 130*f*
  voice recorders and activity logs, 129
compression brake, 102
computer-aided dispatch (CAD), 128–129, 129*f*
confined-space turnaround exercise, 78, 80
contact lenses, 44
control zones, 119
coolant temperature gauge, 60
corner safe areas, 109
counseling and critical incident stress, 12–14, 13*f*
crash scene, 28*f*. *See also* collisions
  ambulance, procedures following, 158–159, 158*f*
  civilian vehicle, 21*f*
  investigation, 54*f*
crew members, educating, 5
criminal law, 50
  legal entanglements, avoiding, 54, 54*f*
  liability in cases of collisions, 54
critical incident stress debriefing (CISD), 13
critical incident stress management (CISM), 12–13
critical speed, 101
cultural brainwashing, 14
curves, control on, 100–101, 101*f*

D

DBMS. *See* driver behavior monitoring systems
deaths and injuries
    among fire fighters
    causes of, 6*f*, 6–7, 6*t*, 7*f*, 112, 112*t*
    reducing, 7
defendant, 50
defensive driving practices, 99–100
digital radio systems, 141
digital technology, 141
diminishing clearance exercise, 78–81, 82
direct channel, 140, 140*f*
direct-line telephones, 132
disc brakes, 64, 64*f*
dispatch, 93–94, 93*f*, 134
dispatcher. *See also* telecommunicators
  additional information from, 94
distracted driving, 41–42, 41*f*
DOT. *See* U.S. Department of Transportation
DriveCam, 151
driver behavior monitoring systems (DBMS), 151, 151*f*
driver monitoring devices, 151
driver/operator, 2
  familiarity with agency's SOPs, 155
  general rules for, 156
  NFPA 1002
    general requirements, 20, 20*f*
    medical and physical requirements, 20
  qualifications for, 159
  roles of
    educating crew members, 5
    lead by example, 15–16
    maintaining safe work environment, 14–15
    promoting safety, 3–5, 4*f*
    trust and team building, 5–6
  selection of, 21–23, 23*f*
  training of, 21, 21*f*
drivetrain, inspection, 63
driving distractions, 41–42, 41*f*
driving emergency vehicle apparatus
  confined-space turnaround, performing, 78, 80
  digital display for open compartment doors, 73, 75*f*
  diminishing clearance exercise, performing, 78–81, 82
  getting under way, 73, 75–77, 75*f*
  inspection before leaving, 73, 75*f*
  issues pertaining to, 79
  returning to station
    reversing the apparatus, 81–84, 83–85*f*, 86
    shutting down the apparatus down, 85, 87–88, 87*f*
  seat belt safety, 73
  serpentine maneuver, performing, 78, 79
  starting, 71–73, 72*f*, 73*f*
  360-degree inspection, 70, 71
driving operations, fire apparatus, 19
driving range, safety on, 157–158
drowsy driving, signs of, 29
Drug and Alcohol-Free Awareness (IAFC), 160
drum brakes, 63, 64*f*
due regard, 16, 51, 78, 98
duplex channel, 140

E

EAPs. *See* employee assistance programs
electrical system, inspection, 62–63
electromagnetic retarder, 102
emergency, type and location of, 94
emergency calls, 136

emergency incident, steps in processing
call classification and prioritization, 133
call receipt, 130–132, 131*f*, 132*f*
dispatch, 134
location validation, 132–133, 133*f*
unit selection, 133
emergency light, 60. *See also* warning lights
color of, 113
emergency response, 52
emergency scenes
approaching, 103–104
address/location, identification of, 104, 104–105*f*
recognizing potential hazards, 105
slowing down as, 104, 104*f*
medical, positioning at, 118–119, 120
special, positioning, 119
emergency services communications, 126–127
communications center, 127*f*
communications facility requirements, 128
computer-aided dispatch, 128–129, 129*f*
telecommunicators, 127–128
voice recorders and activity logs, 129, 130*f*
communications center operations
call classification and prioritization, 133
call receipt, 130–132, 131*f*, 132*f*
dispatch, 134
location validation, 132–133, 133*f*
operational support and coordination, 134
status tracking and deployment management, 134, 136
taking calls, 136, 137
touring communications center, 136, 138
unit selection, 133
radio systems
radio equipment, 136–139, 138–139*f*
radio's operation, 139–141, 140*f*
using radio, 141–143
emergency traffic messages, 142–143
emergency vehicle driving
bridges and overpasses, 102
defensive driving practices, 99–100
emergency medical scene, positioning at, 118–119, 120
emergency scenes, approaching, 103–104
address/location, identify, 104, 104–105*f*
recognizing potential hazards, 105
slowing down, 104, 104*f*
emergency vehicle laws, 97–98
fire scene positioning
ambulances, 111–112
command vehicles, 111
engines and ladders, 108–111, 110–111*f*
proper positioning, 105–106, 106*f*
specialized fire apparatus, 111
staging, 106–108, 107–108*f*
working fire, 106
intersections, 102–103
level of response, 98–99
maintaining control on hills, turns, and curves, 100–101, 101*f*
manual on uniform traffic control devices, 114–116
motor vehicle accidents, 116, 118, 118*f*
mounting and dismounting apparatus, 96–97
night driving, 101–102
passing vehicles, 99, 99*f*
pre-emergency vehicle response
dispatch, 93–94, 93*f*
maps, 94–95, 95*f*
railroad crossings, 103
special emergency scene positioning, 119
traffic safety on the scene
high-visibility reflective vests, wearing, 114
motorist vision impairment, reducing, 113–114, 113*f*
never trust traffic, 112–113
positioning at intersection or on highway, 112, 112*t*
proper protective parking, engage in, 113, 113*f*
emergency vehicle operation and law, 97–98
collisions, types of, 53–54, 54*f*
criminal and civil law, 50–51
legal entanglements, avoiding, 54, 54*f*
liability in cases of collisions, 54
legal terms, 51–52
lights and sirens, use of, 52, 52*f*
responding safely, 52–53, 53*f*
Emergency Vehicle Technician (EVT) Certification Commission, Inc., 67
emergency warning devices, 52. *See also specific devices*
emitter, 103
emotional preparedness, 40, 43
emotions, loss of control, 30
employee assistance programs (EAPs), 14
engine
inspection, 61–62, 62*f*
and ladders, positioning of, 108–109
auxiliary appliances, 111
exposures, 109
fire conditions, 109
overhead obstructions, 11*f*, 110–111
rescue potential, 109
slopes, 110
terrain and surface conditions, 110
water supply, 109–110
wind conditions, 110, 110*f*
Engine 207 example, 141
enhanced 911 systems, 132
envisionCAM, 151
evacuation signal, 143
Everyone Goes Home Program, 7
exhaust brake, 102
exposure protection, 109
exterior inspection, of vehicle, 58, 60

F

FBHA. *See* Firefighter Behavioral Health Alliance
Federal Communications Commission (FCC), 131
fire apparatus and equipment, 9. *See also* driving emergency vehicle apparatus
and civilian vehicle crash scene, 21*f*
cleaning, 18, 18*f*
functions and limitations, 16
inspections, 18, 18*f*
safety across board, 18–19
security, 32
storage of, 4, 4*f*
fire conditions, 109
fire department
connection, 105, 106*f*
vehicle, 20

fire fighters
deaths and injuries
causes of, 6–7, 6*f*, 6*t*, 7*f*, 112, 112*t*
reducing, 7
personal health and well-being
cancer, 11, 11*f*
counseling and critical incident stress, 12–14, 13*f*
employee assistance programs, 14
heart disease, 10
hydration, 10
nutrition, 10
physical fitness, 9–10, 10*f*
sleep, 10
tobacco, alcohol, and illicit drugs, 12
regulations, standards, and procedures, 7–9
safety, as responsibility, 2–3
16 Fire Fighter Life Safety Initiatives, 8*t*
fire response mode, determining, 95
Firefighter Behavioral Health Alliance (FBHA), 14
Firefighter Cancer Support Network, 11
freelancing, 9, 105
frequency, radio, 139
fuel gauge, 60, 72

G
gasoline-powered equipment, 15
gastrointestinal distress, 30, 45
gauges and meters, inspection, 60
gear, securing, 32
General Industry Standards, Occupational Noise Exposure guideline, 43
geographic information system (GIS), 128
global positioning system (GPS), 95, 128, 148–149, 149*f*
global system for mobile communications (GSM), 148
GPS. *See* global positioning system
gross negligence, 51
group stress debriefings, 13*f*
GSM. *See* global system for mobile communications

H
hazardous materials incident, 119
head restraints, 32
headaches, 30, 45
headrests. *See* head restraints
health and safety program, 9
health and well-being
cancer, 11, 11*f*
counseling and critical incident stress, 12–14, 13*f*
employee assistance programs, 14
heart disease, 10
hydration, 10
nutrition, 10
physical fitness, 9–10, 10*f*
sleep, 10
tobacco, alcohol, and illicit drugs, 12
hearing aids, 43
hearing loss, 43–44
hearing testing, 43, 44*f*
heart disease, 10
heating system, vehicle inspection of, 66
helmets, 32
high-visibility reflective vests
roadside safety and, 36, 36*f*
wearing, 114
highway, positioning at, 112, 112*t*, 118
hills, control on, 100–101
hot zone, 119
hour meter, 60
hydration, 10
hydraulic brakes, 64

I
IAFC. *See* International Association of Fire Chiefs
ICS. *See* Incident Command System
ignition switch, 72
illicit drug use, 12. *See also* substance use
incident
description of, 94
space, 116
Incident Command System (ICS), 9, 105, 126
inflation, tire, 60, 66
inspections, 18, 18*f*. *See also* vehicle inspection and maintenance
interior compartments, vehicle inspection of, 60
intermediate traffic incidents, 115
International Association of Fire Chiefs (IAFC), 160
International Safety Equipment Association, 115
intersection, 102–103
collisions, 53
positioning at, 112, 112*t*, 116, 118
inverters, 63

J
job aids, 15
job-related stress, 30
signs of, 14
jump-starting, of vehicles, 63
jumper cables, 60

K
knee bolsters, 31

L
"Lane + 1 blocking," 35
large-diameter hose (LDH), 110
lead by example process, 2, 15–16
leg sprain/strain, 30
legal entanglements, avoiding, 54, 54*f*
Level I staging, 107, 107*f*
Level II staging, 107–108, 108*f*
Levick, Nadine, 32
liability
in cases of collisions, 54
defined, 51
liquid surge, 100
location validation, 132–133, 133*f*
low air warning test, 64
LUNAR, 142

M
major traffic incidents, 115
manual on uniform traffic control devices, 114–116
motor vehicle accidents, 116, 118, 118*f*

maps, 94–95, 95*f*
marijuana use, policy with regard to, 47, 47*f*
mayday, 142
MDCs. *See* mobile data computers
MDTs. *See* mobile data terminals
mechanical components and systems
  vehicle inspection
    braking system, 63–65, 64*f*
    drivetrain, 63
    electrical system, 62–63
    engine, 61–62, 62*f*
    heating and air-conditioning system, 66
    suspension system, 66
    tires, 65–66, 65*f*, 66*f*
mechanical failure, 36–37
  collisions, 53–54
  precautions to protect in event of, 37
medic catcher, 157
medication use, 46–47, 46*f*, 47*f*
mental preparedness, 40–41
  meaning of, 40
  paying attention to detail, 42
  safety-first attitude, 42–43, 42*f*
  technological distractions, avoiding, 41–42, 41*f*
minor traffic incidents, 115
mircosleeping, 45
mirrors
  adjustments, 72, 72*f*
  inspection, 60
  positioning, 32
mobile data computers (MDCs), 60, 150
mobile data terminals (MDTs), 41, 93, 93*f*, 129, 139, 150, 150*f*
mobile radios, 136, 138*f*
mobile repeater systems, 140
mobile tracking devices, 136
morbidity, 31
mortality, 31
motor vehicle accident (MVA), 105, 116, 118, 118*f*
motorist vision impairment, reducing, 113–114, 113*f*
mounting and dismounting apparatus, 96–97
multiplex channels, 140
muscle injuries, 45
MVA. *See* motor vehicle accident

N

National Automotive Sampling System (NASS), 28
National Emergency Number Association (NENA), 127
National Fallen Firefighters Foundation (NFFF), 7, 79
National Fallen Firefighters Memorial Weekend, 7
National Firefighter Life Safety Summit, 7
National Highway Traffic Safety Administration (NHTSA), 29, 156
National Incident Management System (NIMS), 141
National Institute for Occupational Safety and Health (NIOSH), 11, 81
National Sleep Foundation's (NSF) 2009 Sleep in America poll, 29
Near-Miss Reporting System, 7
negligence, legal sense of, 51
NENA. *See* National Emergency Number Association
next-generation 911 systems, 133
NFFF. *See* National Fallen Firefighters Foundation
NFPA 1002, 78–79, 119
  general requirements, 20, 20*f*
  medical and physical requirements, 20
NFPA 1061, 128
NFPA 1071, 67
NFPA 1221, 128
NFPA 1451, 21
NFPA 1500, 7–8, 73, 97
NFPA 1561, 106
NFPA 1582, 8
NFPA 1620, 111
NFPA 1901, 102
NFPA 1911, 67
NFPA 1917, 67
NHTSA. *See* National Highway Traffic Safety Administration
night driving, 101–102
NIMS. *See* National Incident Management System
911 system, 127, 130, 131
  enhanced, 132–133
  next-generation, 133
NIOSH. *See* National Institute for Occupational Safety and Health
no distractions while driving policy, 159–160
non-emergency response, 52
nonemergency calls, 136
nutrition, 10

O

Objective Safety and Research Director of EMS Safety Foundation, 32
Occupational Safety and Health Act, 67
Occupational Safety and Health Administration (OSHA), 8, 43
odometer, 60
OEMs. *See* original equipment manufacturers
oil pressure gauge, 60, 73
on-scene operations, fire apparatus, 19
operational support and coordination, 134
original equipment manufacturers (OEMs), 100
OSHA. *See* Occupational Safety and Health Administration
over-the-counter (OTC) treatments, physical awareness and, 30, 43, 46–47, 46*f*, 160
overhead obstructions, 110–111, 111*f*
overpasses, fire apparatus, 102

P

parking brake, 71, 103
  test, 64–65
parking collisions, 53
passenger safety, 33–34
passing other vehicles during emergency response, 99
patient safety, 32–33
paying attention to detail, 42
pedestrian collisions, 53
pediatric patient, 157, 158*f*
personal attitude, 30–31, 42
personal calls, 136, 137
personal commitment
  being safe as, 32
  to use seatbelt, 31

personal preparedness
attitude, 30–31
emotions, 30
physical awareness, 30
sleep deprivation, 29–30
stress, 30
personal protective clothing, 4, 11*f*
personal protective equipment (PPE), 4
requirements, 16
personnel, safety, 9
physical ailments, 45
physical awareness, 30
physical fitness, 9–10, 10*f*
physical preparedness, 40
hearing testing, 43, 44*f*
medication or substance use, 46–47, 46*f*, 47*f*
physical ailments, 45
tired driving, 45–46, 45*f*
vision testing, 44–45, 44*f*
plaintiff, 50–51
portable radio, 136, 138*f*
potential hazards, recognizing, 105
pre-emergency vehicle response
dispatch, 93–94, 93*f*
maps, 94–95, 95*f*
preemption priority, 150
preincident plan, 111
preponderance of the evidence, 51
pressure gauge, 60
preventable collision, 53–54
preventive maintenance, vehicle inspection, 66–67
proper protective parking, 113, 113*f*
public safety answering point (PSAP), 127, 130
public safety communications center, 127
pump/water supply operator, 93, 94, 98, 105, 112. *See also* fire fighters
dismounting stopped apparatus, 114
prohibited practices, 98
radio, using, 142
receiving call and initiating response to emergency, 137
riding fire apparatus, 96–97
safety, as responsibility, 2–3
touring communications center, 138

R

radio systems
radio equipment, 136–139, 138–139*f*
radio operation, 139–141, 140*f*
using radio, 141–143
radios, use of, 41
railroads, 118
crossings, 103
reaction distance, braking and, 100
rear-end collisions, 53
rear-mounted camera, 84, 85*f*
reasonable doubt, criminal cases and, 51
receiver, on traffic signals, 103
repeater channel, 140, 140*f*
repeater systems, 140–141, 140*f*
rescue potential, 109
response, 93
restraints. *See also specific restraints*
inspection, 60
use of, 156–157, 157–158*f*
returning to station, fire apparatus
reversing, 81–84, 83–85*f*, 86
shutting down, 85, 87–88, 87*f*
reversing, fire apparatus, 81–84, 83–85*f*, 86
rewarding personnel, 151, 151*f*
riding assignments, 5
road performance, vehicle inspection, 67
road rage, 42
Road Safety monitoring system, 151
roadside safety
high-visibility apparel, 36, 36*f*
safe work zone, 34–35
vehicle positioning, 35–36
warning lights, 36
rollover airbags, 31
run cards, 133

S

safe work environment, maintaining, 14–15
safe work zone, roadside safety, 34–35
safety equipment
airbags, 31–32
equipment security, 32
headrests or head restraints, 32
helmets, 32
mirrors, 32
seatbelts, 31, 31*f*
safety-first attitude, 29, 42–43, 42*f*
safety vests, classes of, 115
Safety Vision monitoring system, 151
SCBA. *See* self-contained breathing apparatus
seatbelts, 31, 31*f*
alarms for wearing, 73
inspection, 60
safety, 73
as safety device, 3–4, 4*f*
use of, 156–157, 157–158*f*
self-contained breathing apparatus (SCBA), 5, 139
serpentine maneuver exercise, 78, 79
service brake test, 65
shutting down, fire apparatus, 85, 87–88, 87*f*
side curtain airbags, 31
side-mounted camera, 84, 85*f*
simplex channel, 139
sirens
during gridlock, 80
noise from, 97
speaker, 44
use of, 52, 52*f*
16 Firefighter Life Safety Initiatives, 7
size-up, positioning for better, 105
skidding, fire apparatus, 100
sleep, and health and performance, 10
sleep aids, 46
sleep deprivation, 29, 45
symptoms of, 45
"sleep driving," 46
sloping surfaces, 110

SMART objectives, 155
SMARTER project, 10
smoke
  effect on fire apparatus positioning, 110, 110*f*
  for locating incident, 104, 105*f*
SOGs. *See* standard operating guidelines
SOPs. *See* standard operating procedures
specialized fire apparatus, 111
speedometer, 60
spotter, 32
  arm placement for directing fire apparatus, 83–84, 83–84*f*
  defined, 82
  in driver/operator's full view, 82, 83*f*
  flashlights, use of, 85
  general rules for, 156
  procedures for, 83
spring brake test, 64–65
staging, 106–107
  goals of, 107
  Level I staging, 107, 107*f*
  Level II staging, 107–108, 108*f*
  objective of procedures, 107*f*
staging area, 108
staging area manager, 108
standard operating guidelines (SOGs), 3
standard operating procedures (SOPs), 3, 154
  development of, 154–155
  familiar with agency's, 155
  for global positioning system, 149
  policies, recommendations of, 155
    backing of EMS vehicle, 156
    driving range, safety on, 157–158
    new emergency vehicle operators, qualifications for, 159
    no distractions while driving policy, 159–160
    procedures following a crash, 158–159, 158*f*
    seatbelts and restraints, use of, 156–157, 157–158*f*
    visibility at scene, 159
    zero tolerance for alcohol and drugs, 160
starter switch, 72
state laws, governing fire apparatus, 98
status tracking and deployment management, 134, 136
stress, 30
  managing, 43
stressors, to driver/operator, 14
stretcher restraints, 32–33, 33*f*
substance use, 46–47, 46*f*, 47*f*, 160
suicide, awareness and prevention, 13–14
suspension system, inspection, 66
system check sequence, 72

T

tachometer, 60
tactical benchmarks, 5
tactical radio frequency channel, assigning, 94
talk-around channel, 140
team building, 5–6
teamwork, 9
technological aids
  driver behavior monitoring systems, 151, 151*f*
  global positioning system, 148–149, 149*f*
  mobile data terminals, 150, 150*f*
  next generation of EMS technology, 152
  traffic preemption systems, 149–150, 150*f*
technological distractions, avoiding, 41–42, 41*f*
telecommunicators, 127–128
telephones, 130–132, 131*f*
  interrogation by, 131
ten-codes, 141
termination area, 116
terrain and surface conditions, 110
terrorism, 119
Texas State Fire Marshal's Office Fire Fighter Fatality Investigation Report, 75
text devices, 131, 131*f*
text-to-911 messages, 131
texting while driving, 41, 41*f*
3-second rule, 99
311 system, 131
360-degree inspection, 70, 71
TIM system. *See* Traffic Incident Management (TIM) system
TIMA. *See* traffic incident management area
tired driving, 45–46, 45*f*. *See also* drowsy driving
tires, inspection of, 58, 60, 65–66, 65*f*, 66*f*
tobacco use, 12
tool set, for basic maintenance, 60
total stopping distance, 99
traffic blocking, 34, 34*f*
traffic control, 115
traffic incident, 115, 115*f*
Traffic Incident Management (TIM) system, 34–35, 35*f*
traffic incident management area (TIMA), 115
traffic lane encroachment collisions, 54
traffic preemption systems, 149–150, 150*f*
traffic safety on scene
  high-visibility reflective vests, wearing, 114
  motorist vision impairment, reducing, 113–114, 113*f*
  never trust traffic, 112–113
  positioning at intersection or on highway, 112, 112*t*
  proper protective parking, engage in, 113, 113*f*
traffic signal preemption systems, 103
traffic space, 116
training
  driver/operator, 21, 21*f*
  fire fighter, 9
transition area, 115
transmission, of vehicles, 63
  retarder, 102
trench collapse, 119
true emergency, 51, 52–53, 130
trunked radios, 141
trunking systems, 141
trust and team building, 5–6
TTY/TDD systems, 131, 131*f*
turnout pants and boots, 75
turns, control while making, 100–101

U

ultrahigh-frequency (UHF) band, 140
unit selection, 133
U.S. Department of Transportation (DOT), 20
  Federal Highway Administration, 114

V

valve stem, 65
vehicle dynamics, 16
vehicle fires, 118, 118*f*
vehicle inspection and maintenance
  checklists, 58, 59*f*
  exterior inspection, 58, 60
  guidelines and organizations, 67
  interior compartments, 60
  mechanical components and systems
    braking system, 63–65, 64*f*
    drivetrain, 63
    electrical system, 62–63
    engine, 61–62, 62*f*
    heating and air-conditioning system, 66
    suspension system, 66
    tires, 65–66, 65*f*, 66*f*
  preventive maintenance, 66–67
  road performance, 67
vehicle intercom system, 5
vehicle locator systems, 136
vehicle positioning, roadside safety, 35–36
VHF band. *See* very high-frequency (VHF) band
visibility at scene, 159
vision testing, 44–45, 44*f*
Voice over Internet Protocol (VoIP), 132–133
voice recording system, 129, 130*f*
VoIP. *See* Voice over Internet Protocol
voltmeter, 60, 72–73, 73*f*

W

walk-ins, 132, 132*f*
warm zone, 119
warning lights
  roadside safety, 36
  use of, 52, 52*f*
water supply, 109–110
wind conditions, 110, 110*f*
windshield wipers, 60

Z

zero tolerance policy, 160